LACAN AND MARX

Lacan and Marx: The Invention of the Symptom provides an incisive commentary on Lacan's reading of Marx, mapping the relations between these two vastly influential thinkers.

Unlike previous books, Bruno provides a detailed history of Lacan's reading of Marx and surveys his references to Marx in both his writings and seminars. Examining Lacan's key argument that Marx "invented the symptom", Bruno shows how Lacan went on to criticize Marx and contrasts Marx's concept of surplus-value with Lacan's surplus-enjoyment. Exploring the division between Marxist and psychoanalytic perspectives on social and psychological need and Lacan's formalisation of the capitalist discourse, the book compares the positions of Althusser, Deleuze and Guattari, and Žižek on the relations between Lacan, Marx and capitalism, using a wide range of cultural examples, from Stevenson's Dr. Jekyll and Mr. Hyde to Brecht's Joan Dark and Pierpont Mauler. Through these readings, Bruno also elaborates an extended commentary on Lacan's central idea of the division of the subject. His focus is not only on showing how we can exit from capitalism but also, and just as importantly, on showing how we can make capitalism exit from us.

This book will be of great interest to scholars and readers of Lacan and Marx from across the fields of psychoanalysis, philosophy and political economy, and will also appeal to Lacanian psychoanalysts in clinical practice.

Pierre Bruno is a psychoanalyst based in Paris. He is a former professor of psychoanalysis at the University of Paris 8 Vincennes-Saint-Denis, and he is a member of the psychoanalytic association *Le pari de Lacan* (Lacan's Wager) and the editorial board of the journal *Psychanalyse*.

The Centre for Freudian Analysis and Research Library

Series Editors:
Anouchka Grose, Darian Leader, Alan Rowan

CFAR was founded in 1985 with the aim of developing Freudian and Lacanian psychoanalysis in the UK. Lacan's rereading and rethinking of Freud had been neglected in the Anglophone world, despite its important implications for the theory and practice of psychoanalysis. Today, this situation is changing, with a lively culture of training groups, seminars, conferences, and publications.

CFAR offers both introductory and advanced courses in psychoanalysis, as well as a clinical training programme in Lacanian psychoanalysis. It can provide access to Lacanian psychoanalysts working in the UK, and has links with Lacanian groups across the world. The CFAR Library aims to make classic Lacanian texts available in English for the first time, as well as publishing original research in the Lacanian field. www.cfar.org.uk

Recent titles include

The Marks of a Psychoanalysis
by Luis Izcovich

Obsessional Neurosis
edited by Astrid Gessert

Lacan Reading Joyce
by Colette Soler

The Law of the Mother
An Essay on the Sexual Sinthome
by Geneviève Morel

For more information about this series, please visit: https://www.routledge.com/The-Centre-for-Freudian-Analysis-and-Research-Library/book-series/KARNACCFARL

LACAN AND MARX

The Invention of the Symptom

Pierre Bruno

Translated by John Holland

This translation was supported by House of Publications.

Routledge
Taylor & Francis Group
LONDON AND NEW YORK

HOUSE OF PUBLICATIONS

First published 2020
by Routledge
2 Park Square, Milton Park, Abingdon, Oxon OX14 4RN

and by Routledge
52 Vanderbilt Avenue, New York, NY 10017

Routledge is an imprint of the Taylor & Francis Group, an informa business

This translation was supported by House of Publications.

British Library Cataloguing-in-Publication Data
A catalogue record for this book is available from the British Library

Library of Congress Cataloging-in-Publication Data
A catalog record for this book has been requested

ISBN: 9780367334000 (hbk)
ISBN: 9780367334017 (pbk)
ISBN: 9780429319686 (ebk)

Typeset in Bembo
by Apex CoVantage LLC

CONTENTS

TRANSLATOR'S PREFACE

Pierre Bruno's *Lacan, passeur de Marx: l'invention du symptôme* was published in France during the winter of 2010 and was the culmination of a long process of research concerned with relating psychoanalysis to the work of Karl Marx and the critique of capitalism (see Bruno, 1993, 2003; Roudinesco, 1986, pp. 535–536). Since that time, a number of texts on this subject have appeared in English, and not only because of the continuing crisis of capitalism. For example, in a far-reaching study, Samo Tomšič (2015, pp. 49, 97) has argued that the "unconscious production of *jouissance* and the social production of value follow the same logic" and has pointed to the existence of a "social non-relation"; Alenka Zupančič (2017, pp. 30, 33) has written that the "social relations of power – domination, exploitation, discrimination – are first and foremost forms of exploitation of th[is] non-relation", one that, as Marx understood, is "built into the capitalist mode of production"; David Pavón-Cuéllar (2017, p. 7) has treated both Marxism and psychoanalysis as forms of resistance to the discipline of psychology, with its "dualist distinction between the psychic-mental-behavioural and the physical-somatic-environmental"; and Jodi Dean (2012, p. 187) has advanced the concept of a resurgent "communist desire", which "recognizes the impossibility of reaching the object" – the people as object *a* – "and holds on, refusing to cede it". Much of this work carries the influence of the teaching of Slavoj Žižek, who during this period, has sought to rework dialectical materialism in a way that would include psychoanalysis (Žižek, 2014), and like Tomšič, has provided a reading of Lacan's capitalist discourse that differs markedly from Bruno's (see Tomšič, 2015, pp. 219–229; Žižek, 2017, pp. 208–209).

Bruno's book approaches the connections between Lacan and Marx in a different way; instead of drawing out the relations or nonrelations between Marxism and psychoanalysis, it argues that Lacan's work is marked by a process of transmission, one in which his reading of Marx produced decisive effects on both his teaching and his practice. As the title of this book indicates, the area in which Marx affected psychoanalysis most significantly is the concept of the symptom. In his seminar of 1970–1971, *D'un discours qui ne serait pas du semblant*, Lacan (2006, p. 164) states that it was not psychoanalysis that introduced the "notion of symptom", for the figure "who was responsible for this is Marx". In the same seminar, Lacan argues that:

> if there was a moment when Freud was revolutionary, it was in the way that he highlighted a function that Marx also brought out – it's even the only element that they had in common: that of considering a certain number of facts as symptoms.
>
> *(ibid., p. 24)*

Two years earlier, in his seminar of 1968–1969, *D'un Autre à l'autre*, Lacan had recalled how, during the 1920s, he had read the first volume of *Capital* while he was riding the métro in Paris (see Appendix 1), and his statement in his later seminar locates something of the effect that Marx had on him. For Lacan, Marx, like Sigmund Freud, pursued truth: Lacan applies the psychoanalytic (and medical) term "symptom" to Marx's method because he was struck by the latter's way of examining capitalist phenomena; the critique of political economy, as Jacques Rancière (1965, p. 88) had already written, treats them as "hieroglyphs, which have to be deciphered".[1] One of Marx's effects was to aide Lacan to explore and extend this concept within his own field; Lacan's own work bears witness to the impact and resonance of this encounter with Marx's desire.

I

The importance that Bruno accords to Lacan's statement about Marx, like his own diagnoses of capitalism in this book, is inseparable from his analysis of a series of questions raised by psychoanalytic practice and theory: questions that concern the status of the subject, the end of an analysis and the real father. These concepts are sometimes presented allusively or elusively, in part because this book does not shy away from pushing relations to the point where they become paradoxical; it is not by chance, for example, that Russell's paradox appears at two crucial points in the argument. It is also the case that, like many Lacanians of his generation, Bruno developed his reading of Lacan in the context of an oral teaching; his published texts sometimes serve as "quilting points" or "button ties" for certain aspects of this reading, providing more or less definitive formulations of certain concepts, while taking others as already established, and providing broad outlines of others, which would then be developed more fully elsewhere.[2]

The understandings of both the subject and the end of analysis that are developed in these pages are closely connected to Lacan's seminar of 1967–1968, *L'acte psychanalytique*, which is both unpublished and unfinished; with the outbreak of the revolutionary events of May 1968, Lacan suspended it, thereby leaving the conclusions of his argument undeveloped. Bruno suggests that this seminar and other works related to it have a decisive effect upon the way in which we are to understand the status of the "divided" subject in Lacan: the French word "*division*" corresponds to the German term, "*Spaltung*", a word that Freud brought to the forefront in his late, unfinished paper, "The Splitting of the Ego in the Processes of Defence (*Die Ichspaltung im Abwehrvorgang*)". Division is to be understood as splitting.

Without undertaking a thoroughgoing analysis of Lacan's use of these terms, one can recall that in his seminar *Anxiety*, he approached the "division" of the subject in its mathematical sense. The $\$$, or barred subject, comes into existence in a separation that involves a "fall[ing]-away" of the object *a* (Lacan, 2004, p. 167); this separation is theorised, at the beginning of the seminar, as a mathematical operation in which the $\$$ emerges as a "quotient" and the object *a* as a "remainder" (ibid., p. 27; also see p. 160).

This equation of division and splitting is puzzling, in large part because Freud's presentation of the "splitting" of the ego is very different from the division of the subject. For Freud, this splitting is a consequence of the mechanism of disavowal (*Verleugnung*), which serves as a way of maintaining two contradictory positions: it sets up a fetish as a way of both recognising and denying the mother's castration, of "preserv[ing]" the belief in her penis, while also giving it up (Freud, 1927, p. 153). Near the end of his life, in the paper on the splitting of the ego and in related passages in "An outline of psycho-analysis", Freud develops this concept by defining splitting as the characteristic of the psychic agency – the ego – that must bear the effects of this contradiction. The ego is concerned with recognising reality while defending itself against the insistence of the drives. Such a defence may involve choosing not to acknowledge certain aspects of reality; it can even choose simultaneously to acknowledge and to refuse such aspects. Freud (1940b, p. 275) writes, for example, of a patient who "rejects reality", while "in the same breath, he recognizes the danger of reality". In such situations, "the *disavowal* of perceptions" is "supplemented by an acknowledgement of them" and the "splitting of the ego" results from this co-existence of "two contrary and independent attitudes" (Freud, 1940a, p. 204).

Lacan's theorisation of splitting involves several decisive shifts of emphasis; first, not surprisingly, this disavowal will be related more to the subject than to the ego. As Bruce Fink (1995, p. 45) has noted in reference to Lacan's teaching from this period, the subject can be said to be "split between ego . . . and unconscious . . ., between conscious and unconscious, between an ineluctable false sense of selfhood and the automatic functioning of the unconscious. In such a context, the subject can be defined a being *nothing but this very split*".

In *L'acte psychanalytique* and related texts, the splitting that is emphasised is the one between the $\$$ and the object *a*. In a lecture that Lacan gave one month after his suspension of *L'acte psychanalytique*, he indicates that this distancing involves a very particular form of "disavowal". He notes that

> for years, I have held . . . in reserve . . . the term *Verleugnung*, which Freud . . . brought out in relation to an exemplary moment of the *Spaltung* of the subject, I wanted to make it live where it is . . . pushed to its most touching point, at the level of the analyst him/herself".
>
> *(Lacan, 1985, p. 5)*

The end of analysis includes a "disavowal" that is important, in part, because it will enable us to see retroactively that the primal "division" between subject and object was also a splitting between them. This disavowal is related to the act referred to in the seminar's title, the act that enables the analysand to move to the position of analyst. Within analysis, as the analytic discourse indicates, the object *a* has served as a cause; it has provided the impetus for the analysand's production of a series of signifiers and constructions that are attempts to symbolise it. Now, however, this procedure comes to a halt and the analysand's position changes; s/he approaches the *a* as something that is real through and through, and therefore radically resistant to symbolisation. The newly self-authorised analyst thereby assumes a discordant and even contradictory relation to the object; it serves both as the basis of her/his psychic and libidinal position and as something that s/he can, and must, discard, in a process that can be painful and almost melancholic.

This disavowal, unlike the one that occurs in the splitting of the ego, is not located at the level of reality, and has nothing in common with the fetishistic conception of the mother as simultaneously castrated and uncastrated. Instead, what is in question is what Bruno (2013, p. 96) has referred to elsewhere as a "disavowal of the real", an expression that can be taken in two senses. First, the object that is disavowed – which is simultaneously vitally important and is also capable of being discarded – is real. Second, something of the real is also involved in accomplishing this disavowal: the "*sinthome*", an archaic French word that Lacan adopted in order to designate the symptom with which the analysand has been able to identify at the end of analysis, and which acts to bring about this distancing from the object. By means of such a "disavowal", the subject is able to experience as fully and radically as possible the "splitting" between $\$$ and *a* that had already been operating since their primal "division".

The "real father", another term that recurs throughout this book, originated in Lacan's seminar of 1956–1957, *La relation d'objet*, where it figured in a complex combinatory inspired by Claude Lévi-Strauss; the "real" father is the figure who imposes upon the subject a "symbolic castration" that bears on an "imaginary object" (Lacan, 1994, p. 269). The term reappears thirteen years later, at a crucial moment in *The Other Side of Psychoanalysis*: the point at which Lacan approaches Freud's three myths of the father – the myths of Oedipus, the primal horde and Moses – subjecting them to a critique that would open the path towards the formalisation of sexuation that would be developed in 1971 and 1972, in *. . . ou pire* and *The Psychoanalyst's Knowledge*. In the formulas of sexuation, the father arises as a necessary logical supposition, one that can be written as a propositional formula – $\exists x.\overline{\Phi x}$, the at-least-one term that is not subjected to the phallic function of castration (see Lacan, 2011, p. 22) – thus stripping this figure of many of the imaginary associations that are inevitable when words such as "father" or "mother" (to say nothing of "man" or "woman") are used.

The term "real father", as Bruno employs it, is closely related to this matheme; it is distinct from the Name-of-the-Father, which in Lacan's (1959, p. 481) early definitions, is a signifier that can arise in response to the neurotic's call or "summon[ing]", serving as a foundation for his/her desire. Both the real father's position and what it produces are different. It is located outside the realm of the signifier and Bruno will argue that this externality is the source of the difficulty that Freud's analysands experienced in recounting the fantasy that he discusses in "A Child is Being Beaten". They are unable to remember its second, crucial phase – in which "*I am being beaten by my father*" (Freud, 1919a, p. 198) – because the father in question is too close to the real father, who resists being integrated into the symbolic. This fantasy seeks to stage the action of the real father in order to provide a sort of "myth" of the imposition of castration, which has already been thrust upon the subject by the fact that s/he speaks; a figure who cannot be symbolised becomes, nevertheless, the "agent" (Lacan, 1994, p. 269) of this imposition.

Bruno tends to use the term "real father" instead of the matheme because it serves as a way of highlighting certain qualities of the figure of the exception: there is something living in it, something that is far from being abstract. As Isabelle Morin (2009) has argued, the expression "real father" emphasises, first, a crucial distinction between the Freudian and Lacanian fathers. For Freud, the father whom we encounter is, to a great extent, the dead father; Freud's reading of the Oedipal myth presents us with what Lacan, in *The Other Side of Psychoanalysis*, calls a "crude schema", according to which the "murder of the father" leads to the "*jouissance* of the mother" (Lacan, 1991, pp. 117, 113). In the other two myths Freud discusses, the dead father is not only the foundation of the law, but is also the figure who "holds the key to jouissance" and his death will provide the sons with "access to it" (Morin, 2009, p. 365). Much of Lacan's work, on the other hand, emphasises the living father; it seeks to locate in this figure a trait of jouissance, one that enables him to be seen as the agent of the subject's castration. It is partly in relation to this exceptional quality that the subject is then able to locate him/herself either as "wholly" or as not entirely submitted to castration. Bruno's use of the term "real father" underscores the idea that, however unsayable this trait may be, it can nevertheless be located within a particular figure in the family romance (ibid., p. 367).

II

Lacan's conception of analysis as terminable rather than as interminable serves as a basis for Bruno's treatment of both capitalism and Marx's role as the inventor of the symptom. For Bruno, capitalism is the most radical of all attempts to undo the splitting of the subject. This position is the result of his reading of Lacan's enigmatic rethinking of his theory of discourse, which Lacan had first presented systematically in 1969–1970, in *The Other Side of Psychoanalysis*. Two years later, in 1972, he added an important modification to this theory by introducing a fifth discourse, the capitalist discourse, which is characterised by a "foreclosure" of castration. According to Lacan's conception, the discourse of the master is a way of theorising the effects, within specific social practices, of his own formulation that a "signifier represents the subject for another signifier"; by 1972, he was writing this discourse as follows:

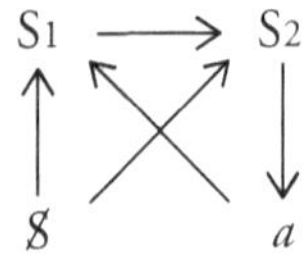

The capitalist discourse involves a "twist" that reverses the two terms on the left:

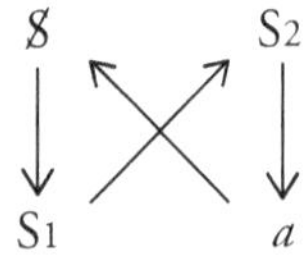

This reversal has two crucial effects. The first is that the master-signifier no longer represents the subject for another signifier, and this change disrupts the relation between knowledge and the subject of the unconscious (Holland, 2015, pp. 99–112). As Bruno shows, in the discourse of the master, the $\not{S}$ is able to communicate directly with the S_2, but this is no longer the case with the capitalist discourse, where the $\not{S}$ can only reach the S_2 through the mediation of S_1, the capitalist. He develops the consequences of this distancing through an analysis of two literary works, both of which involve attempts by the central characters to separate themselves from characteristics with which they are ill at ease: Bertolt Brecht's *Saint Joan of the Stockyards* and Robert Louis Stevenson's *Strange Case of Doctor Jekyll and Mr. Hyde*. In Brecht's play, Pierpont Mauler, the "meat king" of Chicago situates himself in the place of a form of knowledge that would include unconscious knowledge, while also attempting to distance himself from his own goodness, which he locates as $\not{S}$, in the figure of the missionary Joan Dark. In Stevenson's short novel, Henry Jekyll also locates himself in S_2 and seeks to separate himself from the pure "evil" of the drives, which becomes embodied in Edward Hyde, in the place of $\not{S}$. For Bruno, Stevenson thereby inaugurates a modern myth, distancing his work from the tradition of the double, a figure that represents something like the repressed aspects of the main character: his "suppressed acts of volition" (see Freud, 1919b, p. 236). Hyde, however, is not Jekyll's unconscious; instead, the opposite is the case. Jekyll, in the place of knowledge, embodies what would be Hyde's unconscious if the two figures were not radically separated. Jekyll, through his use of technoscience, has entered the capitalist discourse in order to effect and maintain a radical distance between the unconscious and the drives, which he wants to know nothing about.

The rigid distancing of the subject from knowledge goes hand-in-hand with a second effect of the capitalist discourse, one whose outlines can already be discerned in Jekyll's reaction to Hyde. Whereas the structure of the discourse of the master had rendered it impossible for the object *a* to communicate with the barred subject, the capitalist discourse nullifies this impossibility; a vector goes directly from *a* to $\not{S}$, thereby inducing the expectation that there can be a jouissance that satisfies this subject.

Bruno's construction of the capitalist discourse enables him to locate what he considers to be certain limitations in Marx's analysis of capitalism: this analysis, he claims, does not provide a fully adequate account of our psychic subjection to capitalism. In revealing the hidden and causal role of surplus-value, Marx produced a fundamental concept, which remains indispensable if we are to understand the character of capitalist exploitation. This concept does not, however, lay bare the nature of capitalism's libidinal and psychic hold over us. Bruno makes a similar argument in relation to Marx's analysis of the fetishism of commodities, which masterfully lays bare their concealed social character but fails to explain their libidinal force.

Instead, Bruno suggests that the capitalist discourse provides the key by which we can understand our relation to jouissance within this mode of production. Although the vector that leads directly from the object *a* to the barred subject promises jouissance, it also inevitably disappoints us. Todd McGowan (2016, p. 11) has argued that "capitalist subjects experience satisfaction itself as unsatisfying"; Bruno suggests that the vector from *a* to $\$$ actually creates what Lacan (1970, p. 455) describes as a thirst, the "thirst of the lack-in-jouissance [*manque-à-jouir*]". It is not only the case that "the more I drink, the thirstier I get" (p. 140); we also develop an appetite precisely for this thirst, and the jouissance that we derive from lack becomes itself insatiable. As Bruno points out, such formulations strike at the heart of the fundamental assumptions of marginalist economics. Vilfredo Pareto had argued that levels of satisfaction can be calculated: consuming one commodity of a particular type will be more satisfying than the immediate consumption of a second, which in turn will be more enjoyable than a third. Once, however, the question of jouissance comes to contaminate that of satisfaction, it becomes impossible to envision an end to consumption.

According to this perspective, therefore, "*it is not possible to exit from capitalism through a new distribution of surplus-value*"; this goal, instead, "*can only occur through a mutation in the subject's relation to jouissance*" (p. 162). This mutation, however, is extraordinarily difficult to accomplish, precisely because of the same structural condition that had made Jekyll believe that he could separate himself completely from Hyde: the capitalist discourse has made any direct relation between the subject and its unconscious impossible. Capitalism thus sustains and reproduces itself not through ideology or by "formatting consciousnesses", but by a specific discursive operation: "*by cutting the bond between the subject and the unconscious*", between $\$$ and S_2 (p. 165). This cut prevents the unconscious from providing the slightest treatment or amelioration of the lack-in-jouissance that is located in $\$$. Our inability to lessen this particular lack entraps us more and more within a capitalist libido.

It is in this context that the symptom becomes important. Bruno argues that the capitalist discourse stands as the most impenetrable obstacle to what analytic practice can achieve and does so precisely because the direct relation between $\$$ and *a* renders the disavowal of the real impossible. The symptom, however, moves in precisely the opposite direction, and for this reason, Marx re-enters the argument. Bruno proposes that Lacan's encounter with Marx's treatment of the symptom – both its theoretical advances and its supposed limitations – would enable him to develop a theory of the symptom that would have radical effects upon analytic practice. The beginning of this development can be found in Lacan's text of 1966, "*On the subject who is finally in question*", in which he alludes to Marx's relation to the symptom:

> it is difficult not to see that even before the advent of psychoanalysis, a dimension that might be called that of the symptom was introduced, which was articulated on the basis of the fact that it represents the return of truth as such into the gap of a certain knowledge.
>
> *(Lacan, 1966, p. 194)*

Bruno notes how, in almost the same breath, Lacan goes on to demarcate the limits of Marx's approach:

> Symptoms remained somewhat vague when they were understood as representing some irruption of truth. In fact they *are* truth, being made of the same wood from which truth is made, if we posit materialistically that truth is what is instated on the basis of the signifying chain.
>
> *(ibid., p. 194)*

In this passage, the symptom is not simply the index of truth, in a way that a strike would point to the existence of exploitation; instead, because the signifier is a part of it and creates surprise when we grasp its presence, the symptom *is* truth. The development of this implication would lead Lacan, in the 1970s, to his new theory of the symptom, and this theory bears witness to the impact of his encounter with Marx, even if certain aspects of it also clearly situate his formulations outside Marx's concerns.

For Bruno, this new theory also arose from an axiom related to clinical practice. At the beginning of our psychic lives, we are guided by a double determination; on the one hand, "I want to get off on the Other", but on the other hand, "I don't want the Other to get off on me" (p. 191). A series of theses unfolds from this axiom, and it is a measure of the complexity and ambiguity of Lacan's clinical and theoretical legacy that some of these stand in direct opposition to other prominent readings of Lacan's work on the symptom. For example, Bruno explicitly criticises Colette Soler's (2003, p. 275) view that the symptom acts to mask the nonexistence of the sexual relation: "The symptom is . . . what makes up, in every case, for the absence of a sexual relation that can be written". His position is that the symptom instead arises first as a primal manifestation of the impossibility of the sexual relation, in the form of the infant's refusal to become One with the mother. He also disagrees with Jacques-Alain Miller's judgement, made in the light of Lacan's discussions of James Joyce, concerning the relation between the symptom and the Name-of-the-Father. As a psychotic, Joyce had foreclosed the Name-of-the-Father, but his symptomatic use of writing enabled him to make up for this foreclosure and avoid a psychotic break. For Miller (2005, pp. vii – viii), this analysis indicates that Lacan's examination of the "limits of the Oedipus complex and of the paternal myth" culminated in the reduction of the "Name-of-the-Father to the level of a symptom and utensil"; the Name-of-the-Father becomes nothing more than a particular form of the symptom. Bruno counters that such a formulation is correct as a reading of Joyce, but that it misses the more general role of the symptom: to provide a far more radical way of making up for the limitations of the Name-of-the-Father.

The symptom enables the subject to surpass the Name-of-the-Father's – and, for that matter, the real father's – inability to open onto the right – feminine – side of the table of sexuation: the side where "phallocentrism fails, and where poetry becomes possible" (p. 166). This can occur with the emergence of the *sinthome*, which would also embody more fully a position that is already present in our symptoms. The *sinthome* here provides a place outside the deadlock between subject and Other that results from the initial clinical axiom: the *sinthome* is neither subject nor Other but instead a third element, one that enables us to experience a new relation between knowledge and truth, and meaning and the real. A certain kind of knowledge comes to be located in neither the subject nor the Other, but in this form of the symptom; this knowledge will not, however, exclude the disruptive effects of truth. The symptom will also be the place of a *jouis-sens*, in which meaning and the real are no longer, as they usually are, mutually exclusive (Lacan, 1974–1975, p. 11); instead, "*the symptom, through an inconceivable circuit* [*tour*]", will "*kno*[*t*] *them together*" (p. 152).

Such considerations do not, in themselves, show us how we can exit from capitalism; Bruno does argue, however, that analytic practice and the *sinthome* that results from it are antithetical to the capitalist discourse. While the radical disjunction between the unconscious and the drive establishes a direct connection between *a* and $\$$, thereby heightening the subject's subjection to surplus-jouissance, analysis seeks to induce the subject – through the disavowal of the real – to cast away the object. The final sections of this book explore various aspects of the hope, which is admittedly razor-thin, that identifying with the symptom will provide sufficient numbers of people with a capacity to leave capitalist jouissance behind. Two sections in particular – the discussions of problems within psychoanalytic schools and of Catherine Millot's quasi-mystical experience of the not-all – call for a fuller explanation of certain of his references.

The emergence of the *sinthome* can have numerous effects; it can serve as a basis for a new kind of social bond among analysts and it can also open up an access to a jouissance that goes beyond the limitations imposed by castration. In examining the character of the bonds among analysts, Bruno develops a distinction between "institution" and "association", an opposition based on certain indications that are found in the "Letter of Dissolution" of 5 January 1980 – in which Lacan declared that he was dissolving the *École freudienne de Paris*[3] – and his seminar, "The Other is Missing", which followed ten days later.

In the "Letter of Dissolution", Lacan (1980a, p. 130) defines an "institution" as the "effect of a consolidated group", thus linking it directly to Freud's analysis of the army and the church in *Group Psychology and the Analysis of the Ego*. He then sets such institutions in opposition to the analytic discourse, arguing that the Freudian school had been working "at the expense of the discursive effect that is expected from an experiment, when it is Freudian. One knows what price was paid for Freud's having permitted the psychoanalytic group to win out over discourse, becoming a Church" (ibid., p. 130). Suffering from the effects of the "deviations and compromises" that had "blunt[ed] its progress while degrading its use" (ibid., p. 129), this school had failed "to produce Analysts within it who would be of the requisite level" (Lacan, 1980b, p. 133). Hoping to found a new school, Lacan (1980a, p. 130) called for members who would "Demonstrat[e] through acts" that the institutionalisation of the *École freudienne* "is not of their doing" (ibid., p. 130). He asked those who were willing to take part in this school to write to him, "declar[ing] to me that [they are] interested in continuing with me" (Lacan, 1980b, p. 134). If they did "so in terms that do not, to my mind, contradict the assertion in advance, they will be accepted by me to *associate* with [anyone who] does the same" (ibid., p. 134, emphasis added).

Bruno bases the distinction between institution and association on these statements, arguing that Lacanian schools have not been exempt from the pernicious effects of leaders who are determined to turn an association into a group. On the other hand, he also argues that an association can become an institution through the effects of "envy", a term that he borrows from Melanie Klein (1957, pp. 183, 186), who understood envy as the libidinal force that "spoil[s] . . . the object" and the "capacity for enjoyment", thus creating a situation in which "the envied person is felt to possess what is at bottom most prized and desired . . . a good object, which also implies a good character and sanity" (ibid., p. 203). For Bruno, in cases in which envy "threatens to undo the associative foundation", then "the solution becomes dissolution" (p. 178). This argument is related directly to his explanation that the identification with one's symptom at the end of analysisinvolves the acceptance of one's own radical singularity. The effect of this singularity is to "rende[r] null and void all forms of comparison"; it thus constitutes the "only way to get out of envy" (p. 167, note 8). Envy here becomes a sign that one has not yet identified with the symptom.

In the section entitled "*Gelassenheit*", Bruno treats the more or less mystical experiences that Catherine Millot recounts in *Abîmes ordinaires* (2001) as an instance of the symptom's ability to open up access to aspects of the not-all, aspects that would not – or would no longer be – impeded by the limitations imposed by the Name-of-the-Father. In Millot's own case, these "ordinary abysses" began before, and precipitated, her entry into analysis; at the beginning of her book, she recounts three of them. The first occurred when she was six, after her father, a diplomat, had been posted to a position in the French embassy in Hungary and her family was moving into a villa near Budapest. Asked to find something on a lower floor, she began to walk down the stairs, when "suddenly the world emptied out. In an instant, it had become deserted. No longer any before, no longer any afterwards, no longer any parents, no longer anyone. For several seconds, I was absolutely alone" (Millot, 2001, p. 11). To write of her experience in this way, however, is already too coherent: "it is even too much to say 'I', or rather it would have to be said that it was an 'I' without qualities, a pure stain of bare existence. On the empty staircase with nothing around" (ibid., p. 11).

Something of this sense of "bare existence" recurred six years later, shortly after Millot and her family had arrived in another city, Helsinki. Alone in a room filled with packing boxes, she again suddenly experiences a

> void, and even more, the infinity of a sidereal space that was opening up. A sudden cutting had snatched [*arrachée*] me from myself and sucked me into light-years, leaving a self [*moi*] that was no longer anything like me, in this strange room, reducing me with extraordinary quickness to a ridiculously small point: the "I", no longer with any identity, was vertiginously carried away – more abducted [*raptée*] than spirited away or ravished [*ravie*] – to cosmic heights.
>
> *(ibid., pp. 11–12)*

In this state of bewilderment, Millot seeks refuge by invoking her "own proper name, the effect of which was to call me back to common realities" (ibid., p. 11).

Her third such experience occurred after she had reached adulthood, when she was moving once again to a new place, this time alone. Having been assigned to a teaching post in a village whose name began with "*Mort* [Death] . . .", she was driving a rented car when a tyre exploded, nearly propelling her into an oncoming truck. Her first reaction was to feel that she had survived only by a miracle; "almost dying on the road to *Mort* . . ." became a sort of "obscure verdict and a no less obscure early release" (ibid., p. 13). Then, during the next few days, "A great void set in" (ibid., p. 13). She felt as if "an invisible lid" had been lifted from the sky, "allowing a bottomless hole to be seen". Shortly afterwards, the void "extended" and became

> an almost material, interstitial, separating void. It reigned in the intervals between things like a crystal in which each thing shone in isolation, for it was a magnifying void. It gave birth to another space and another time of vibrant immobility, in which one ceased to be ahead of oneself [*d'être en avant de soi-même*], always a bit elsewhere. Everything was there, simply, and nothing was lacking, where the nothing had become obvious, and presence was made more acute by a background of absence, so that what was beyond was dissipated. It was as if the world was lit by a more intense light.
>
> *(ibid., p. 15)*

At the end of this period, she left *Mort* . . ., and shortly afterwards, began an analysis with Lacan. When she described her experiences, "He answered me with a word that did not have the appearance of an interpretation and was still less a clinical label. What I had described to him, he told me, was *Gelassenheit*" (ibid., p. 16). "*Gelassenheit*", as Bret W. Davis (2010, p. xi) notes, is a word commonly used in German, where it refers to a "sense of 'calm composure'", especially in an "existential or religious experience of letting-go, being-let, and letting-be". Millot recognised this word from her reading of Meister Eckhart, but Lacan's reference was especially to Martin Heidegger's rethinking of the concept. Translators of Heidegger commonly render it in English as "releasement" (ibid., p. xi). Releasement involves leaving behind our common mode of thinking, which is a "willful representation, an objectification that transcends – climbs over – things to determine a transcendental horizon which determines the forms through which things can only appear as objects to subjects" (ibid., p. xiii). With releasement, one lets go not only of such representations, but also, and especially, of the "will-to-representation" that underlies them (Heidegger, 1995, p. 71). Accordingly, "releasement lies – if we may speak of lying here – outside the distinction between activity and passivity", since such an opposition depends upon the "domain of the will" (ibid., p. 70 also see Davis, p. xi). This sense of releasement gives us a way to theorise the experience of the not-all, which is located on the feminine side of the table of sexuation. Bruno, in turn, seeks to connect the not-all to the *sinthome* and to see in it something that is at the furthest remove from capitalist jouissance.

III

Translating Lacanian terminology is frequently difficult, and translators are often obliged to leave a number of fundamental terms in French or to stretch – or dismember – them on the Procrustean bed of the foreign language. In the present case, this dilemma began with the French title of the book, which presents Lacan as Marx's "*passeur*", a reference that has had to be lopped off in the English translation. The word is the technical term for one of the participants in the "*passe*", a term that itself, in this context, refers not to the analysand's movement to the position of analyst, but rather to the procedure in which s/he testifies about what has made this change possible. The term "*passe*" is translated here, as elsewhere, as the "pass", a term that needs to be approached with some caution. To Anglophone ears, to "pass" is too often understood as to "succeed" – in, for example, a competitive examination. To understand the verdict that the pass has occurred as a success and the opposite judgement as a pure and simple failure is to cover over the more complex sense of the term: the pass is an attempt to transmit something about the movement of change that has occurred. In this procedure, a *passant*, the analysand who has authorised him/herself to become an analyst, explains to two *passeurs* the changes that enabled this to take place. The *passeurs* then, in turn, seek to convey the character of the change to a committee of analysts; the indirect character of the testimony is part of an attempt to ensure that the effect of the testimony will not be produced, for example, by personal magnetism. Instead, something in the *passeurs*' words may perhaps allow the contours of the analytic act to be grasped. Stuart Schneiderman (1983, p. 67) and others have translated "*passeur*" as "passer", a word that I have also used. For "*passant*", I have chosen the rather inelegant term, "passand", on the basis of its analogy with the only slightly more elegant, but much more familiar term, "analysand".

Following Bruce Fink (2006, p. 764) and others, I have used the direct English cognate of the French word "*signification*" in order to translate it. "*Sens*", which is itself related to Freud's term "*Sinn*", has been translated as both "meaning" and "sense". In using the latter word, I am following the practice of the *Standard Edition* of Freud's works in English translation, which entitles the seventeenth lecture of the *Introductory Lectures on Psycho-analysis* "The Sense of Symptoms". It is this lecture that Bruno discusses in the first chapter of the final section of this book, and which gives this chapter its title.

In the French version of this book, Bruno uses the verb "*scinder*" in a new way: it names the capitalist discourse's operation of breaking the direct linkage between knowledge (S_2) and the barred subject ($\$$). I have rendered this term as "sunder".

– John Holland, Nantes, August 2018

Notes

1 One can also remember that in the same collective work, *Reading Capital*, Louis Althusser (1965, p. 27; also see Althusser, 1993, p. 170) had argued that Marx performed a "symptomatic" reading" of the texts of classical political economy.
2 It can be noted, for example, that Bruno's seminar in 1998–1999 at the department of psychoanalysis of the University of Paris 8 was devoted to the capitalist discourse and included readings of the *Strange Case of Doctor Jekyll and Mr. Hyde* and *Saint Joan of the Stockyards*. The present work serves as a way of nailing down and situating some of the developments of that seminar.
3 The questions that have been raised concerning the provenance of the "Letter of Dissolution" (Roudinesco, 1986, pp. 651–653) will not be addressed here.

References

Althusser, L. (1965). From *Capital* to Marx's philosophy. In D. Fernbach & B. Brewster (Trans.), *Reading Capital: The Complete Edition* (pp. 9–72). London: Verso, 2015.
Althusser, L. (1993). *Writings on Psychoanalysis: Freud and Lacan*. (O. Corpet & F. Matheron, Eds., J. Mehlman, Trans.). New York: Columbia University Press, 1996.
Bruno, P. (1993). Partition: Marx, Freud, Lacan. *Barca! 1*: 19–53.
Bruno, P. (2003). L'anticapitalisme féminin. In *La passe* (pp. 225–236). Toulouse: Presses universitaires du Mirail.
Bruno, P. (2013). L'invention de la fin. In *La psychanalyse: du rébus au rebut* (pp. 85–97). Toulouse: Erès.
Davis, B. W. (2010). Translator's foreword. In M. Heidegger & B. W. Davis (Trans.), *Country Path Conversations* (pp. vii–xxii). Bloomington, IN: Indiana University Press.
Dean, J. (2012). *The Communist Horizon*. London: Verso.
Fink, B. (1995). *The Lacanian Subject: Between Language and Jouissance*. Princeton, NJ: Princeton University Press.
Fink, B. (2006). Translator's endnotes. In J. Lacan & B. Fink (Trans.), *Écrits: The First Complete Edition in English* (pp. 759–850). New York: Norton.
Freud, S. (1919a). A child is being beaten. *The Standard Edition of the Complete Psychological Works, 17*: 179–204. London: Hogarth, 1955.
Freud, S. (1919b). The uncanny. *The Standard Edition of the Complete Psychological Works, 17*: 217–252. London: Hogarth, 1955.
Freud, S. (1927). Fetishism. *The Standard Edition of the Complete Psychological Works, 21*: 147–157. London: Hogarth, 1961.

Freud, S. (1940a). An outline of psycho-analysis. *The Standard Edition of the Complete Psychological Works, 23*: 144–207. London: Hogarth, 1964.

Freud, S. (1940b). Splitting of the ego in the process of defence. *The Standard Edition of the Complete Psychological Works, 23*: 275–278. London: Hogarth, 1964.

Heidegger, M. (1995). Ἀγχιβασίη: A triadic conversation on a country path between a scientist, a scholar, and a guide. In B. W. Davis (Trans.), *Country Path Conversations* (pp. 1–104). Bloomington, IN: Indiana University Press, 2010.

Holland, J. (2015). The capitalist uncanny. *S: Journal of the Circle for Lacanian Ideology Critique, 8*: 96–124.

Klein, M. (1957). Envy and gratitude. In *Envy and Gratitude, and Other Works, 1946–1963* (pp. 176–235). New York: Free Press, 1984.

Lacan, J. (1959). On a question prior to any possible treatment of psychosis. In B. Fink (Trans.), *Écrits: The First Complete Edition in English* (pp. 445–488). New York: Norton, 2006.

Lacan, J. (1966). On the subject who is finally in question. In B. Fink (Trans.), *Écrits: The First Complete Edition in English* (pp. 189–196). New York: Norton, 2006.

Lacan, J. (1970). Radiophonie [Radiophony]. In *Autres écrits* (pp. 403–447). Paris: Seuil, 2001.

Lacan, J. (1974–1975). *Le séminaire XXII: R.S.I., 1974–1975*. Retrieved from http://staferla.free.fr/S22/S22%20R.S.I.pdf

Lacan, J. (1980a). Letter of dissolution. In J. Copjec (Ed.), D. Hollier, R. Krauss, & A. Michelson (Trans.), *Television/A Challenge to the Psychoanalytic Establishment* (pp. 129–132). New York: Norton, 1990.

Lacan, J. (1980b). The other is missing. In J. Copjec (Ed.), D. Hollier, R. Krauss, & A. Michelson (Trans.), *Television/A Challenge to the Psychoanalytic Establishment* (pp. 133–135). New York: Norton, 1990.

Lacan, J. (1985) Conférence du mercredi 19 juin 1968 [Lecture Given on 19 June 1968]. *Bulletin de l'Association freudienne, 35*: 3–9.

Lacan, J. (1991). *The Other Side of Psychoanalysis* [*Seminar XVII*]. (J.-A. Miller, Ed., R. Grigg, Trans.). New York: Norton, 2007.

Lacan, J. (1994). *Le séminaire de Jacques Lacan, livre IV: La relation d'objet* [*Object Relations*], *1956–1957*. (J.-A. Miller, Ed.). Paris: Seuil.

Lacan, J. (2004). *Anxiety: The Seminar of Jacques Lacan, Book X*. (J.-A. Miller, Ed., A. R. Price, Trans.). Cambridge: Polity, 2014.

Lacan, J. (2006). *Le séminaire de Jacques Lacan. Livre XVIII, D'un discours qui ne serait pas du semblant* [*On a Discourse that Would Not Be of a Semblance*]*: 1971*. (J.-A. Miller, Ed.). Paris: Seuil.

Lacan, J. (2011). *Le séminaire de Jacques Lacan. Livre XIX, . . .ou pire* [*. . . or Worse*]*: 1971–1972*. (J.-A. Miller, Ed.). Paris: Seuil.

McGowan, T. (2016). *Capitalism and Desire: The Psychic Cost of Free Markets*. New York: Columbia University Press.

Miller, J.-A. (2005). Foreword. In J. Lacan & B. Fink (Trans.), *On the Names-of-the-Father* (pp. vi–viii). Cambridge: Polity, 2013.

Millot, C. (2001). *Abîmes ordinaires* [*Ordinary Abysses*]. Paris: Gallimard.

Morin, I. (2009). *La phobie, le vivant, le féminin* [*Phobia, the Living Being, and the Feminine*]. Toulouse: Presses universitaires du Mirail.

Pavón-Cuéllar, D. (2017). *Marxism and Psychoanalysis: In or Against Psychology?* (P. Kersey & D. Pavón-Cuéllar, Trans.). Abingdon-on-Thames: Routledge.

Rancière, J. (1965). The concept of critique and the critique of political economy: From the 1844 Manuscripts to Capital. In D. Fernbach & B. Brewster (Trans.), *Reading Capital: The Complete Edition* (pp. 73–174). London: Verso, 2015.

Roudinesco, É. (1986). *Jacques Lacan & Co.: A History of Psychoanalysis in France, 1925–1985* [*Histoire de la psychanalyse en France (Vol. 2)*]. (J. Mehlman, Trans.). Chicago, IL: University of Chicago Press, 1990.

Schneiderman, S. (1983). *Jacques Lacan: The Death of an Intellectual Hero*. Cambridge, MA: Harvard University Press.

Soler, C. (2003). *What Lacan Said About Women: A Psychoanalytic Study*. (J. Holland, Trans.). New York: Other Press, 2006.

Tomšič, S. (2015). *The Capitalist Unconscious: Marx and Lacan*. London: Verso.

Žižek, S. (2014). *Absolute Recoil: Towards a New Foundation of Dialectical Materialism*. London: Verso.

Žižek, S. (2017). *Incontinence of the Void: Economico-Philosophical Spandrels*. Cambridge, MA: MIT Press.

Zupančič, A. (2017). *What Is Sex?* Cambridge, MA: MIT Press.

INTRODUCTION

> "The problem of descending from the world of thoughts to the actual world is turned into the problem of descending from language to life."
>
> Karl Marx and Friedrich Engels, *The German Ideology*

> "Marx was also a poet, a poet who had the advantage of having succeeded in starting a political movement."
>
> Jacques Lacan, 15 November 1977

> "Warning to non-communists: All is common property, even God."
>
> —Charles Baudelaire[1]

Psychoanalytic causality and the resilience of capitalism

Each day, as it perpetuates itself ever more completely, capitalism shows its inability to construct a civilisation that would break, definitively, with its prehistory. The fall of the Berlin Wall in August 1989 marked the end of a credible communist alternative, at least in the form of what is known as "real socialism". Correlatively, and even for those who take issue with it not only as a mode of production but as a form of social organisation, capitalism has come to seem endowed with a resilience that has forced us to break with earlier judgements that its ascension was resistible. The question of its possible replacement remains abstract, purely formal and only becomes truly urgent for those who fear that capitalism may end up as the worst of all "utopias": an "end of history" that could really put an end to history. Furthermore, even if we suppose that capitalism could be replaced, what its replacement could be must still be determined, and this may make us wary of some blind "deconstruction" of it. To take up these two questions, we must first, as a prerequisite, ask whether all civilisation is in league with progress. When "progress" refers to cultural triumphs that have come to seem definitive – the development of the productive forces of science and technology – as long as their expansion does not harm nature, then there is no reason to stigmatise it.

However, in this sense, progress is more a means than an end. Authentic progress would involve the extension of human rights and putting them into practice, an equitable distribution of wealth, a lifting of the barriers of segregation, a satisfactory mixture of individual freedoms, respect for others and so on. Yet, even if communism were to come about as a sort of addendum to the current situation, this would not suffice. There is effectively no guarantee that such an optimal social state, balanced between the golden age and the communist promise of a better life, would be anything more than a fantasy; no one is certain that we would not end up under the "black sun of Melancholy" (Nerval, 1851, p. 41) or the grey clouds of ennui.

What matters is not simply to renounce the diabolical underside of progress: in concrete terms, capitalism's mad "kinetics", to use Sloterdijk's (2007) expression. There is little doubt that in the twenty-second century, and, let us hope, even before then, people will feel the same dismay about financial bubbles – which serve only to concentrate money and impoverish people – that we feel about the Mayan religious practice of human sacrifice. What we deem to be inevitable today may come to seem unthinkable.[2] Progress must nevertheless be called into question, for even in its least dubious ethical ambitions, it disregards the nature of satisfaction and remains a serf to attempts to evaluate levels and degrees of jouissance.

The pre-eminence of jouissance over satisfaction is all the more difficult to contest because satisfaction is itself defined by a threshold of jouissance, one that must be attained in order to reach the point at which something is "enough". The "discontents" of civilisation: that was Freud's name for the ferocity of the superego, which insists that we are guilty for being alive, something punishable by the forfeit of jouissance. In the light of this diagnosis, how can we exit from this structural malaise, which has its origins in the inventiveness of language and the mortification of the thing through symbolisation? How can each of us have the opportunity to depose the "dark God" that is the superego (Lacan, 1973d, p. 275)? This God is nothing more than a paper tiger, but it is precisely its lack of flesh and blood that makes it so difficult to defeat. We may not want to propose any utopian vision of a satisfaction that would either be devoid of all jouissance or – and this amounts to the same thing – would procure an absolute jouissance. Yet how can we envision a satisfaction that, even if it is not relieved of the burden of the superego, would, at least, be distant *enough* from the superego that its virulence would be deactivated? A solution would lie not in some general askesis that would do away with jouissance, but rather in *devaluing* jouissance. In what follows, we shall attempt to define this devaluation, but here, at the outset, it is already possible to note the pivotal role of the notion of value, which is fundamental to Karl Marx's thought, but which is also found, more discreetly but just as decisively, in Jacques Lacan's work.

What allows one to say that psychoanalysis, which has so little influence in the world in general and in politics in particular, is precisely what we cannot do without? It enables us not so much to take leave of the fantasy of progress, but to take it apart, in order to adjust the levers and dials of jouissance. Jouissance is neither pleasure nor pain. It is what Baudelaire was talking about: that exquisite, intoxicating scent that changes unexpectedly when we seek to concentrate it, to make it "divine". Then it becomes a horrible stench, the stink of rot, since jouissance attains its nirvana in death.[3] Psychoanalysis undertakes to liberate the body that has been colonised by jouissance, so that this jouissance can make way for satisfaction. This does not imply that jouissance must be renounced; instead, it will no longer be subjected to an endless and unreasonable attempt at escalation, and this change would not be to the taste of those who traffic in a marketable jouissance. Lacan himself said that psychoanalysis would lay down its arms when faced with "civilisation's increasing impasses", although he did add that this would lead people to consult "the instructions in my *Écrits*" (1968a, p. 349). Psychoanalysis can hope to play such a role because of the very texture of its experience, which rejects every possible combination of biological, sociological, and psychological determinants. Other approaches combine these determinants in varying degrees – on a scale that goes from zero to just about everything – in order to arrive at a satisfying explanation. It would be a mistake to deduce, on the basis of Freud's resolute determinism, a concept of the subject, who, at the end of analysis, would "know" her/himself. To put this in more modern terms, such a subject would be transparent to her/himself, once s/he had made a complete circuit around the biological, sociological and psychological variants that determine her/his history.

Let us say, at the outset, why this would be a mistake.

Suppose that a particular analysand's father and mother are political refugees from Spain, while another analysand is a victim of paedophilia and incest. A third has excellent parents and a close family and has never experienced any events that could be thought of as traumatic, whereas the father of yet another analysand was regularly cheating on his wife and leading a double life. The grandfather of a fifth analysand was a Nazi collaborator, who apparently tortured members of the resistance, and so on. Whether these realities are viewed as sociological ("her parents are political refugees"), psychological ("his uncle sexually abused him"), or even in terms of Saint DNA, and regardless of the consequences that – as the analysand believes – they have had on him/her, these realities cannot be changed.

How is it possible to change the *effects* of what cannot itself be changed unless we have a novel conception of causality? In other words, the fact that a person has parents who are political refugees (or rich capitalists), has an uncle who is an incestuous paedophile, or has a developmental disorder does not make that person blameless in relation to the symptomatic result of these experiences, whatever they may be.

The paradox is that renouncing this innocence enables an analysand to wash away her/his feelings of guilt, by recognising the part that s/he had played in constructing the symptom. Having acknowledged this, the analysand can then subtract her/himself from the status of someone who, at birth, was the object of his parents' jouissance (this is the basis of the passivity that Freud (1915a) considers to be one of the poles of the drive). The jouissance that they obtain from the subject can go to the point of making her/him nothing more than the puppet of their desire.

Once he had discovered repression, Freud wasted no time in drawing attention to resistance (*Widerstand*), the force that opposed its lifting. Freud provided several hypotheses about where this force comes from: the unconscious, the id, the ego and the superego. All of these may well be correct, but perhaps it would be better to define resistance in an even more general way: as a force that uses reality in order to allow repression to remain intact, for the sake of a refusal of knowledge. As Lacan noted, resistance comes from neither the analyst nor the analysand, but rather from the inertia that reality opposes to any rift between the cause (which concerns how a subject grasps what he or she is an effect of) and determinism (which concerns reality). From this point of view, we can say that *resistance neutralises the cause in favour of determinism, while psychoanalysis is supposed to liberate the cause from determinism.*[4] By distinguishing among biological, sociological and psychological determinants, and by trying to weigh the respective importance of each, we place an ideological mask over the fact that *reality can only be defined by including its subject-effect.*[5] Consequently, the subject, in making itself a response to this effect, confronts reality with what Lacan calls the *real* of this response, which takes the form of the symptom. These initial considerations are certainly not self-evident, and they will be drawn out and developed in what follows, but we also cannot ignore them; if we were to do so, it would be, as Robert Musil (1930, p. 494) puts it, "like trying to hammer a nail into a fountain's jet of water". The same problem arose in this form just before the birth of psychoanalysis: was a particular hysterical symptom produced by a direct physical action (a particular accident) or by the fear provoked by this accident? There is no "either/or" answer to this question because, even if fear – an effect of the subject – did not provoke the appearance of symptoms, another consideration remains. When we encounter an hysterical symptom, we should suppose that the subject has played a part, unconsciously in this case, in its appearance; we should not settle simply for speculating on a cause-and-effect relationship, which, as a result of as-yet-undiscovered chemical pathways, would be responsible for a paralysis that has no known organic basis. Similarly, if an analysand tells you that when s/he leans out the window, s/he can hear the roofs talking to her/him, it is only through self-discovery and through coming to accept that s/he actually is the voice of the roof that this analysand can come to distance her/himself from the hallucination.

An erratic practice

Psychoanalysis is an erratic practice. An "erratic" is one of those irregular blocks of ice that breaks away from a glacier when it is melting. This was already happening during Freud's lifetime. Without getting caught up in the many deviations that were explicitly rejected by Freud, yet still continue, in some cases, to lay claim to the name of psychoanalysis (Alfred Adler, C. G. Jung, Wilhelm Reich), nor in the brazen shamelessness of old-fashioned hypnosis when it tries to present itself as some sort of neo-psychoanalysis, let us note that, after Freud, there has been a kind of dispersion and dislocation of psychoanalysis (to limit ourselves to the most neutral of terms). This has not at all slowed down and, in the absence of Freud's speech [*dire*], confusion has, at least for a while, become the rule.

In an unpublished lecture given in San Francisco in 1946 under the title "Social science and sociological tendencies in psychoanalysis" (published in French as *La psychanalyse revisitée* [1972]), Theodor Adorno – someone who, incidentally, was never an ardent Freudian – provides a compelling critique of revisions of Freud's work, especially those of Karen Horney, who, in the 1930s, was one of the first to oppose Freud in the "Jones – Freud controversy" concerning feminine sexuality in the 1930s (see Guillen, 2007). Adorno was taking aim at a psychoanalysis that had been "culturalised" in the wrong way, skipping over infantile sexuality and completely misunderstanding the implications of Freud's introduction of the death drive. By way of Horney (whose dubious friendship with Matthias Göring, Herman's elder cousin, should suffice to discredit her approach), Eric Fromm also came in for criticism, although he had been working intermittently with Max Horkheimer's Institute of Social Research.[6]

The ensuing post-war period was monopolised by the confrontation between Anna Freud and Melanie Klein. These two theorists injected divergent approaches into analytic practice, which remain active today in the International Psychoanalytic Association (IPA). The first of these approaches overestimates the ego, which is thought to be able to master the conflict between the id and the superego; the second provides an over-interpretation of the unconscious, thus understanding transference in the present as the resurgence of something much earlier: the initial "I love you ... me neither"[7] of the mother-child relationship. Both of these neglect any examination of the role of the symptom, a primal rebellion against the sense that this relation has no exit [*huit clos*]. In both cases, the theory leaves behind an aporia for practice: for Anna Freud (1936), analytic treatment ends with the subject's "adaptation" to a "way of life", without having drawn the necessary conclusions from his/her symptom; for Melanie Klein (1957, p. 234), it ends with envy, the destructiveness of which could only be overcome "to some extent", as she had the honesty to acknowledge in her final book.

When Lacan burst onto the analytic scene at the end of the 1950s, his work provided a new way of understanding analysis and introduced a new era. Lacan began as a Kleinian and continued to have great respect for two British psychoanalysts who followed in her footsteps, D. W. Winnicott and Michael Balint, even if he also criticised their work. Lacan is often credited with having been the first to provide a psychoanalytic interpretation of the mirror stage, in a presentation given at the 1936 International Congress of the IPA in Marienbad.[8] It is true that this revitalising and innovative theory served as the basis for his critique of ego-psychology (and, by extension, of Anna Freud), for it argues that the ego, as a result of the way it takes shape, is a form of imaginary misconception [*méconnaissance*] and that it is pointless to make its strengthening and reinforcing the desired outcome of psychoanalysis. However, an exaggerated emphasis on this theory of the ego leads one to neglect what is at least as decisive for Lacan's ensuing theory: his article, "Logical time and the assertion of anticipated certainty" (Lacan, 1945), written when the tide of World War II had turned against the Nazis. In this text, Lacan argues that the act precedes knowledge and is its basis, and not the reverse. This rather abrupt rejection of the French tradition of spiritualist philosophy, which held that action is the result of a cognitive process, would become the cornerstone of the dialectic to come: the enunciation [*énonciation*], as act, goes beyond the statement [*énoncé*]. Consider this admirable formulation: "The point is not to know whether I speak of myself in a way that conforms to what I am, but rather to know whether, when I speak of myself, I am the same as the self of whom I speak" (Lacan, 1957c, p. 430).

The anticipation that characterises the act would only take on its full significance after Lacan had theorised "structure", a term borrowed from linguistics and Lévi-Straussian anthropology. Here again, there is room for misunderstanding: during a certain period, Lacan was classified as a structuralist (as were Roland Barthes, Michel Foucault and Louis Althusser). This is a theoretical blunder because, for Lacan, structure was not a subset of the universe; instead, it enables us to grasp a real that the concept of "universe" can neither exhaust nor even approach without falsity. In a certain sense, Lacan got himself out of structuralism by taking a door opened up by twentieth-century mathematics, and especially Gödel, who came along at just the right moment with his demonstration of formal undecidability (see Nagel & Newman, 1986). This demonstration destroyed the possibility of creating a mathematics that could cover the universal.[9]

Even worse, Lacan's reading of Freud's death drive has been misunderstood. He characterises it not as some mysterious biological force, but rather as the power [*puissance*] of symbolic nihilation [*néantisation*] through language, thus stripping language of its instrumental, communicative function and making it the condition of the existence of the unconscious.[10] The unconscious is a form of knowledge that is, in part, real, which is based on the fact that its status as unconscious is confirmed as one goes about interpreting it. This would serve as the basis for some decisive and unprecedented statements during the 1970s, in particular in reference to feminine jouissance and the symptom.

This is an abbreviated survey, but it at least enables us to pinpoint the essential isomers of psychoanalysis. To go further, we would need to start making a list of the misinterpretations that are continuing to squander Freud's discovery. I shall only mention two examples of them here.

Freud is often considered as the source of the idea that the prohibitions that a subject sets itself involve internalising (or "introjecting", to use the technical term) prohibitions established by the parents. So be it. We could use Freud's texts on the superego as the basis for this position. To do so, however, would be to put the cart before the horse. We forget that, according to this thesis, parental prohibitions do not fundamentally explain why children submit to them, in a servitude that is both voluntary and unconscious; instead, they are *what generate desire*. In *Totem and Taboo*, Freud (1912–13) states that it is the prohibition communicated to the sons by the father or the father's wives that leads them to turn murder into the first epiphany of desire; only then, *secondarily*, do they internalise the parental prohibitions. In other words, the prohibition is the condition that enables desire to emerge. How are the daughters involved in this? This question is more delicate: for them, the prohibition concerning the father is a prerequisite, but it makes the prohibition that bears on the mother more uncertain. This accounts for both the "ravaging" character of the mother-daughter relation, and, more positively, the detour through homosexual initiation that often paves the way for the encounter with a man. Lacan conceptualised Freud's immense work in this area in order to shed some light on questions that had, until then, remained shrouded behind prejudices of all kinds: he posited that "law and repressed desire are one and the same thing" (Lacan, 1963, p. 660). In other words, the law gives form to desire; this wipes out the ideologies (whether they are libertarian or restrict freedom) that make the opposition between desire and social repression a sort of universal passkey.

The other example is more bibliographical. It is common knowledge that a certain Mikkel Borch-Jacobsen has distinguished himself by his persistent efforts to destroy psychoanalysis, especially with his contribution to the famous "black book" dealing with the field (see Meyer, 2005). It should perhaps also be noted that this same author, who was interested in hypnosis, had already perpetrated a book intended to introduce Lacan to Anglophone readers, entitled *Lacan, The Absolute Master* (Borch-Jacobsen, 1990). This book should not be underrated, because it presents a serious reading of Lacan's *Écrits* and seminars (with the important exception of the later seminars). However, a strain is put on the book by the author's excessive taste for philosophy, which leads him to make himself the absolute master of the "absolute master". In the chapter on the phallus, after having done a good job of explaining Lacan's (1958) article "The Signification of the Phallus", Borch-Jacobsen (1990, p. 217) turns to some of Lacan's much earlier texts in order to state that, in the final analysis and "in spite of all Lacan's negations", the phallus is fundamentally imaginary:

> it is not surprising that the phallus, actually penile and masculine, is simultaneously so asexual in Lacan. It is nothing but the object in which the subject, before any sexual characterization, represents himself to himself, in his fixed, permanent, substantial identity. The phallus, erected and majestic, is the statue of the ego . . ., the *Vorbild* or *Gestalt* typical of humanity in general.
>
> *(ibid., p. 218)*

After this pedantic rigmarole, we could begin to think that Lacan's style is a paradigm of Boileau's vision of the poetic arts. How, on the basis of a reading of Borch-Jacobsen, can we understand the cutting edge of Lacan's views on the phallus, namely, that it is a symbolic operator that, unlike every other signifier, has no signified, but instead conditions the signified-effects of every other signifier?

Psychoanalysis and science: an impossible *glasnost*

After the era in which the "absolute master" was exalted, we have now reached the moment when the alleged "guru" is being put to death, with greater and lesser degrees of brutality. Freud was subjected to similar misfortunes; in France, for example, he was accused of being a coarse German, so that speakers of the more refined and subtle romance languages had no reason to involve themselves with psychoanalysis.[11]

Following the looting of his legacy in the university, Lacan is certainly no longer the darling of the French media, as he once was. There has been an obscurantist regression, which needs to be examined analytically and understood as a symptom. Rather than focusing nostalgically on the once-mighty Lacanian empire, which had its own problems, we ought to try to decipher this situation.

Before doing so, however, we must consider whether Lacan established psychoanalysis, which Freud discovered, as a science. Freud himself never gave up on its scientific, or even scientistic, character. The keenness of his observational skills and the rigour of his reasoning were as outstanding as his inventiveness. Lacan had another objective: to raise the question of the singularity of psychoanalysis in relation to science, while also retaining its scientific character, as Freud had conceived of it.

This singularity can already be grasped in the caesura between experience and structure (see Bruno, 2000). In "*L'étourdit*", Lacan (1973b, p. 483) defined structure as "the aspheric that is contained in the articulation of language, inasmuch as an effect of the subject can be grasped through it".[12] This is another way of saying that the subject of the enunciation, the subject that is speaking about itself in the present, is heterogeneous to the subject that it is speaking about ("spheri*cal*"). It also highlights how the subject, in the psychoanalytic sense of the term – the divided subject – is a consequence of language; at the same time, this subject is only an effect to the extent that it can grasp itself in the "aspherical" revealed by language. This theoretical assertion gives a good sense of the division that exists within psychoanalysis: it is divided between a doctrine (the knowledge developed by Freud and subsequent psychoanalysts) and the singular experience constituted by each analytic treatment. Could it be said that the doctrine is ever "applied" to the treatment? Perhaps, but only on the condition that we do not forget that such an application always leads to the aspects of the case that cause problems for the theory, a situation that also occurs frequently in hard science. The originality of psychoanalysis lies elsewhere. If the purpose of treatment is the emancipation "of", or "from", desire, we must look into just what the possessive term "of desire" implies; it means both "desire is emancipated" and "I emancipate myself from, or of, desire". This is one of the key aspects of the method Lacan has given us.[13] In its first sense – "desire is emancipated" – there are no objections: it is liberated when it is allowed to be recognised and accepted in terms of what "I" say and do. Thus, in one of Freud's (Breuer & Freud, 1895, p. 135) first cases, Elisabeth von R. came to recognise that the "painful fatigue" of her left thigh was a masked indicator of her desire to be loved by her brother-in-law, the husband of a sister who had just died. In its second sense, in which "I emancipate myself from, or of desire," it is something else. Desire is metonymic, like the ferret, which runs from object to object, without ever being satisfied[14]; it is maintained only as unsatisfied (this is another thesis that the study of hysteria enabled Freud to set forth). Thus, in order for desire to stop recycling itself through endless and precarious demands and for the subject to stop always putting off the act until tomorrow, analysis seeks *also*, and especially, to get him "to know if he wants what he desires", as Lacan (1961, pp. 571–572) writes in his "Remarks on Daniel Lagache's Presentation". This game between will and desire signals a dialectic that is opposed both to an indecisive desire – as we have just seen – and to a desire that would veer into a monomania that would denature it. What enables desire to be satisfied and not to lose itself in a headlong rush is the alternation between disappearance and resurgence. One must thus be careful not to confuse a "resolute desire" with a frozen desire.

The subject who begins an analysis is indeterminate, in the sense that what has determined her/his particular history is, to a large extent, unknown. Free association, and even more fully, *Durcharbeitung*, "working through" (see Freud, 1914) – if we take "through" to mean both a lateral movement and a movement beyond – will enable the subject to reconstruct the succession of determinations that have produced her/him as s/he is. It happens that, at the very point at which the subject could finally see her/himself as a whole, s/he discovers that s/he is not the product of these determinations, which have nevertheless been proven and experienced. S/he exists only as a process of detaching her/himself from them, a process during which s/he rewrites her/his history. It cannot even be said that this crucial process is simply a matter of mourning "who I was"; instead, it involves a "new love", and through it – whether s/he yields to her/his desire or not – s/he adopts the symptom that s/he now makes into her/his cause.[15] This border defines her/his history as a past that can never be rebuilt, and in order to make it perceptible, Freud and Lacan paid great attention to poets; through them, freedom, which is a kind of ethical synonym for infinity, finds its true place, a place to which the judiciary will make a civilising accomodation, but always much later.

Two additional comments must be added to this decisive remark. The first concerns transference. One of the fundamental achievements of Lacan's return to Freud lay in his separation of repetition and transference. The latter is not reduced to what had originally characterised the subject's relation to her/his parents, since it also enlists a sexual reality that is aroused by the analyst's presence. In other words, the real of the analyst prevents the analysand's relation to her/him from being an exact reproduction of the old relation with the parents. This is the case whether the analytic relation is approached in terms of love ("I could never do without you") or of distrust, which is more difficult to confess; it took several months for the Rat Man to tell Freud (1909, p. 285) that he suspected him of being the brother of a criminal who was also named Freud and who had just been condemned to death. Both love and distrust are ways of trying to reach what had first been missed in the relation with the parents: a knowledge of whether the Other's love was authentic or duplicitous. Nevertheless, analysis will always only have one outcome: the discovery and verification that there is no Other who can definitively guarantee to us what the Other wants. The analyst's only function is to allow her/himself to bear the consequences of this failure, and this authorises Lacan to define satisfaction as what puts an end to the mirage of truth.[16] This is a way not of giving in to scepticism, but of showing that truth cannot be said completely, and that this truth is known only in the unconscious.

The second comment is connected with what Freud began to specify with the processes of primal identification, and which Lacan, in "*Radiophonie*" (1970), treated as the incorporation of the symbolic body into the bodily organism. It is common today to observe that before speaking, and even before being born, the child is spoken of. We could then think that when s/he begins to speak, the subject may well be offered every latitude – although this is not always the case – to rectify what does not suit her/him in the way that s/he has been spoken of.

This supposes that s/he could free her/himself from suggestion. Yet this supposition forgets that in this structural incorporation, the whole grammar of the drive is set up, and this takes place in the form of "it speaks [*ça parle*] about her": it manifests itself in Dora's thumb-sucking, in the Wolf Man's constipation, and even in Schreber's transformation of the gaze into sound. The addiction to the objects of the drive dates from this. To believe that it could be abolished by de-conditioning the drive is to ignore an important fact: such de-conditioning does not operate when it is confronted with the grammar of the drives because this grammar does not result from conditioning. Thus, subjects can act on this grammar in another way: by deciphering – more often through construction than through interpretation – the way in which this grammar has been inscribed on their bodies.

These considerations can suggest a more concrete way of approaching the relation between science and psychoanalysis, especially by enabling us to set aside the petty and malevolent criticisms that focus on the mote in the other person's eye, without any awareness of the beam in our own. Almost at the midpoint of his teaching, Lacan wrote a text about this problem (1966g).[17]

His central concern was to bring out two new theses: 1) the subject involved in analytic practice is none other than the "subject of science" and 2) the subject of science is none other than the Cartesian subject of the cogito, or even, instead, of the "*dubito sum*". This subject is distinguished by rejecting all knowledge, as obvious as it may be (2 and 3 make 5, for example) in order to allow a certainty about being to emerge. What is illuminating here is its homology with analysands' experiences: their being as truth emerges by disassembling the family romance, screen memories, the fundamental fantasy, etc.

Lacan makes only a slight correction to Descartes' extraordinary formulation: instead of writing, "I think, therefore I am", he writes "I think: 'Therefore I am'", "with quotes around the second clause, it is legible that thought only grounds being by knotting itself in speech where every operation goes right to the essence of language" (Lacan, 1966g, p. 734). By being *speech*, "therefore I am" escapes from the objection that it is only one more thought. There is no doubt that the failure of science to consider speech as something that is said disables science, or at least makes it problematic, in the eyes of psychoanalysis. The irruption of speech makes this division of the subject manifest. This division or splitting, in turn, can be said – and I am seeking to phrase this in a way that preserves psychoanalysis from any burdensome psychologising appropriation – to place the unconscious outside, rather than in the "depths" of the subject.

Once he had been "excommunicated" from the IPA in 1963, Lacan put a great deal of energy into clarifying the relations between science and psychoanalysis.

Our contemporary amnesia has covered over this excommunication, making it just one more item in a chronology; the intensity of this subjective cataclysm can no longer be measured. Yet if you are a psychoanalyst yourself, try to imagine the effect of being erased from the map of "Freud country", disqualified as a psychoanalyst, denounced as a dissident theorist, reviled and *Berufsverboten* – forbidden to teach or to train analysts – by the entire analytic "fraternity", including by a few psychoanalysts who deserved to be considered true Freudians. The only exception was a handful of students, almost all of whom were nearly unknown, whose transference to Lacan had resisted the institutional transference to the IPA. The tacit complicity that was and remains the rule of the analytic establishment, as may well be the case for every establishment, was also involved, and silently covered over a mass cowardice.

This may be one of the reasons that led Lacan (1973d), in his 1964 seminar *The Four Fundamental Concepts of Psychoanalysis*, to align himself with a scientific method, one that was connected epistemologically to the philosophy of the Enlightenment, and then to devote "Science and Truth" (1966g) to a more subtle and dialectical elucidation of the relations between science and psychoanalysis. It should be noted that people tend to modify the tense and mode of the verb that Lacan used when suggesting a definition for science. He writes that "science would not want-to-know-anything about the truth as cause" (Lacan, 1966g, p. 742, translation modified). The use of the modal "would" indicates, beyond a shadow of a doubt, that science does not succeed in what it tries to do. Another definition of science appears in "*Radiophonie*": it is the "ideology of the suppression of the subject" (Lacan, 1970, p. 437), a definition that is congruent with this reading, since the term "ideology" refers to science's misrecognition of itself.

In this same text, he notes that mathematical logic, which is difficult for science to wash its hands of, "brings us back to the structure in knowledge" (ibid., p. 437). A programme has thus been opened up, one that would involve – here the modal appears again but is now turned towards the future – an entrance into a new age of knowledge, because of psychoanalysis. Without seeking for the moment to go beyond this formulation, we can deduce that, whatever the other criticisms that Lacan would make later concerning the discourse of science and its affinity with the capitalist discourse, the fate of science has never been sealed. Today, numerous facts invite us to consider that, if we set aside ideologies and technosciences and concentrate on the sciences that are the least contestable, the question of the place of the subject has now become inevitable (see Klein, 2004). We can thus catch ourselves dreaming that, in a new scientific age, psychoanalysis will be in the driver's seat. This may well be a dream, or even a fantasy; perhaps it is also how we should understand the term "ascience" (see Briest, Le Fur, & Tajan, 2006).

The topology of the final seminars can point in this direction. Topology, like psychoanalytic theory, can be made to say anything. A bit of string passes above or below another bit of string, and this is independent of the unconscious relation between the person who is manipulating it and his own servitude. If we keep to their topological properties, a hand is a cord and the organism as a whole is a torus (the volume constituted by the inner tube of a tyre). The electron microscope can certainly give us a less "figurative" idea of a body's composition, especially with its helices, but this does not make topology obsolete, because the same topological mode can be appropriated at two levels. It can be added, as a supplementary step, that the Borromean principle – two cannot come together without a third – may only be a local property, but one that could possibly introduce us to the principle that could make topology the universal science of "fabric", whether physical or psychical.

Let us, however, bring these motley ideas to a stop before we get too far afield, and just retain the following idea: psychoanalytic knowledge, as a textual knowledge, only comes to life within an analysis, and such analyses must be approached one by one. Each analysis, in its structure, involves an objection to the textual knowledge of psychoanalysis. This is why psychoanalysis cannot be included within the scientific paradigm: the analysand can end her/his treatment only by extracting her/himself as an exception from the totality of statements that have constituted the treatment, and which are articulated with one another in a way that conforms to the textual knowledge of psychoanalysis. S/he only exits from her/his treatment through an act, rather than by adding one more element of knowledge. S/he renounces the hope of finding the truth of the knowledge that s/he has accumulated throughout her/his treatment; this is the meaning of her/his acceptance of division. This renunciation creates a boundary to the knowledge that has been produced. Let us be clear, however: this act can only really occur in a situation in which the knowledge that has been produced is not just any knowledge; if this is not the case, then what takes place would only be a false act, in which the subject would lose her/himself.

Situating Lacan's references to Marx

Let us now approach the figure who is Lacan's partner, or even his sparring partner.

One only has to consult the index of proper names for the *Écrits* (Lacan, 1966b), the *Autres écrits* (Lacan, 2001a) and the seminars (see Krutzen, 2003) to notice something that speaks volumes: Marx is mentioned seven times in the *Écrits*, twelve times in the *Autres écrits* (Lenin is only referred to four times). This may not seem to be many references, but they are rarely mere allusions. For the most part, Marx's name is connected to decisive theoretical developments. A comparative and relatively unselective analysis of these references will provide an appropriate framework for our research.

Let us begin with references to Marx's name in the *Écrits*:

- Marx, like Socrates, Descartes and Freud, has a passion for truth (Lacan, 1947b, p. 157). Such a statement is not simply praise, either for Marx or for the others, since the passion for truth can mask the real.
- Marx's "reversal" of Hegel consisted in the "materialist return" of "the question of truth" (Lacan, 1966c, p. 194). This return involves marking out the "symptom's proper operation", an operation to which Freud would later give its definitive status.

- Marx, like Jacques-Bénigne Bossuet, Arnold Toynbee or Auguste Comte, discovered a meaning and direction in history (Lacan, 1956b, p. 216). Lacan then suggests that what we can retain from this concerns the theory and philosophy of history rather than history in a more conventional sense.
- What is propagated in our culture "in Freud's name" is not unlike what is carried out in Marx's name (Lacan, 1957a, p. 70).[18]
- Finally, the last reference to Marx's name in the *Écrits*, in "Science and Truth", may be the most significant. Lacan criticises the naivety of Lenin's formula: "Marx's theory is omnipotent because it is true!" He continues by saying that, "An economic science inspired by *Capital* does not necessarily lead to its utilisation as a revolutionary power and history seems to require help from something other than a predicative dialectic" (Lacan, 1966g, p. 738). This rather caustic remark prefigures what Lacan would develop concerning the primacy of the real over the true – which is the single condition for a materialism that would be more authentic than its Marxist version – and echoes the false praise for the passion for truth, which he attributed to both Marx and Freud.

Turning next to the *Autres écrits*, we note that the references to Marx's name occur in works that were written after the final texts of the *Écrits*. The first is found in "Response to Students of Philosophy Concerning the Object of Psychoanalysis" (published in English in *Television* [1974b]); these students were from the *École normale supérieure*, and, after May 1968, they became one of the sources of the enormous media attention devoted to both Lacan and Marx. Lacan casts doubt on the possibility of the "subject's revolutionary praxis of going beyond his alienated labor" (ibid., p. 110). This would be, he says, like wanting to go "beyond the alienation of discourse" (ibid., p. 111). He then adds, pointing to the students' adherence to a questionable Marxist vernacular:

> All I can see as transcending that alienation is the object sustaining its value, what Marx in a homonym singularly anticipatory of psychoanalysis, called the fetish, it being understood that psychoanalysis reveals its biological significance.
>
> *(ibid., p. 111)*

The five following references, which I shall examine more closely in the course of this book, are in "*Radiophonie*" (1970). Lacan notes first that the French Revolution would have been reduced to the "return of the masters" – a reduction that was as true "for Bonaparte as for Chateaubriand" – if Marx had not put it back "into the structure that he formulates it in: a discourse of the capitalist" (Lacan, 1970, p. 424). Yet this salutary change is undone because this structure "foreclosed the surplus-value by which it motivates this discourse". Lacan continues:

> In other words, it is with the unconscious and the symptom that he claims to extend the great Revolution: it is by discovering surplus-value that he

> precipitates the consciousness that is called class consciousness. Lenin, through his *passage à l'acte*, obtained nothing more than what is called regression in psychoanalysis: which is the time of a discourse that has not been given in reality, first of all because this discourse is untenable.
>
> *(ibid., p. 424)*

As I shall discuss below, it is the status of surplus-value that is questioned. This is not a repudiation of Marx's essential discovery, which constitutes the foundation of his critique of classical political economy. Instead, as we shall see, the problem is that he did not take jouissance into account in his calculations. The other references concern the way in which Marx's desire was involved in his discovery of surplus-value. Hence this striking formula: "*Mehrwert* [surplus-value] is *Marxlust*, Marx's surplus-jouissance" (ibid., p. 434).

In the "*Postface au Séminaire XI*" (Lacan, 1973c, p. 506), there is a passing reference to the "gospel according to Marx" and then in *Television*, Lacan (1974b, p. 14) refers to the "ideal worker", who, with Marx would "take over the discourse of the master". Finally, in the first appendix to the *Autres écrits*, there is a comment about the insufficiency of Marx's views of Jewish people, "so as to repay the debt incurred by the constitutive segregation of this ethnic group" (Lacan, 1978a, pp. 588–589).

When we move on to the twenty-seven years of Lacan's seminar (1953–1980), Henry Krutzen's (2003) concordance identifies sixteen references to Marx's name, and this is to say nothing of his references to communism and communists, capitalism and capitalists, revolution, Marxism and surplus-value. The references to his name, however, offer us some relevant starting-points. These references are various and disparate, touching several times on the concepts of use-value and exchange-value. In this context, I would like to highlight several stumbling blocks. Let us consider a session from the seminar, *La logique du fantasme*, where Lacan (1966–1967, 12 April 1967) sets up an opposition between use-value and "jouissance-value", which he places beside exchange-value. He does this because jouissance is only thinkable if something is subtracted from it. Exchange-value does not realise use-value, for it suspends use in order for exchange to take place. From this perspective, Lacan sets up a homology between the psychoanalytic and the Marxist concepts of the fetish: the fetish is a use-value, "extracted" and "frozen – a hole somewhere". In Freud, the fetish is the substitute for the penis that a woman does not have, and thus fills a "hole". It happens that this hole in jouissance *establishes* jouissance. In a comparable way, Marx, in order to explain the relations between commodities, treats the fetish as presenting commodities as relations between things rather than between people. This very astute and subtle intuition leads to a definition of commodity-fetishism as the setting up of a substitute, the commodity, as having an intrinsic value as a thing; it then allows us to disavow the fact that this thing-value does not exist and is only the result of a social relation between people who are working during a determinate time. The hole that is masked in this case is the gap between the working time necessary to reproduce labour-power and surplus-labour.

Let us also take note of the seminar that followed May 1968 directly. In the first four sessions of *D'un Autre à l'autre*, Lacan (2006a) reminds his audience that surplus-value depends on a renunciation of jouissance (ibid., p. 18), alludes to Althusser's work on Marx (ibid., pp. 16–17, 29–30) and refers to the passage in *Capital* where Marx speaks of the capitalist's laughter (ibid., p. 65; also see Marx, 1867, pp. 300–301). Finally, he talks about his memory of reading *Capital* in the Paris metro when he was twenty (ibid., p. 64).

Lacan's relation with Marx is expressed in its densest form in *The Other Side of Psychoanalysis*. Here we find the thesis that the Soviet Union is directed by the discourse of the university: a bureaucracy has appropriated for itself the place of a knowledge that is defined as a whole (Lacan, 1991, p. 206). This is a consequence of Marx's inability to find a way out of the discourse of the master, the discourse that is the other side (or underside) of psychoanalysis. The discourse of the university derives from it, with the difference that, in the university, the master is hidden.[19] I shall come back to this.

Two points, in particular, are taken up in this seminar. Lacan notes that surplus-value corresponds strictly to Marx's concept of "surplus-labour": surplus-value comes from the socially necessary labour-time over and above the labour-time that is affected in order to maintain labour-power. Such labour is paid for in the same way that any other commodity is (ibid., p. 20). Instead of workers, who have sold their labour-power, being paid more, their surplus-labour pays for a bonus of jouissance, a surplus-jouissance, which "it is very urgent that one squander" (ibid., p. 20).[20]

The second point concerns the objective of the session that deals with the "Lacanian field", the "field of jouissance" (ibid., p. 81). What Lacan posits here concerns the transformation of the discourse of the master into that of the university. In the first of these discourses, the master is in the dominant place, while in the second, it is knowledge. According to Lacan, Marx calls this rotation a "spoliation" because the key to exploitation involves reducing labour-power to a commodity that has a particular value, a reduction that is permitted by knowledge (ibid., p. 81).

A pivotal thesis is also found in the next seminar, *D'un discours qui ne serait pas du semblant*, where Lacan (2006b, p. 164) says that Marx is "responsible" for the notion of the symptom. This passage situates Marx as the figure who denounces the fetish as a semblance, unlike Hegel, who constitutes the acme of a tradition in which the semblance is taken at face value.

In following these signposts, it is striking to note that, for Lacan, while Marx and Freud are similar in that "they don't bullshit" (Lacan, 1991, p. 71), Marx reinforced the discourse of the master by calling it into question. In his 1971–1972 seminar *. . . ou pire*, Lacan (2011a, p. 118) states that Marx's discourse "includes a protest, which happens to consolidate the discourse of the master by completing it, and not only with surplus-value – I feel that this is going to create some turmoil – by inciting woman to exist as an equal". This is not simply a criticism, since by "crystallising the discourse of the master" (ibid., p. 224), Marx takes a decisive step, but this is not the same as Freud's.

What is the difference between Marx and Freud? An answer – one that, in this case, does not fluctuate very much – is given in two of his later seminars. In *RSI*, Lacan reiterates Marx's primacy as the inventor of the symptom and then comments on how he analyses this symptom: because the proletarian is the one who has been "stripped of everything" (Marx, 1877, p. 201), Marx transforms this figure into the "Messiah of the future":

> If we treat man no longer as what may convey a future ideal, but if we determine him in terms of the particularity, in each case, of his unconscious and of the way that he gets off on it, the symptom remains in the same place where Marx placed it, but it takes on another meaning. It is not a social symptom; it is a particular symptom.
>
> *(Lacan, 1974–1975, 18 January 1975)*

This judgement is confirmed on 18 March 1980 during the seminar *Dissolution*, one of Lacan's final public presentations:

> I have paid homage to Marx as the inventor of the symptom. This Marx, however, is someone who restores order, simply because he breathed the *dit-mension* of meaning [*sens*] back into the proletariat. The proletariat was enough for him to do this, and he says this. This was a lesson to the church.... Know that religious meaning is going to go through the kind of boom that you can't imagine. . . . I'm trying to go against this, so that psychoanalysis won't be a religion, as it tends irresistibly to be, as soon as we imagine that interpretation only operates through meaning. I teach that the mainspring of interpretation is elsewhere, namely in the signifier as such.
>
> *(Lacan, 1980c, pp. 18–19)*

This passage is a superb statement of the blind spot in Marx's work – the impasse concerning jouissance – which dilutes his intrinsically revolutionary conception of the symptom, transforming it into a political gospel that is irrevocably counter-insurrectionist. QED.

Lacan "*vs.*" Marx?

This book is neither a sword-and-sandal epic nor a horror film along the lines of "Godzilla *vs.* Frankenstein". The preposition "*vs.*" or "against" [*contre*]" is to be understood in the sense that it takes on in the expression "helpmeet against", which can be found in Lacan.[21] The playing field thus levelled, a new temptation can be born: the temptation to create a new couple – Lacan-Marx – which can be substituted for another couple – Marx-Freud – which has long been divorced. In itself, there would be no contradiction in giving in to this temptation. It is clear that, for Lacan, Marx is a major thinker whose work is at least the equal of the thought of those who, apart from Freud, have opened up our understanding of what exists and have done so in ways that have never been surpassed. Plato, Aristotle, Dante, Rabelais, Galileo and Descartes are our authentic contemporaries. Such figures are not intimidated by the idea that history always delegates the task of knowing to future generations, making former "contemporaries" into outmoded figures in relation to what the truth of knowledge could be. Lacan certainly felt close to Marx's adventure, and even to planet "Marx". To take a single example, in one of the final texts of the *Écrits*, "Position of the Unconscious", Lacan (1966e, p. 706) mentions the communists' mistrust of psychoanalysis and says that "I . . . consider justified the prejudice that psychoanalysis encounters" – note the use of the present tense – "in Eastern Europe". His sympathy for Georges Politzer or Lev Vygotsky, like his "lukewarm" attitude (a euphemism) towards Jean Piaget goes in the same direction. He even chose his favourite poets, such as Louis Aragon and Paul Éluard, from what could be called a certain (i.e. the communist) camp.

These considerations are neither off-topic nor anecdotal. They enable us to deduce the existence of a discreet yet real "comradeship" between Lacan and the children of Marx, as well as a no less perceptible irritation at the doggedness with which communists sought to transform Marx's saying [*dire*] into a catechism. The consequence of such a tendency is to reduce Marx to being nothing more than a philosopher of history.

The borderline is located here. Freud (1933, pp. 176–177) used the term *Weltanschauung* to pin down and stigmatise Marxism and wanted to prevent psychoanalysis from suffering the same fate. Perhaps one key to the differences between the lineages of Freud and Marx can be found in the fact that the term "Freudianism" has not been substituted for "psychoanalysis" and that "dialectical materialism" has not supplanted "Marxism". In French, for that matter, the use of the word "*lacanisme*" remains both limited and pejorative. We could perhaps even question whether "psychoanalysis" – in the singular – exists at all, because of the extraordinary differences and divergences that can be found within it, even if we set aside flagrant shams such as Jungianism and "psychoanalytic" psychotherapy. Should we therefore speak of "psychoanalyses"? Yes and no. No, because psychoanalysis as a form of knowledge cannot refuse to question itself about its borders: which statements can be called "non-psychoanalytic" or "anti-psychoanalytic"? Do the various tendencies within psychoanalysis come together, in a more or less unified or consistent way, to explain difficult phenomena? To speak not of "psychoanalysis" but of "psychoanalys*es*" would be to admit that there has been a diaspora and that there is no longer any common denominator among analysts; this would eliminate any common reference to the radical difference that is named "Freud". It would be better to speak of "psychoanalyst*s*" to the point of daring to say, as Lacan (1973b, p. 454) did: "There is not the slightest access to Freud's words that has not been foreclosed – and without any possibility of return in this case – by the choice of such an analyst".

The degradation of Marx's work could perhaps be imputed partially to his disciples – or rather to sectarians – but to do so would be to promote a repetition of the same failure: the failure in which the key contained in his work is used to open the wrong door. Marx, as Althusser (see 1965, p. 334) judiciously emphasised, defines the subject as the bearer [*Träger*] of the relations of production. He thus transforms the subject into an agent. The concept of groups or masses – which Freud (1921) deals with in *Group Psychology and the Analysis of the Ego* – relies on the postulate that agents can be treated as a collective. To say then that the masses make history is neither incoherent nor shocking. What *is* damaging is that, in Freud and in a way that has an even stronger foundation in Lacan, the subject is neither a bearer nor an agent. It is still less the subject of psychology, the homunculus that only reflects the really restricted span of its creator: it is not enough to add conflict or the unconscious in order to transform the pumpkin into a coach. It would be better, instead, to turn the coach into a pumpkin, for the pumpkin – the divided subject – is real.

The division or splitting of the subject ($) is the element without which psychoanalysis would collapse. As we shall argue, this subject is linked to two considerations. First, the sexual drive, which is somatic and psychical rather than organic, consists in the very failure that results from the incorporation of language by the physical organism. Second, the unconscious has a "navel", a kernel that remains irreducibly unconscious, since speech cannot itself speak. It is this double discovery that Freud brings together in his final conception of the *Spaltung* – the splitting of the ego between a recognition and a disavowal of the mother's castration – a conception that Lacan then takes up as the division of the subject.

It turns out, as a result, that divided subjects, unlike subjects who are "bearers", cannot be grouped into a set [*ensemble*], and that social psychology can exist only on the individual level, in which each subject is taken one by one; at the intersubjective level, the relations between subjects can only lead to an authentic dialogue in extremely rare occurrences. Thus communist millennialism leaves the stage (see Delumeau, 1995), and what enters is evil (or in more secular terms, jouissance) as the only possible bond with my neighbour (the *nebenmensch*). The idea that "it feels good to do evil", rather than being a postromantic whim, is what Sade, still a bit too apprehensively, was able to theorise (Lacan, 1963, p. 646). Only by recognising the evil within jouissance and by understanding that this evil is permanent does it become possible to envision a way of devalorising it.

Perhaps, finally, the most relevant way of measuring the gap between Lacan and Marx might be their relation to Jeremy Bentham. In *L'homme économique: essai sur les racines du néolibéralisme*, a book that immediately became the reference in its field when it appeared in France, Christian Laval (2007) paints an historical portrait of "*homo oeconomicus*", a portrait to which, significantly, Marx contributed nothing, while Bentham brought a great deal. This might seem surprising, for Marx is often presented as the figure who imposed an economist dogma in which everything that is "human" is determined by the base concern of putting food on the table or, at best, by "material" needs. In reality, what emerges from this book is the ingenuity by which everyone – from Bentham to Walras, and even to Keynes – uses a psychology of desire to cover over the quantitative measurement of value, a form of measurement that must be made manifest if exploitation is to be recognised.

In relation to Bentham and his utilitarianism, Lacan, who always lauded the discovery of surplus-value, had first adopted a position that was very close to Marx's absolute condemnation:

> With the dryest naiveté he assumes that the modern petty bourgeois, especially the English petty bourgeois, is the normal man. Whatever is useful to this peculiar kind of normal man, and to his world, is useful in and for itself. He applies this yardstick to the past, the present and the future. . . . If I had the courage of my friend Heinrich Heine, I should call Mr Jeremy a genius in the way of bourgeois stupidity.
>
> *(1867, p. 759, note 51)*

Lacan then changed his opinion in *The Ethics of Psychoanalysis*, indicating that Roman Jakobson had led him to read Bentham in a new way (Lacan, 1986, p. 12). What he now finds attractive in Bentham's work is that he is "the man who approaches the question at the level of the signifier" (ibid., p. 228). Bentham's guiding intuition, to which Lacan pays homage, is that pleasures and pains can only serve as an arithmetic that can regulate the functioning of society if they are approached as "fictions": not as phenomena that can be quantified naturally, but as phenomena that are shaped symbolically by language. This is the great difference between Bentham and naturalist utilitarianism, and this may be why Marx himself applied the word "genius" to him. Anyone who uses the term "symbolic" is saying that the cathexis of the signifier involves taking into account the body's relation to jouissance, and not simply to needs, whether these needs are said to be natural or historical. Because he did not recognise the beach of jouissance under the paving stones of surplus-value, Marx failed, for example, to give a satisfying account of the gap between the exchange-value and the price of works of art, thereby underestimating the monstrous development of financial capital and of credit as a *fiction*.

Youthful questions

This is not to disqualify history, just to consider it still early days, although this fact should not stop us from following Walter Benjamin in bringing out those chapters that have been forgotten, as they were vanquished, as it were, smothered in their cribs. History should not only be written by the victors, and this procedure is analogous to what serves as the true cutting edge of analysis. As Benjamin (1950, p. 256) writes in his extraordinary, "Theses on the Philosophy of History", "There is no better way of characterising the method with which historical materialism has broken. It is a process of empathy whose origin is the indolence of the heart, *acedia*". *Acedia*, or sadness, affects historians who empathise with the victors. One of the consequences of doing so, as Benjamin notes, is to prevent us from seeing that the most eminent conquests of culture could not have been accomplished without barbarism: they depend on the "anonymous toil" of the people who lived through and suffered from these conquests (ibid., p. 256). This "*acedia*" is quite precisely the "moral failing" that, in *Television*, Lacan (1974b, p. 22) treats as the equivalent of sadness. When the historian identifies with the victor, this cowardice returns in the form of sadness; similarly, when the subject identifies with repression, the result is the affect of sadness.

These remarks enable us to be more precise: the dominant modes of production are what benefit from this empathy, and *today*, the forgotten histories are the ones that have challenged the capitalist discourse, which is an avatar of the discourse of the master. This other side of history remains to be explored, but we can already wonder whether beginning to write this history may not be a symptom, one that indicates that this discourse is being questioned and is beginning to decay.

As soon as the back of the page is written, it turns out to have an other, front side, which is what Lacan made visible by crediting Marx as the inventor of the symptom. In saying this, Lacan was making a strong interpretation, because the term itself is rarely present in Marx. One notable exception is to be found in the speech Marx gave for the anniversary of the *People's Paper*:

> There is one great fact, characteristic of this our nineteenth century, a fact which no party dares deny. On the one hand, there have started into life industrial and scientific forces, which no epoch of former human history had ever suspected. On the other hand, there exist *symptoms of decay*, far surpassing the horrors recorded of the latter times of the Roman Empire.
>
> *(Marx, 1856, p. 299, emphasis added)*[22]

Here, Marx is sketching out the problem that defines political space. What is the meaning of the decay that is located at the very heart of progress, and which serves as a symptom? The correlation between symptom and decay can help us theorise not only the very real opposition between the forces of progress and of reaction, but also something that is much more important: the question of what does not work in progress. Progress can open up a margin for this "decay". In other words, does the invention of the symptom only involve theorising the polarised distribution of wealth produced by the growing production of this wealth in capitalism? Perhaps the symptom also calls into question one of the ways in which a socialist or communist alternative to capitalism has been constructed: the tendency to conceive of "progress" as a consistent whole. Of course, according to this perspective, a symptom such as a workers' strike would take on a meaning in whatever political context it may take place, whether in a regime that is overtly capitalist or that claims to serve the working class.

In any case, doesn't this "decay", taken as a symptom, always work in opposition to a tendency towards idealisation which would aim simply to eradicate every symptom? Wouldn't this set a limit to any understanding of progress as an asymptotic approach (see Lacan, 1956b, p. 251) towards a paradise on earth? At this level, an examination of what a symptom is for psychoanalysis can throw light on this question.

The symptom is out of pace with progress, with the idea that history can have an end, and therefore can be said to have instituted the field of politics. Today, politics can only be approached in terms of its relation to democracy. How, then, can we understand the sort of compass constituted by democracy today? In his stimulating book, *Hatred of Democracy*, Jacques Rancière (2005) creates and defends a thesis that has a fortunate stereoscopic effect upon any attempt to grasp what is at stake in this problem. He uses a striking formulation to criticise the foregone conclusion that democracy can only be "representative democracy": "'Representative democracy' might appear today as a pleonasm. But it was initially an oxymoron" (ibid., p. 53). His thesis is that:

> Democracy is neither a type of constitution nor a form of society. The power of the people is not that of a people gathered together, nor of a working class. It is simply the power peculiar to those who have no more entitlements to govern than to submit.
>
> *(ibid., pp. 46–47)*

This thesis has strong Freudian resonances: "democracy" becomes the name of the impossibility of governing. If we grant this comparison, however, it gives rise to an objection. Democracy becomes detached from any historical reference; from this perspective, the requirements of democracy have been present since the dawn of politics.

In *Democracy in Europe: A History of an Ideology*, Luciano Canfora (2004) uses a different method. Canfora is an historian and locates his work explicitly within the Marxist tradition. History is the single cultural field in which this reference truly remains current, although the historians marked by Marxism – including Moses Finley, Eric Hobsbawm, Albert Soboul and Michel Vovelle – come from a generation that was born before the Second World War. If we were to follow only Canfora's subtitle, we could be led to believe that he is interested in the concrete historical avatars of democracy. This assumption, however, sets aside what is really at stake in the book. Although Canfora begins by relativising the belief that democracy began in Greece during the fifth century BCE, and is closely concerned with ideological uses of this term, the fundamental aim of his detailed study is to demonstrate that democracy has been subordinated, as superstructure, to historical configurations that can be analysed in terms of class struggle. Even more significantly, in refusing, like Rancière, to reduce democracy to "political forms" or "forms of government", he comments on a passage in Herodotus that highlights its scandalous character: it is founded on the requirement of equality (Canfora, 2004, pp. 248–249).[23] This formulation may well be vague, yet it succeeds in emphasising the insurrectionary character of the famous slogan, "One man, one vote", a slogan that, until the end of Apartheid, struck fear into the hearts of most white South Africans.

It is regrettable that the rectification that distances the reader from a fascination with the history of the victors – for the moment, capitalism – can throw less light on why the Soviet political system became the greatest enemy of communism. Yet this immediately raises a question that keeps recurring throughout history: the question of Caesarism and the lethal attraction exercised by power on both those who hold it and those upon whom it is exerted. Lacan (1973a, p. 379) speaks of "The proven impossibility of a pulverulent discourse is the Trojan horse by which the master who is the psychotic returns into the city of discourse" (the cult of the One prevents the psychotic's delusion from crumbling). Such a remark immediately calls to mind Wilson and Hitler, Stalin and Ceausescu, Saddam Hussein, and more recently, the dynamic duo of "B." and "B.", etc. We may well wonder whether, among the "great men" who have made their careers in politics, psychotics might not be the rule, rather than the exception. This observation is not made to stigmatise psychotics. Instead, it forces us to confront a major question: why today, at every level of the social hierarchy, including psychoanalytic associations, is the place of *Führer* the preferred place that enables psychotics to treat their wandering [*errance*] by mistreating their neighbour? This was not the case in other societies, where the psychotic could find a less harmful place – that of shaman, for example. A second question, correlative to that of the status of the symptom, needs to be asked here. What sort of civilisation would enable the genius of psychotics to flourish, while permitting them to renounce their tyranny? Conversely, what would help neurotics to rid themselves of their lethal fascination with psychotic tyranny (Freud (see 1905b) had already noticed the hypnotic effect that the pervert exercises upon the neurotic)? The entire work of Michel Foucault – however we may judge his solution – was devoted to producing a shift in this terrible cartography.

These preliminary remarks would be pointless if the question of Freud's relation to the transcendent had not already been raised directly, and such a question is interesting since religions claim that only they can provide a suitable place for transcendence. Freud opted to break this presumption: one has only to read his correspondence with Oskar Pfister (1963), with its sometimes fierce dismantling of the temptation to turn psychoanalysis into a gospel, and analysands into experimental catechumens. As Ernest Jones (1957) noted and sometimes even criticised, Freud's relation to occultism was more complex and troubled. Should Freud's papers on the occult and telepathy be considered as bits of refuse that need to be swept away? Should we note, instead, that in these tortuous works, even while seeking a scientistic explanation of phenomena that are called supernatural or paranormal, Freud also allows an intimate bond between infinity and discourse to show through, in the very place of his own symptomatic vulnerability? I am not going to analyse these texts, because I shall take a more classical approach; I believe, however, that my approach will be just as effective in questioning the border that gives religions the monopoly on the transcendent and reduces the symptom to the field of medicine. Freud's response to Romain Rolland concerning the "oceanic feeling",[24] for example, suggests that beyond his atheistic motives and his ambition for giving metapsychological explanations, Freud tends to close off problems of this kind. It is also true, however, that any way of opening up these problems that would arouse the anxiety of a "negative" oceanic feeling – today, we would call it a bad "trip"[25] – must be excluded from the start.

To lay my cards on the table, I shall argue that the foreclosure of the transcendent, which can certainly be connected to the scientism endemic among scientists and scholars, and which can go hand-in-hand with an indulgent attitude towards parapsychology, must be rethought. The enunciation always stands in an ex-centric relation to the statement, since the "I" cannot be grasped simultaneously in its statement and in its act of enunciation. For this reason, Freud could legitimately reproach both metaphysics and every ontology for aggrandising themselves by suggesting that there is a being whose enunciation would be included in its statement. These would be avatars of the celebrated assertion, "I am the one who is, or who will be". If this is correct, it may well be through the saying [*dire*], which, as we shall see, transforms the symptom into the sinthome, that the transcendence connected with the real can pierce the virtuality of the linguistic: this is the promise of a world without boredom.

There has indeed been some misdealing of the psychoanalytic cards, which – to change the metaphor – has made the ship of analysis sail and sink in an area located between ecclesiastical atheism and positivist spiritualism. Psychoanalysis can only have both a meaning and a direction if it does not shrink from connecting the infinite quality of the mystery of existence to the relative character of discourse – while recognising the effectiveness of science. In referring to the "infinite quality of mystery", I mean what critical philosophy has restored to us, on the basis of a crisis of transcendence, in the form of the aporias of reason. "Where do we come from?" What follows this is an echo that does not stop answering this question but does enable each singular language to compose its own version of the eternal song: "From where nothing knows everything".

The expression "infinite quality of mystery" might seem overblown, and arouse the objection that we are in danger of regressing from Freud's metapsychology to metaphysics. This phrase is, however, brave enough not to allow certain kinds of questions to be diluted in the hypocritical shadow of medicine: these are the questions asked by the psychotic, whom I am calling upon again, and who, in this respect, is more courageous than the neurotic and the pervert. The psychotic welcomes such questions, considering them to be fundamental, for they contain the enigmas that religion and philosophy seek to sterilise. Freud's sometimes reluctant discovery restored these questions, which opened up the issues of the *Heimlich* and the *Unheimlich*, as well as of *das Ding*, the thing that the Other cannot tame. Lacan himself does not hesitate to place his *Écrits* on the same shelf as what he calls "mystical jaculations" (Lacan, 1975c, p. 76). For psychoanalysis, the outcome of this questioning is not a doctrine but an effect *in* the body, and even an effect *of* the body: the lifting of inhibition, the disappearance of anxiety, the reversal of jouissance in relation to the symptom. (Such a remark indicates the Rubicon that psychoanalysis has crossed within culture.) These results of treatment are corporeal responses to the "infinity of mystery". Saint Theresa, at the end of a transference that transcended the object that was called God – an object that could only be represented inadequately – experienced what Marguerite Duras would have called a "ravishing". This ravishing enabled her to disencumber herself from the horror of doubt, which had led her to wonder whether she was being possessed or being enraptured, and which had provided so much painful jouissance for her.

What defines the prehistory that we are perhaps now in the painful process of leaving is the absence of any emancipation from the death drive.[26] This drive, which Freud discovered and named so aptly, is the consequence of language: in killing things, language also kills the things that are called "human beings", who then continue the ideal of language by reducing themselves to their names. They prefer glory and death to life and dishonour, and administration to psychoanalysis, for what matters above all else is to extract oneself from the fate of being unimportant human beings. The result of this primary allegiance to the rites of the virtual is that the real – which is to be distinguished from reality – is always encountered only by chance or, on the contrary, is brought out through practices – including psychoanalytic, poetic and political experience – when the act has not been appropriated by and for a thirst for power.

A three-part division

Before venturing into the "French" jungle that is opened up by this kind of psychoanalytic questioning, I would like to make several clarifications. I would like to claim, first, that this entire book belongs to the field of psychoanalytic knowledge. To this end, I shall develop a thesis that will have certain consequences for analytic experience, for it involves the interpretation of structure: *the division of the subject constitutes the subject*. Beginning with his 1962–1963 seminar, *Anxiety* (2004), the barred subject is said to be produced as the quotient that results when a subject that does not yet exist is divided by the Other: the place occupied by language and from which speech originates. This can occur if there is a living agent or bearer to carry out this division. The symptom, in its primal emergence, is the ineffaceable mark of this division. It is what objects to any pseudo-jouissance that would aim to annul this division. In psychoanalytic practice, we encounter the very early appearance of symptoms that testify to an almost innate discord between mother and *infans*.

On the basis of this thesis, a new understanding of castration and its complex becomes necessary. This will enable us to clarify Lacan's otherwise incomprehensible proposition that capitalism is the "foreclosure of castration". To give the reader a foretaste of this clarification, in a form that is as compressed as Lacan's own thesis, we shall say that castration is what makes it possible to produce the semblance in which the Other would not itself be divided by the subject who proceeds from it. In other words, even when castration operates, it maintains the fiction that there is at-least-one who would not be castrated. Lacan resolves this paradox by identifying what founds this fiction: the fiction of a real father, who is exempt from the phallic function's requirement that we be castrated, whether or not we have the phallus. For a man, "having" the phallus requires that he had once not had it, and that it was then given to him. Lacan's advance in this area is related to another aspect of his teaching, which also calls into question some claims of certain currents of feminism: a woman is not entirely submitted to the regime of castration, and, like her, a man can be exempted from this regime. Division, on the other hand, holds for everyone. As we can see, there is a risk of confusion, if castration is considered as the equivalent of division. An analysis can dissipate this confusion and bring out the division of the Other, the matheme for which is S(Ⱥ). It can also put an end to the culture of lack and the anxiety which accompanies this. In helping the subject no longer to play with castration, it enables the subject to put an inaugural loss – that of the invention of language – behind him/her, and to discover that it is fullness, rather than the void, which can be frightening.

Finally, the specific character of psychoanalysis is exemplified by the bizarre encounters that often take place in the analyst's waiting room: a psychiatrist may meet her patient there; an analyst can run into another analyst, who is seeing him for supervision. Yet all of them are in this room as analysands, and their very presence contradicts any arrangement of discourse that would be based on hierarchy. The bond between analyst and analysand, except in the fantasy of one of them, is not set up in the same way that the connection between other pairs – master/slave, professor/student, patient/doctor – is arranged. The hysteric, in reversing the conventional hierarchical order, creates a symptom, which analytic discourse can then throw light on. The final word here is always the analysand's.

I have therefore started by bringing out the subject's inescapable division (part I) and then what could be qualified as either its apogee or its opposite: the capitalist accident, which involves a filling in of this split, an operation that I have called the "sundering" of the subject. Hyde/Jekyll, Dark/Mauler. The spectre of paranoiac sincerity hangs over these two couples; this sincerity can lead such characters to strangle with one hand and bless with the other. Then, immediately afterwards, I shall examine four thinkers who did not hesitate to confront Lacanian psychoanalysis: Louis Althusser, Gilles Deleuze and Félix Guattari, and Slavoj Žižek, each of whom, in his own way, produced a reading of the Freudian subject. Precisely because their undertakings are rigorous and well argued, it is necessary to show how they diverge from the path of psychoanalysis. If castration means that the mother has no phallus, whereas division and splitting concern every subject, whether a man or a woman, we can explain what division is by starting with its mathematical sense: the Other, the place of language, is divided by the subject, and this division gives rise to a remainder that Lacan calls the object *a*, which cannot be symbolised, and which constitutes the failure of language to represent all of the real.[27] In the first part, I seek to make this pared-down algebra more concrete.

The second part is more difficult. It will sometimes require the reader to become a re-reader.

I have tried to present Lacan's concept of discourse in a fluid prose that would almost resemble the style of classic adventure novels as retold for children. I would even have preferred, paradoxically, not to use Lacan's mathemes. This is paradoxical because the explicit function of these mathemes is to favour the transmission of knowledge.[28]

I would have liked to be able to explain intrinsically difficult matters directly and simply. Finding myself unable to do so, I have adopted a two-stage procedure:

1 I present the clothes;
2 I present the man whom they do not make.

In other words, first I provide an exposition of the matrix of the discourses, its formal functioning and its descriptive relevance; then I examine the consequences of these discourses and what is at stake in the battles that have arisen over Freud's discovery. I am not simply trying to make my work readable, however legitimate this requirement may be. Instead, I am trying to verify that I have mourned the primal language, which is Lacan's, the figure who brought us into psychoanalysis. Here, concerted mourning precedes and precipitates loss. In other words, if we call ourselves Lacan's students, we should not remain vassals to his signifiers; students should preserve only the concepts that they have reconstructed themselves. This even implies that because the concepts themselves turn out to flatten the experience that connects the infinite to the finite, only the axioms should be retained. Such axioms enable us precisely to bend structure to experience. Do these axioms exist? Have they existed from time immemorial, just waiting to be discovered? Are they created by someone, or are they ultimately only conventions? The investigation is still taking place.

Lacan provided us with various means – graphs, mathemes, topology – of transmitting the aspects of psychoanalysis that can be transmitted in a way that can be verified. Whatever the validity of these means, this transmission can only take place in a process that must not remain formal – in the sense of a calculation that could be affected by the "scientist's" computer. If this process were simply formal, it would risk being disqualified, for it would not involve the analyst's desire. In relation to this desire, we cannot do anything other than to note its presence: it manifests itself in this questioning of the primal language. It involves a rethinking, at its own expense, of psychoanalysis.

Finally, part III seeks to reformulate, in terms of the fundamental vector of the symptom – which is a sort of insurrection or uprising – questions that have been worked on from every conceivable angle in a field that had ended up being sterilised. It has been sterilised by the hypothesis that there is a lack of division between Marx and Freud. At the present moment, the land has been left fallow for a certain period, and new growth seems both possible and desirable.

This part is entitled "On the Symptom" because it re-examines Lacan's major thesis: the symptom is a "clip", in both senses of the term: it both fastens the work of Marx and Freud together and cuts them apart. Lacan repeatedly paid homage to Marx for his invention of the symptom. As we shall see, although Freud's treatment of the symptom is fundamentally different from Marx's, there is an intersection between the two, which enables us to discern their common epistemic atheism. For both of them, the symptom is what does not work well. Marx presents it as being both the first and the last obstacle to Hegelian idealism, which ultimately promotes the rationality of the real and sketches out a contradiction that, at the ever-delayed end of history, will itself be absorbed in order to produce a totalisation of knowledge in a truth with a capital "T". For Freud, the symptom sets up an obstacle to a miracle: one that would dissolve polymorphous perversion – the "bad start" of sexuality – in the acid of the genital relation. With the symptom, Freud rids us of the illusion that sexuality would be something like a little peg that will fit comfortably into a little hole.

If we held on to a bit of the philosophy of history, we could remark that the slow death of the Bolshevik revolution was the history of the forcing, and then the disappearance, of this contradiction contained in the symptom, thereby enslaving the revolution to a teleological conception of communism. People were then awakened from this history by the fall of a wall – which is a symptom par excellence. A parallel could be established between this and the slow degradation of psychoanalysis after Freud's death and the American exile of his students, a degradation that Lacan condemned. This is also the history of a forcing, one that set itself in opposition to the pranks of an *infans* who was seen both as pre-Oedipal and as insufficiently Oedipal. This forcing was undertaken to make genitality the norm for the beast with two backs, even if, in the fullness of time, these backs were permitted to be of the same sex. The symptom made its force felt not with the fall of a wall, but with the excommunication of a psychoanalyst, an excommunication that would liberate him.[29]

We should bear in mind the following observation: a contradiction, which only language can bring out as real, can only become a (dialectical) motive force by making black equal white. It thereby allows the human act the privilege of making contingent good emerge from necessary evil. We owe this salutary discovery of cruelty to Antonin Artaud.

On this basis, we shall try to offer a few scraps of an answer to the question of how to leave capitalism. We can do so, first, by giving up our tendency to think of socialism and communism – to use these words again – as the movement beyond a contraction between productive forces and the relations of production; such a movement would then get rid of the private ownership of the means of production (which certainly needs to be abolished), the market and the financialisation of capital. These actions are necessary but not sufficient. When we take a retrospective look at the daily life of the countries that practised "real socialism" – an unconsciously ironic expression – what is striking is that once revolutionary enthusiasm had passed, apathy invaded public space. Although there have been no subtle social-psychological investigations to back up this hypothesis, the endemic debate, in these countries, on the respective importance of material and ideological *stimuli* points incontestably to societies in which, in the best of cases, a certain material security, a relative sexual liberation and a strong encouragement of culture were powerless against the syndrome of small differences. This syndrome gave the advantage to the smoke and mirrors of the capitalist countries. Freedom of movement, less official censorship, a greater diversity of consumer goods, and even risks: all of these conferred upon this capitalist world the semblances that maintained a more lively enthusiasm for jouissance.[30]

I have sufficiently emphasised the way in which the stumbling block of the symptom becomes a token of life (*Eros*). Now I would like to highlight – as a counterpoint and in a way that surely falls short of the symptomatic being by which each subject separates and distinguishes him/herself from the social and parental Other – the requirement that generational being be respected. This is the celebrated Name-of-the-Father, which one must either make do with or make up for in order to allow the symptom to heal with a scar and thus keep the subject from becoming a skinless, tormented being. In the developed capitalist countries, civil religion, like religion itself, can easily take the form of the primal fabric or tissue onto which semblances can be grafted. Unlike this situation, the more recent epic of revolution and its rites in real socialist countries was skewed by a fraudulent materialism, which foreclosed the transcendent. In order not to succumb to the complaint, "What good is jouissance?" such an epic required a society that would have been composed exclusively of poets. Vladimir Mayakovsky's suicide marked the death knell of such a hope.

The easiest task of the book is to show the impact of Marx and Freud's kinship in terms of the insurrectional character of the symptom. In the final part, I have tried to do something much more difficult. Instead of prolonging the negative remarks that I have just made concerning the malaise of real socialist countries, I have sought to approach, in a more positive light, the question of how to leave capitalism. Instead of providing a definitive answer, I give a few preliminary scraps of a response to this question, one whose currency and urgency is always before us.

Very early, in his 1945 article, which I have already quoted, on logical time, Lacan takes a gamble: through a "logical" problem – the parable of the three prisoners – he seeks to elaborate a collective logic that is removed from both Freud's *Massenpsychologie* (1921) and Jean-Paul Sartre's sense that there is *No Exit* (1947). What he brings out, in particular, is that the solution to the problem can only be envisioned if each of the three prisoners trusts the reasoning of the other two; in such a case, as soon as one of the three finds the solution and is freed, the same will occur for the others. Can this ideal model be applied in this context? We know that in the postwar years, Lacan (see 1947a) was very interested in the psychiatric experiments of Wilfred Bion and John Rickman, who overturned a number of assumptions about the discourse of the master and the ideology of selection, assumptions that had, until then, been considered self-evident. Lacan always considered this to be an inexhaustible axis of research, and it may well have been a priority for him. When he founded the *École freudienne de Paris* [Freudian School of Paris] in 1964, he was seeking to create an association that would be based on the bond of the analytic discourse. His dissolution of the school in January 1980 was an attempt not to allow this experiment to collapse. During this period, he invented the pass and several years later, in 1974, tried to form a school on its basis. I shall argue that Lacan's work of the 1970s suggests that he may well have hoped that an association of "saints" could succeed where the *École freudienne* was failing.

During the same period, and especially in *Television*, Lacan (1974b, p. 15) examined what a saint is, defining this figure as the one whose actions involve "*trashitas*" and seeking to bring the saint closer to the psychoanalyst, even making them counterparts. *Trashitas* goes against the ecclesiastical tradition and is closer to the line of François Fénelon than of Jacques-Bénigne Bossuet. It involves subtracting oneself from worldliness and the wish to repair, or at least to reduce the unjust distribution of goods, and thus of money. The impulse towards *trashitas* leads the saint to abstain, first and foremost, from the theological virtue that would treat God as the supremely expensive or dear (*carus*) being, the figure that no one can do without.

Can capitalism be rendered obsolete by making psychoanalysis as widespread as literacy? To ask this question is, at the very least, to forget that no one is born psychoanalysed. Is my aim then to attain a majority of saints? It is unlikely that Lacan would have appreciated this adulterated conception of a theologically-inflected democracy. After the dissolution of 1980, he wagered on whether persons who were – or were not – saints could create the conditions for a psychoanalytic association that would finally not be afraid to guide psychoanalytic discourse: to do so in a way that would prevent it from falling back into the ruts of group "obscenity."

This final section will close by examining the dialectic between association and institution; it will test the idea that culture does not necessarily need to be legalist in order to be active and that law, as necessary as it may be, is only positive if subjects mark out the boundaries of its empire.

Finally, by approaching the decisive question of the transcendent in psychoanalysis (see Lacan, 1974b, pp. 111, 112), my objective is not only to refine the separation between psychoanalysis and psychotherapy, but to suggest a stereoscopic presentation: one that will include both the sinthome and the requirement not to fill in the gap between the Name-of-the-Father and the symptom. This Name guarantees a law that a father, as Other, has the task of seeing that it be respected; the symptom objects to this guarantee and founds, at its own risk, the division of the subject.

Notes

1 Marx & Engels (1932), p. 446. Lacan (1977–1978). Baudelaire (1897), p. 92.
2 This question has been specifically addressed in *Le nouveau mur de l'argent* by François Morin (2006) and *La finance mondialisée*, edited by François Chesnais (2004).
3 See, for example, Charles Baudelaire's (1869) prose poem "Dog and Flask"; the structural caprices of jouissance as regards pleasure (and unpleasure) are perhaps most intelligible in relation to the sense of smell.
4 In a footnote added to the *Interpretation of Dreams* in 1925, Freud (1900, p. 517, note 1) writes:

> The proposition laid down in these peremptory terms – "whatever interrupts the progress of analytic work is a resistance" – is easily open to misunderstanding. It is of course only to be taken as a technical rule, as a warning to analysts. It cannot be disputed that in the course of an analysis various events may occur the responsibility for which cannot be laid upon the patient's intentions. His father may die without his having murdered him; or a war may break out which brings the analysis to an end. But behind its obvious exaggeration the proposition is asserting something both true and new. Even if the interrupting event is a real one and independent of the patient, it often depends on him how great an interruption it causes; and resistance shows itself unmistakably in the readiness with which he accepts an occurrence of this kind or the exaggerated use which he makes of it.

5 [*Translator's note*: see, for example, Jean-Louis Baudry (1986, p. 59).]
6 [*Translator's note*: on Fromm and the IPA, see Paul Roazen (2001).]
7 [*Translator's note*: this is a reference to the Serge Gainsbourg song "*Je t'aime . . . moi non plus*".]
8 This text was published in the *Écrits* as "The mirror stage as formative of the *I* function as revealed in psychoanalytic experience" (Lacan, 1949); its initial version, presented at the Congress 1936, has not survived.
9 For more on Gödel, also see Pierre Cassou-Noguès' excellent *Les démons de Gödel: logique et folie* (2007). The work of the logician Charles Sanders Peirce also played an important role in Lacan's distancing of himself from structuralism.
10 Lacan's *Écrits* were published in 1966, and then in 1970, Jean Laplanche's *Vie et mort en psychanalyse* (translated into English as *Life and Death in Psychoanalysis* in 1976), was published by Flammarion. Although the section of this work that deals with "life" is interesting, the

section on "death" gets caught up in a reading of Freud that accentuates the opacity of his text. This book is the beginning of Laplanche's movement away from Lacan's teaching, a distancing that culminates in his claim that the unconscious is the condition of language; this is, essentially, the most succinct antithesis possible of Lacan's teaching.

11 In an early writing, Georges Politzer (1939, p. 13) attributed this view to Charles Blondel.

12 [*Translator's note*: Unless otherwise noted, the citations in English of texts published in French have been translated for this edition.]

13 Lacan translated several of Freud's terms with *désir* [desire]: *Wunsch* [wish], which was commonly used by Freud, but also *Begierde* [desire or craving] and *Begehren* [desire or avidity], which Freud used very rarely but which is found in *The Phenomenology of Spirit* (Hegel, 1807). This double meaning must be included in any serious reading of what Lacan meant by *désir*.

14 [*Translator's note*: This is a reference to a game in which a small object – a "*furet*" or ferret – is passed around from one person to another while a person standing in the middle tries to guess who is holding it. See Fink (Lacan, 1966a, p. 787, note 259,1).]

15 Michael Turnheim (2001) correctly emphasises the gap between "Mourning and Melancholia", where Freud (1917) treats mourning as a process that can be completed, and his letter of 12 April 1929 to Ludwig Binswanger, where he states that there is something beyond mourning, something that remains "inconsolable" (E. L. Freud, 1975, p. 386). Also note that the expression "*Qui je fus*" is the title of a collection of poems by Henri Michaux (see 1997, pp. 3–5).

16 As Lacan (1973d, p. viii) writes in his preface to the English translation of *The Four Fundamental Concepts of Psychoanalysis*: "The mirage of truth . . .] has no other term than the satisfaction that marks the end of the analysis.

17 This article, "Science and Truth", is a reworking of the first, introductory session of Lacan's (1965–1966, 1 December 1965) seminar, *L'objet de la psychanalyse*.

18 [*Translator's note*: This reference comes from the discussion that followed Lacan's presentation of "*La psychanalyse et son enseignement*" at the *Société française de philosophie* on 23 February 1957 (see 1966a, p. 866). The discussion itself is not reprinted in the *Écrits*; it only appears in the original version published in the *Bulletin de la Société française de philosophie* (Lacan, 1957a).]

19 Would this imply that Stalin was a hidden master? There is no reason not to reply in the affirmative, especially if we suppose that he was presented as the custodian of the line as it was supposedly determined by the Party.

20 We could however add that such squandering has to be supervised, so that the capitalist can invest part of the surplus-labour in the process of production. It is worth noting that Lacan had read and appreciated Weber's (1905) *The Protestant Ethic and the Spirit of Capitalism*.

21 For example, Lacan (2005b, p. 20) states: "My starting point is my condition, which is that of bringing to Man what the Scripture states, not as *an help meet for him*, but as an helpmeet *against* him".

22 Also see Rubel's (1994) introduction to volume IV of the French *Pléiade* edition of Marx's collected works.

23 Incidentally, Herodotus locates the origin of democracy here with the Persians rather than the Greeks.

24 In *Civilization and its Discontents*, Freud (1930, p. 64) explores the oceanic feeling (*Gefühl*), a feeling that Rolland held was the basis of all religious needs, independently of "every belief and every illusion" (p. 64).". After stating that he is not able to discover this feeling within himself, which suggests that it is not universal, Freud provides a metapsychological analysis. He argues that the feeling is the "restoration" of a primary emotional state, specifically one of "limitless narcissism", but he does not agree that such "oneness with the universe" involves any "attempt at religious consolation" (ibid., p. 72). For Freud, religious needs derive from the experience of infantile helplessness (*Hilflösigkeit*) and are a substitute for the need for paternal protection. He thus rules out all forms of religious mysticism, or at least considers them to be secondary matters.

We also note that to express his own views, Freud (ibid., p. 73, note 1) cites Schiller's (1797, p. 48) poem "*Der Taucher* [The Diver]": "Happy they whom the rose-hues of daylight rejoice". It is interesting to note the next lines of the poem, which Freud does not cite: "May the horror below never more find a voice – /Nor Man stretch too far the wide mercy of Heaven!/ Never more – never more may he lift from the mirror, /The Veil which is woven with Night and with Terror!". These lines seem to testify to Freud's need to defend himself against a fear of what is "below". We thus could say that Freud's rejection of the transcendental is related to the fact that he was unable to forgo a recourse to the father as the solution to infantile helplessness. His secularisation of the father, which is the decisive condition for the existence of psychoanalysis, may well not be the final word on the matter. (It is also worth noting that, in a letter written a few years later – "A Disturbance of Memory on the Acropolis" – Freud (1936) put himself in the position of the analysand in relation to his friend Rolland.)

Here, however, Freud did have access to what poets use to free themselves from the lysis of language, as he shows in quoting an extraordinary phrase from Christian Dietrich Grabbe, which he (Freud, 1930, p. 65, note 2) cites without wanting to acknowledge its significance: "Indeed we shall not fall out of this world. We are in it once and for all". He has Hannibal speak these words; this figure, in Western history, is the epitome of an unbeatable loser. A ghost calls out to us: what if Rome, rather than Carthage, had been destroyed?

25 [*Translator's note*: English in the original.]

26 Jacques Derrida (2000, p. 241) asked the right question here, albeit from a philosophical perspective: "can one think this apparently impossible, but otherwise impossible thing, namely, a beyond the death drive or the drive for sovereign mastery, thus the beyond of a cruelty, a beyond that would have nothing to do with either drives or principles?" Although this question can be formulated philosophically, one can wonder whether it can be answered through philosophy or whether analytic experience is required.

27 The subject itself consists in this division, and the end of analysis can be defined as the acceptance of the Other's division, along with the externalisation of the object *a*, which refers to the discovery and acceptance that it is impossible to convey or render it fully with signifiers.

28 For readers who may be unfamiliar with mathemes, here is an example:

$$\begin{array}{ccc} A & \dashrightarrow & B \\ \uparrow & & \downarrow \\ D & & C \end{array}$$

It can be read as follows: an hysteric (such as Anna O., for instance), represented by "A", asks a doctor (such as Breuer), represented by "B", to explain the causes of her troubles to her. The causes are a form of knowledge, represented by "C". However, in the end the doctor fails. The true cause, represented by "D", eludes her (and that is why there is no arrow from "C" to "D").

29 Marxists could say that when Lacan was excommunicated from the IPA in1963, he was the victim of a purge.

30 Regarding the "small-difference syndrome", see the films of directors from the former German Democratic Republic, such as *Good Bye, Lenin!* and *The Lives of Others*.

PART I

The splitting of the subject

1

LONDON/BERLIN

The "division of the subject" is not a warlike expression, although the military sense of the word "division" can introduce the idea that such division is the only weapon at the subject's disposal for becoming and remaining sensitive to the real. This real, indeed, only becomes such by resisting the linguistic domestication that, like time for Baudelaire (1857, p. 20), is an "enemy that gnaws our heart". "Division" and "splitting" are translations of Freud's German term, *die Spaltung*, a word that appears late in his work, in his article, "The Splitting of the Ego in the Processes of Defence" (1940b). The epistemic event signalled by this term went unnoticed for a time; splitting was first understood as a supplementary defence mechanism (although the Kleinians were more perceptive on this point than the followers of Anna Freud). Nevertheless, it prefigures what I do not hesitate to call, in a proposition that owes everything to Lacan, a new treatment of castration. It should be noted that the article on the *Spaltung* is more or less contemporaneous with "Analysis Terminable and Interminable" (1937), the article in which Freud introduced the expression, the "bedrock" of castration.[1]

Post-Freudianism does not distinguish between castration and splitting, and a part of "post-Lacanianism" seems to have repeated this lazy reading. Yet the difference between them is decisive. Lacan (1967–1968) began to theorise this in his 1967–1968 seminar, *L'acte psychanalytique*. What is in question is a difference that is synonymous with that between lack (which opens up the possibility of not lacking) and loss (which is irreversible) and especially between the negativisation of the phallus ($-\varphi$) and the barred subject ($\$$). The latter implies the production of an object, called the object *a*, which has no representation; this situates it radically outside any representation in language. The end of an analysis lies in accepting this division and mourning one's castration, inasmuch as the latter, as we have just seen, preserves the possibility of filling in lack (by sex, money, power). This idea will be decisive for this section of the book: because the capitalist discourse rejects castration, its effect is *a fortiori* to mask the division of the subject.

Two couples – Robert Louis Stevenson's Jekyll and Hyde, in the *Strange Case of Dr. Jekyll and Mr. Hyde* (1886), and Bertolt Becht's Joan Dark and Pierpont Mauler, in *Saint Joan of the Stockyards* (1938) – show us this refusal of subjective division, in the form of a new literary myth that ultimately includes both the material for the ideology of this refusal and a critique of that ideology. It seems incontestable and relatively easy to demonstrate that capitalism, in the form of the individualism that derived from the French Revolution, projected its lethal shadow upon both Stevenson and Brecht. What this myth concerns is not the kind of contradictory debate between libertinism and virtue, which can be set up between Sade and Robespierre, Mirabeau and Saint-Just, figures who exist as entities outside their pairing and each of whom claims the privilege of having been faithful to the revolution. Instead, these couples – Jekyll and Hyde, and Mauler and Dark – constitute a single unit, and their sundering into two separate people prevents either of them from being split; such a splitting would involve accepting the dialectic of the relation to the unconscious. Far from being the recognition that the unconscious has an intangible and inaccessible kernel, it is purely and simply the rejection of the very hypothesis of the unconscious. Hyde, because he has been cut away from his unconscious, which is found in Jekyll, escapes from the latter's control; this proscription of the unconscious enables us to hear the silence of the drives.

Joan Dark has also been cut from her unconscious, which exists in Mauler, to whom she lends her innocence, and she does not want to question her own relation to this innocence. This position leads her to betray the cause that she has sincerely adopted, and she does so without even realising it. Pure evil (Hyde) like pure good (Joan Dark) are fictions of the ideology that enables capitalism – or more precisely, its discourse – to breathe; this discourse is the linguistic armature without which the capitalist mode of production would collapse.

I shall refrain from giving an exposition of the four discourses, as Lacan forged them in *The Other Side of Psychoanalysis*, and the capitalist discourse, which derives from one of these four – the discourse of the master – until a later section, entitled "UMHA [**U**niversity-**M**aster-**H**ysteric-**A**nalyst]". However, in order to make the relevance of its epistemic use in this first part understandable, I must note that the specific characteristic of the capitalist discourse is an exemption from the form of the four discourses. These discourses – of the university, the master, the hysteric and the analyst – are explicitly constructed in terms of the principle of a "barrier" of jouissance (Lacan, 1991, p. 108); within these discourses, this barrier prevents the place of the production from reaching that of truth. In order to forestall any misunderstanding, I shall note that this major thesis does not signify an absolute scepticism; it simply means that truth, which should not be confused with the real, can be touched only through the negative path of falsification. In no case is it possible to say the truth about the truth, or to hope that the "whole truth" can be said, to quote one of Lacan's (1974b, p. 3) canonical formulations.

What characterises the capitalist discourse, on the contrary, is the lifting, or rather the annulment of this barrier. Its spirit is best summarised by the slogans coined by the sinister Prime Minister of the French July Monarchy, François Guizot – "Everyone is a capitalist [*Tous capitalistes*]!" and "Enrich yourselves [*Enrichissez-vous*]!" – who took advantage of the legal equality between individuals in order to authorise the idea of a potential equality that would exist at a level of having possessions, an equality that capitalism would offer. I would like to argue immediately that the secret that provides the foundation for this lie is found in the capitalist discourse: by annulling the barrier of jouissance and thus allowing people to glimpse the mirage of a consumption that would saturate desire (a possible definition of jouissance), this discourse asserts that the object *a* – the surplus object, of which we can fundamentally have no idea – is equal to money, which can be counted and entered into financial records.[2] This enables us to understand why Lacan credits – or discredits – Marx with having given a foundation to capitalism by taking surplus jouissance, the object *a*, as a surplus-value, thus making it subject to an energetics and contradicting the principal axiom of psychoanalysis: there is no energetics of jouissance.[3]

The alchemy of capitalism does not transform desire into jouissance, yet in making the plastic carrot glimmer with desire, capitalism keeps sharpening it until it has been worn down to nothing, as is demonstrated by the various addictions that are responses to this death of desire.

I shall now give the briefest sketch possible of the logical bases of Lacan's discourses. In the matheme of the capitalist discourse, as I shall argue in detail later, there is a vector that goes from *a* (surplus-jouissance) to $\$$, the subject.[4] As with all scientific notions, even when it is possible to give definitions and formulas for them, this relation is not absolutely transparent: it cannot be reduced to a denotation that would make it entirely and eternally intelligible. This same arrow is also found in the analytic discourse, where, however, it is marked as impossible.

$$a \overset{\text{impossibility}}{\dashrightarrow} \$$$

This can be read from right to left: the desire of a subject – in this case, the analysand – cannot (hence the impossibility) find its satisfaction in the object *a* – in this case, the analyst – which nevertheless causes the subject's desire. If analytic treatment can be described as the analysand's mobilisation, through transference, of surplus-jouissance, a "profit" of jouissance that feeds his/her desire to speak, then at the end of analysis, this jouissance proves to be vacuous, and this "profit" becomes the commemoration of an initial and founding absence: that of a jouissance that could saturate desire. In reality, as I shall argue later about the analytic discourse, this absent jouissance is the Other's. The jouissance that I impute to the Other is nothing more than a product of my thought, for any jouissance that I experience can only be what affects my body. I cannot reach jouissance in the Other's body. The genius of obsessional neurosis is to support this jouissance of the Other by pure thought, while the genius of hysteria is to posit that a lack of satisfaction is the condition for desire. The analytic discourse is able to turn these two neurotic creations around by turning the fantasy around, because it is constituted on the basis of the impossibility for the subject to experience the jouissance of the Other (God, the parents, the partner, etc.).[5]

The capitalist discourse presents us with a route that can be repeated indefinitely, a route that, in a certain way, makes repetition present. This discourse derives from the discourse of the master. In the latter discourse, with the vector that goes from S_1 to S_2, the master commands the slave, but the slave is the one who knows, a knowledge that enables him/her to act. In this respect, the transposition of this couple into that of the capitalist and the worker is not unwarranted, since what intervenes in production is the certification (S_2) of labour-power. What gives this S_1 its ability to command is not knowledge but money. This money will be valorised by the investment and cathexis of knowledge in production.

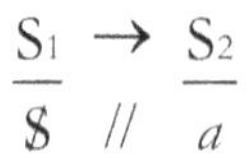

Discourse of the Master

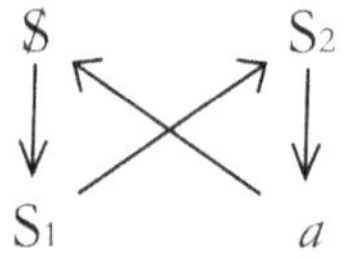

Discourse of the Capitalist

The worker produces, and in the Marxist sense, produces surplus-value. Within capitalism, labour-power becomes a commodity. Thus, surplus-jouissance can take the form of surplus-value. This surplus-value (*Mehrwert*) is the extra value produced by the wage-earner during his/her overall labour time, once the value of his/her labour-power has been reproduced during the earlier hours of the working day. As Marx notes in the *Grundrisse*:

> if the worker needs only half a working day in order to live a whole day, then, in order to keep alive as a worker, he needs to work only half a day. The second half of the labour day is forced labour; surplus-labour. What appears as surplus value on capital's side appears identically on the worker's side as surplus labour in excess of his requirements as worker, hence in excess of his immediate requirements for keeping himself alive.
>
> *(Marx, 1939, pp. 324–325)*

Hyde and seek

In the capitalist discourse, $ (the subject) and S_2 (knowledge) constitute a couple in which each element is *sundered* [*scindé*], rather than *split* [*divisé*] from the other. I am using the term "sundered" as the name of a process in which the dialectic that occurs in splitting is absent. This sundering is the true subject of Robert Louis Stevenson's extraordinary text, the *Strange Case of Dr. Jekyll and Mr. Hyde*. This book appeared in 1886, three years after Marx's death, and two years before the article on hysteria that Freud (1888) wrote for Villaret's medical dictionary. This narrative deserves to be considered as a new myth because it is different from the problematic of the double, which is characteristic of German "dark romanticism". Just as Hyde is not Jekyll's double, so Jekyll is also not Hyde's double. They are two sundered entities rather than a split subject.

It is true that Jekyll himself uses the word, "double" in the succinct notes that he keeps on the experiment in transformation (see Stevenson, 1886, p. 123). Yet there is a decisive reason not to rank Stevenson's story within the enormous body of literature concerning the double produced during the nineteenth century: Hyde and Jekyll never encounter one another, for although they are sundered, they are also the *same*. They are both enclosed within the "fortress of identity", as Stevenson (1886, p. 111) says. Naturally, Jekyll is situated in the place of S_2 and Hyde in $\$$. Jekyll is a doctor, a man of knowledge, like Faust. Yet Doctor Faust triumphs where Jekyll fails. If a diagnosis were required, one could say that Jekyll and Hyde together are a *single* schizophrenic. Yet what is important is that, during the very period when the process of constituting the individual had been achieved and the metaphor of the organic social body had become obsolete, Stevenson's story brought to light an individual sundered from himself, in the form quite exactly of a *subject who has been cut from his unconscious:* $\$ // S_2$.

This is one of the keys to the book: Jekyll is Hyde's foreclosed unconscious. In other words, Hyde should be considered as the hero, whose inability to know anything about his unconscious is the tragic weakness that constitutes the story's motive force and novelty. His access to the unconscious has been radically closed because the barrier of jouissance has been lifted and the unconscious ends up going solo. If the unconscious, like Jekyll, is in S_2, this means that, contrary to the received psychoanalytic idea that Hyde is Jekyll's unconscious, *it is Jekyll who is Hyde's unconscious*. Because Jekyll is the unconscious, which is closed in the capitalist discourse, Hyde becomes the drive. Dr. Jekyll and Mr. Hyde are the emblematic figures of this "sundering". They could even become its eponym, if we keep the game of hide and seek in mind, since Hyde's name is obviously a punning reference to this game.

Stevenson, who came from a family whose men had traditionally been builders or engineers of lighthouses, wrote this tale at the age of 36. The kernel of the story emerged in a nightmare that he had had a year before, from which he had been awakened by his wife, Fanny, frightened by his screams. He wrote a first narrative based on this nightmare, which he then destroyed after a violent argument with her; she objected to it because it did not include any moral.

This tale has a precedent in Stevenson's work: an early play written with William Ernest Henley entitled *Deacon Brodie, or the Double Life* (1892), which was inspired by a real event. By day, Brodie was a deacon and cabinet-maker; by night, he was a burglar. The fact that he is a deacon – and thus charged with the distribution of alms – already indicates that Stevenson is concerned more with questions of money than with neo-romantic narratives of doubles. It is not irrelevant to note both that his father was a rigorous and intransigent Calvinist and that, according to his own statements, he wrote his tale to pay his debts to "Byles the butcher" (see Dury, 2005, p. 9). It is also worth noting that Stevenson was once struck by reading an article on the subconscious. All of these matters converge on an emphasis on a conflict between good and evil, in which problems of money and the "subconscious" come into play in an entirely new way; the result is a new configuration that goes beyond received ethical conceptions.[6]

I have chosen the term "sundering" in order to accentuate the incompatibility between two entities, which belong, nevertheless, to a single personality. *Entzweiung* [division, split, rupture, rift], the term that Freud uses in the article, "Splitting of the Ego in the Process of Defence", would have been appropriate if I were writing in German. "Two divide into one" – a reversal of Mao Zedong's (see 2007, p. 196, note 19) definition of dialectic – could also be appropriated ironically. For that matter, the lacerating "schism [*scission*]" of the French psychoanalytic movement in 1953, in which Lacan and other notables broke away from the *Société psychanalytique de Paris* [Paris Psychoanalytic Society], could be described as an institutional sundering. Lacan, by analogy, would, of course, be Mr. Hyde (the drive) and the *Société psychanalytique de Paris* would just as incontestably be the unconscious. Let us hope that this institute will not lead to Lacan's "suicide" – which, in my little analogy, would involve the transformation of his work into something that would be absorbed into the IPA, if we equate this with a sort of petrification of theory.

Do contemporary myths exist, or must we now resign ourselves to dealing only with ideologies? I am tempted to maintain that myths remain relevant; perhaps we would be better off if we replaced – or regenerated – sociology with an ethnography of our own societies. These societies, although they may be civilised, are nonetheless prehistoric, since writing still does not have its true place in them. Writing was compromised first by the sacralisation that it inspired, and now by an inflation of publications, which resembles what is referred to, in finance, as a money-printing frenzy.

As the very perceptive critic Jean-Pierre Naugrette (1994) notes in his preface to a French translation of Stevenson's story, there is, however, a limit to this sundering: except on one occasion, Hyde never says "I". For this reason, he can never become the radically immoral narrator of the tale. The final chapter is entitled, "Henry Jekyll's Full Statement of the Case", with its equivocal use of the term "case", which can refer to both a police investigation and a clinical case. Jekyll has thus not, at this point, lost the capacity to speak. The loss of his subjectivity will eventually reach the point where he can no longer say "I", and where Hyde will take over from him. This may be the story's sole resemblance to the problematic of the double, but this also may not be a correct assessment. It would be better to ask what the status of this "I" is in analytic experience. A narration of a dream often begins with "I", but we know that the action reported by this "I" also conceals the actual place of desire; this desire is figured, instead, in the third person, in another of the dream's entities. This brings up another question: does waking up have the function of preventing us from articulating the aspect of desire that has to do with pure evil, with Thanatos, freed from its entanglements? It certainly does. Perhaps this means that there could be a satisfying dream, one from which we would never wake up, or at least one that would be brought to an end by our awakening. Such a dream would have to contain a certain cache of Thanatos, some element that would bind Thanatos libidinally. This is Stevenson's story: *disentangled Thanatos*. Mr. Hyde is forbidden an "I". In other words, saying "I" is a minimal libidinalisation of the pure culture of death.

These are the sorts of questions raised by the story of Henry Jekyll, an honourable physician and scientist, who is transformed by a drug into the cruel Mr. Hyde. The latter, after trampling a girl in the street, kills a member of parliament, Sir Danvers Carew, for no reason. Jekyll decides to stop this experiment, but the transformations continue, and he can no longer control them. In order not to become and remain Hyde, Jekyll commits suicide.[7]

From the door to the window

In this story, the choice of various last names involves a certain "predestination" in Stevenson's treatment of his characters. This is obvious with "Hyde", but is also the case with "Utterson", the utter, perfect son, who is also an utter idiot. He is an "incurable" son: one who cannot make himself an exception to the Oedipus complex, whether the latter be positive or negative. Such a son would fundamentally be a sinner, even without killing his father. Utterson thus contrasts with Markheim, the main character of another story by Stevenson. Refusing to believe that he can be reduced to his criminal act, Markheim wants to be judged only on the basis of his interiority, of what exists within himself. Externally, he is determined by his act, but he remains free "within"; this, according to Markheim, is what counts in God's eyes. He is his father's son, but this predicate misses his being. For this reason, he refuses the pact that the devil proposes to make with him.[8] There is another difference between "Markheim" and the *Strange Case*. In the former, the hero resists the devil – or at least the tempter – whereas Hyde is constantly mentioned as a possible figure of the devil. This suggests, as soon as we learn that Hyde *is* Jekyll, that the devil is not an external character: instead, the devil is the part of each of us that involves the drives. If we go a step further, we will reach Freud's thesis that the devil is the equivalent of the father: a representation of the father whom it is possible to hate.

We can now return to Utterson, the strange lawyer who, in apparent contrast with his well-ordered and disciplined life, "incline[s] to Cain's heresy", by "lett[ing] my brother go to the devil in his own way" (Stevenson, 1886, p. 2).[9] His ability to forgive anything makes him an ideal father, which is the fate of a son who is imprisoned for life in the Oedipus complex. In the first part of the story, as investigator, he wants to know who Hyde is: "If he be Mr. Hyde . . . I shall be Mr. Seek" (ibid., p. 21). Yet he starts off by following a false, rather vague lead, which is not exactly the one that was given to him by Richard Enfield, the friend who had witnessed Hyde's trampling of the little girl. Enfield had mentioned the possibility that Mr. Hyde was blackmailing Dr. Jekyll, but Utterson fixates on a somewhat different idea: that Jekyll is concealing an old wrongdoing, which would explain the mysterious will in which he has made Hyde his heir, just as it would explain why Hyde is in possession of his signed checks. Utterson, after seeing his friend and trying in vain to convince him to change the will, ends up in consenting to a request of Jekyll's: that he help Hyde after he himself is dead.

Both these events and those that follow raise a question concerning the reader. As the story progresses, there are numerous clues that Jekyll is indeed Hyde. Unfortunately, it is difficult to locate a particular moment when readers would solve the mystery, since most readers are now aware of the solution from the beginning. Even a reader who does not know the story would probably be a few steps ahead of Utterson, who is unequalled in his capacity to be duped. While we await the revelation, the facts emerge gradually, before being placed in logical order by Jekyll's final confession. Yet a question remains, one whose importance can be emphasised by returning to the question of psychosis: at what point is it possible to know that Jekyll is Hyde, and thus escape from the trap of paranoiac innocence (which is so admirably preserved in the background of authenticity found in paranoid behaviour) as well as the trap of fierce schizophrenic ignorance?

A year after Jekyll's request to Utterson, a crime occurs: it repeats, in an aggravated form, the inaugural scene in which Hyde trampled the little girl. In this second scene, the victim, who does not survive, is a member of parliament, Sir Danvers Carew, who is "trampl[ed] . . . under foot", an action that, because of its repetition, suggests that it had figured in Stevenson's nightmare (ibid., p. 37). In scene I, the witness is Utterson's friend, Enfield. In scene II, the witness is a maid with "romantic" tendencies, whose master was being visited by Hyde (ibid., p. 35). A letter for Utterson is found on the corpse, thus confirming Utterson's status as the key character to whom all the others are connected. This is an important point: Utterson is the ultimate receiver of all the numerous letters in the story, even of those that are not initially addressed to him. This letter is the only one whose content we never discover. It has the status of an exception, and it constitutes a point of incompleteness in the story, like the hand of one of the "*meninas*" in Velasquez's painting. Let us also note, because it confirms that this text is not part of the romantic tradition, the narrative's astonishing modernity. The action involves objects that could be so many clues to help us discover the truth, but which must await the correct interpretation: an example is the cane, which is not only the murderer's weapon, but is also a present given by Utterson to Jekyll. The same could be said for the butt of the cheque book, which had escaped being destroyed by fire in the chimney of Hyde's apartment, and which bears Hyde's name.

Because of this clue, the police inspector and Utterson wait for Hyde at the bank where he has his account, but he never comes. Then Utterson visits Dr. Jekyll, who claims that he no longer has any relation with Hyde. He shows Utterson a letter supposedly written by Hyde (letter 2), in which he assures Jekyll that he has a way to keep from getting caught. Utterson is reassured, but after asking Poole, Jekyll's servant, what the messenger looked like, he learns that there had been no messenger. Returning, worried again, to his home, he shows the letter to Mr. Guest, his head clerk, who also happens to be an expert graphologist, and asks him his opinion about the "murderer's autograph" (ibid., p. 51). After examining the paper, Guest says that the writer is "not mad; but it is an odd hand" (ibid., p. 51). When a servant enters, carrying a letter (letter 3) – an invitation from Dr. Jekyll – Guest recognises the handwriting and asks Utterson for permission to compare Hyde's letter with Jekyll's note, concluding that "the two hands are in many points identical:

only differently sloped" (ibid., p. 52). Later, when alone, Utterson thinks to himself, "What! . . . Henry Jekyll forge for a murderer!" (ibid., p. 52). This episode is interesting because it raises the question of whether Jekyll knew what he was doing in forging a letter. The answer revises this question; the "forgery" is real. A better question would be: who wrote it, Jekyll or Hyde? If Hyde wrote it, he did so not to deceive Jekyll, but to enable Jekyll to deceive Utterson. If Jekyll wrote it, it would still have the same goal. The ruse is the same whoever wrote it.

Thousands of pounds are offered for Hyde's capture, to no avail. Jekyll becomes himself again and renews his relations with his friends. However, Utterson twice finds his friend's door closed to everyone, and worried once again, pays a visit to Lanyon, with whom he had dined at Jekyll's home a few evenings before. He finds Lanyon dying, and the latter, knowing that he has so little time left, confides in him: "I sometimes think that if we knew all, we should be more glad to get away" (ibid., p. 57). In retrospect, we can, of course, explain why Lanyon makes this statement, but upon reading it for the first time, it is enigmatic. Lanyon also tells Utterson that he has broken entirely with Jekyll. Troubled, Utterson returns home, writes to Jekyll to ask him why he is not receiving and why he has quarrelled with Lanyon. Jekyll answers (letter 4) without revealing anything, and only asking Utterson to "suffer me to go my own dark way" (ibid., p. 58). Eight days later, Lanyon dies, leaving Utterson an envelope (letter 5) that contains another envelope (letter 6) marked as "not to be opened till the death or disappearance of Dr. Henry Jekyll" (ibid., p. 60). Utterson is struck by the term, "disappearance", which had already figured in the will that Jekyll had made in Hyde's favour.

Utterson has stopped visiting Jekyll because of his friend's taciturnity, but one evening, while on a walk with Enfield, he finds himself standing under Jekyll's window. Encountering Jekyll, they begin to speak with him, and he seems happy to see them, but then suddenly "the smile was struck out of his face and succeeded by an expression of such abject terror and despair, as froze the very blood of the two gentlemen below" (ibid., p. 64).

From then on, events move quickly. One evening, Jekyll's servant, Poole, visits Utterson and begs him for help, since his master has shut himself up in his laboratory. On knocking on its door, they hear Jekyll say that he does not want to see anyone. Poole remarks to Utterson that Jekyll's voice has changed, and that they are now hearing Mr. Hyde's voice.

The change of voice

It is difficult to resist referring once again to the anomalous matheme of the capitalist discourse. The statement about the voice allows this object to be located at *a*:

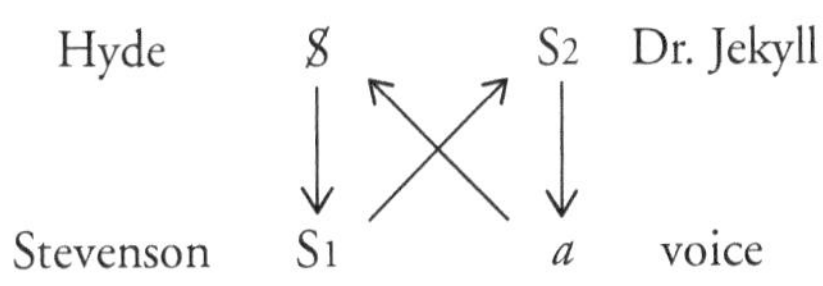

If S_2, knowledge, is Dr. Jekyll, and the subject is Mr. Hyde, then in S_1 we can only place the author himself, Robert Louis Stevenson, the master of the mystery. The transformation of the voice concerns two vectors: the one that descends from S_2 to a, and then the diagonal arrow that moves upward from a to $\$$. Voices are modulated by knowledge. Is it possible, for example, not to recognise the voice of a priest on a radio broadcast? In this context, the consequence of the transformation of Jekyll's voice into Hyde's is to strip it of the knowledge that has clothed it; now the strings of the drive – which had until then been concealed – begin to vibrate. Knowledge has one voice and the drive has a very different one, which betrays the subject. This reading may seem a bit forced, but, more generally, since Lacan defines the object a in this discourse as surplus-jouissance, one might well wonder whether it would be more appropriate to say that money – and especially surplus-value – occupies the place of production. This place could also be taken by the numerous consumer objects, which are intended to saturate the subject's desire; the attempt to use them for this purpose fails, however, since the subject never ceases to be split. This structural requisite will form the centre of the denouement of the "strange case". I shall soon confirm these hypotheses.

Despite these considerations, there is another reason to emphasise the voice as object a. The variation in the voice invites us to locate not only Hyde, but also Utterson, in $\$$. Perhaps, at the end, Utterson, the utter son, is also found here, in a way that resolves the enigma of how two are divided into one. After all, it is Utterson who will be substituted for Hyde in Jekyll's will, a substitution that has never received the emphasis that it deserves.

In the denouement, Poole provides Utterson with new information, giving him a note (letter 7) in which Jekyll complains to his apothecary that a particular powder did not have the same composition as the one that he had bought earlier. (It will turn out that the first powder was *impure* and that this very impurity had probably enabled it to turn Hyde back into Jekyll.) Then Poole tells Utterson that he had once seen his master disguised, as if he were wearing a mask on his face. After having once again produced an incorrect explanation, Utterson finally decides to intervene, as Poole had asked him to. They break down the laboratory door, and find the corpse of Hyde, who has swallowed cyanide.

This time, the reader will certainly have seen further than Utterson, who is still looking for Dr. Jekyll, even after finding Hyde's body. Utterson's time is always, structurally, late. He does not know how to read the clues that he continues to discover, even when he finds a religious text, which is annotated in Jekyll's own hand with "startling blasphemies" (ibid., p. 86). Finally, on the table, Utterson finds three documents: Jekyll's will, in which he is designated as heir in Hyde's place; a letter (letter 9) in which Jekyll enjoins him to read the document that Lanyon had sent to him; and finally, Jekyll's confession (letter 10). The solution to the mystery finally appears in these two last documents.

These two documents bring to an end the story, along with its enigmas and lacunae, its holes in the narrative tissue, its red herrings and the pseudo-explanations produced systematically by Utterson. The action finishes. Lanyon and Jekyll are dead. With the unveiling of what had been hidden, one returns to the present in order to go back over the course of events, which has now become comprehensible.

The devil or science

There is a reason why the two final texts were written by two doctors, custodians of knowledge, who were rivals in the field of science, or rather, disagreed about its powers. One, Lanyon, was a humanist/positivist, while the other wanted to enable human beings to become the equals of their "creator", to borrow the terminology that was used in the second half of the nineteenth century. This theme marks a turning point. In dark romanticism, people turned towards their doubles or their shadows and thought that the Devil was responsible for the coherence of these forms. A pact – which was itself constraining – could be made with the Devil, which would permit access to a jouissance that would otherwise be inaccessible. Goethe was an exception to this scheme, because he subverted the notion of the pact, making Faust the victor and Mephistopheles the vanquished. In this respect, Jekyll is more modern than Lanyon, just as Doctor Moreau is more modern than Brigitte Bardot: they prefigure the biological manipulation that seeks to preserve the animality of the human, rather than to imagine the humanity of the animal. Nevertheless, the gap between Lanyon and Jekyll cannot be more slender. The most blinkered positivism can be compatible with the most credulous spiritualism,[10] but this is not what is really at stake: neither Lanyon nor Jekyll is tempted by spiritualism, and they are not responsible for the return of an interest in astrology under capitalism. Instead, the question is the fundamental one of the limits of science. Does science have a place in the field of jouissance? What is in question is not sexology, which is always stupid and fraudulent, but the intertwining and the disentwining of the drives, of Eros and Thanatos.

The two final documents, particularly Jekyll's statement, throw an interesting light on this problem. Before examining them, I would like to point out a significant discrepancy in Lanyon's text concerning the date of the letter in which Jekyll had appealed to him to follow his bizarre instructions (which were supposed to enable Jekyll, who had been transformed unexpectedly into Hyde while far from home, to procure the drugs necessary to recover his original identity). The date of this letter is 10 December. In his confession, however, Jekyll situates this episode on a "fine, clear, January day" (ibid., p. 131). Perhaps this contradiction results merely from an oversight on Stevenson's part. Yet even if there is some confusion, why not raise this to the level of a symptom, and consider it as the final mark, in the real, of the impossibility of grasping simultaneity? One person's time is never the same as another's, and even if physics can measure both, it cannot situate them on the same continuum, since the space in which they take place is never the same.

More importantly, we learn from Lanyon's narrative that he encountered Hyde and was shocked to see him being transformed into Jekyll. Lanyon tells Utterson about the effect produced by Hyde's presence: an "odd subjective disturbance [was] caused by his neighbourhood. This bore some resemblance to incipient rigour, and was accompanied by a marked sinking of the pulse" (ibid., p. 99). Lanyon makes it clear that his reaction does not result from hatred. Certainly Hyde, as other witnesses have attested, inspires and even catalyses hatred. Yet Lanyon is testifying to something else: perhaps what he discovers in this unalterable alterity is the human being as such.

The effect of Jekyll's reappearance is less shocking, although just as cataclysmic: "My life", says Lanyon, "is shaken to its roots" (ibid., p. 105). The horror of discovering Jekyll's "moral turpitude" and that he is Carew's murderer (note the affectionate use of the name, "Sir Danvers") will push Lanyon to his death. Only ethics can evaluate this situation, since morality, as Dr. Lanyon's death proves, does not provide a sufficient rampart against this discovery.[11]

The central part of Stevenson's edifice is Jekyll's own narrative, his "statement of the case", before Utterson as judge. Jekyll's rather commonplace biography is dominated by the conflict between duplicity and sincerity: objective duplicity and subjective sincerity. Closer to the heart of the ethical question, we find the thesis that "man is not truly one, but truly two" (ibid., p. 108). Perhaps, he wonders, the "fortress of identity" exists only to contain this primal sundering and can be undone by orienting one's scientific studies "towards the mystic and the transcendental" (ibid., pp. 111, 107). Beyond this, Jekyll does not reject the idea that people can be multiple; Stevenson himself kept abreast of the work of psychologists and physicians, who were using an experimental model involving hypnosis to study multiple personalities. The story, however, leaves the question of dualism or pluralism in suspense, and we shall return to it in the chapter on Deleuze and Guattari.

In the case of Jekyll, however, only two entities are confronted with one another: good and evil. These "polar twins" are not divided up in Jekyll and Hyde *partes extra partes*. Although Hyde is indeed presented as pure evil, Jekyll remains torn between the two. Had this not been the case, Jekyll would not have been tempted to become Hyde. Two points need to be noted concerning Jekyll's relation to Hyde. First, isolating evil and transferring it onto Hyde, exonerates Jekyll from his guilt:

> the unjust might go his way, delivered from the aspirations and remorse of his more upright twin; and the just could walk steadfastly and securely on his upward path, doing the good things in which he found his pleasure, and no longer exposed to disgrace and penitence by the hands of this extraneous evil.
>
> *(ibid., p. 109)*

One can only be struck by this prefiguration of the modern, even postmodern subject; nearly half a century later, the character of Pierpont Mauler in Bertolt Brecht's *Saint Joan of the Stockyards* would follow this configuration to an astonishing degree. Yet it should also not be forgotten that this attempt at sundering, which can be criticised for its conformity to the capitalist discourse, was originally a rejection of the doctrine of original sin. Seen in these terms, the conclusion would not be so unilateral, for this ideal goes well beyond its possible uses by capitalism.

Second, in relation to his conception of Jekyll's transformation into Hyde (evil is physically smaller!), Stevenson has an intuition about the immateriality of the body. To translate this intuition without forcing things, I shall quote Lacan's (1970, p. 409) treatment of this question in "*Radiophonie*": "The first body [the body of the symbolic] creates the second by incorporating itself into it. This is where the incorporeal that remains to mark the first comes from, from the time after its incorporation". This is why Hyde is called an "inorganic" creature, which does not contradict, but rather confirms his "love of life" (Stevenson, 1886, pp. 133, 139). This love is not an Eros that has a biological essence; it is the result of an experimentation that had been wanted and conducted by a human being.

This leads us to the heart of Jekyll's practical reason. Whereas Hyde is supposed to be pure evil, Jekyll is a composite of good and evil. Because he rejects this subjective division, he conceives and carries out the "Hyde project", but without succeeding. Jekyll and Hyde are therefore not symmetrical, and we have reason to believe that the myth forged by Stevenson concerns the refusal of the subject's splitting. There are only two ways by which Jekyll can rid himself of the Hyde within him: change himself entirely into Hyde or kill himself. In the same way, *mutatis mutandis*, in *Saint Joan of the Stockyards*, Joan is supposed to be pure good, and Mauler embodies the splitting between good and evil. Thus, it is not very surprising that Jekyll himself had believed that he had made this discovery "under the empire of generous or pious aspirations", and that it would enable him to "come forth an angel instead of a fiend" (ibid., p. 115). This may be an illusion, but it reveals the temptation to rid himself of the ethical question. In this sense, *sundering is an orthopaedic prosthesis that serves to screen off the subject's splitting.*

As I have mentioned, a gnawing preoccupation makes itself felt throughout the everyday life of this bizarre couple: the need for the money that would enable Hyde to survive should Jekyll disappear. At the beginning, there is the will that makes Hyde the heir; then the money demanded by the parents of the girl whom he had trampled; the cheque to them taken from a cheque book in Hyde's name; the fact that the police believe wrongly that they can catch him when he goes to the bank to take out some money, etc. The transfer of personalities requires a transfer of money; with the emergence of the capitalist mode of production, money has become not only the indispensable means of subsistence, but also the standard for measuring value. Hyde's "respectability" can only be guaranteed by Jekyll's fortune. There is no subject without money, no $\$$ without *a*. The entry into language produces a loss of jouissance, which then establishes the requirement for jouissance; in this way, money comes to occupy the place of this loss. In the place of *a* in the capitalist discourse, I first situated the voice, as part-object. Yet the voice, as Stevenson says over and over, changes. Hyde's voice is not Jekyll's. This variability of the objects *a* makes them precarious and signals their inability to ensure surplus-jouissance; this surplus-jouissance, in the capitalist discourse – for an individual who has been *deprived* of his/her unconscious – is expected finally to be able to lift the bar that divides the subject. The full-fledged capitalist discourse would reduce this subject to the status of zero, which would be its status outside its constitutive division. Zero is the value that would be appropriate to the subject as soon as the latter is treated as a pure effect of language. Since, however, the splitting of the subject cannot be eliminated, it is the capitalist discourse that is headed for a blowout.[12]

In the capitalist discourse, money therefore comes to substitute for the part-objects as their general or "universal equivalent", to use Marx's (1867, p. 180) term; it ensures that there will be an invariability in surplus-jouissance, thus preventing this jouissance from failing. Its ability to act in this way in the capitalist discourse supposes that money can be conceived through a parthenogenesis, which would shelter it from devaluation. (This is precisely the illusion that is being maintained by those who have abandoned the real economy.)

The point of no return is reached when Jekyll can no longer control Hyde's transformations into him and vice versa. Jekyll's will is now deactivated. This event occurs on that "fine, clear, January day" mentioned earlier; until then, his will had guaranteed the permanence of his identity (ibid., p. 131). Hyde was merely his "creature", even if the "creator" rejoiced in Hyde's "moral" independence. In this new configuration, Jekyll's panic becomes the signal that he is threatened with depersonalisation: the total loss of identity, which would involve reconstituting his identity in the form of Hyde. In this situation, what comes literally to save Jekyll is a memory: "that of my original character, one part remained to me: I could write my own hand; and once I had conceived that kindling spark, the way that I must follow became lighted up from end to end" (ibid., p. 133).

As we recall, it was Guest, Utterson's first clerk, who noticed that Jekyll and Hyde's handwriting differed only in their slopes. Unlike the voice, writing cannot change; it can only, at a pinch, be forged. Writing is on one side, and the voice and money are on the other. To speak in general terms: what saves Jekyll is what condemns the capitalist discourse. To make this formulation more absolute, I shall add that writing resists virtualisation and is therefore nothing other than the symptom as such. There is no need to treat "writing" as a metaphor to move from handwriting to Stevenson's status as writer. The signature marks the presence of the proper Name, which has a geographical particularity that goes against the globalisation of language; writing becomes the way to exit from the prison-house of language. As Nathalie Sarraute wrote, "Knock, knock, real, open up!"

Finally, on this basis, we can approach the most sensitive question: who dies when Jekyll commits suicide? Is it even a suicide? After all, the body of the person who has killed himself is not the same as the corpse that Utterson and Poole find. In his statement of the case, Jekyll makes a revealing remark: "He, I say – I cannot say, I" (ibid., p. 134). He thus emphasises that when he is Hyde, he can no longer appropriate himself subjectively by speaking in the first person. In a sense, this is a usual and necessary state: the "I" of the enunciation never corresponds to that of the statement. Is Jekyll, however, telling the truth? The final proposition of this narrative is "I bring the life of that unhappy Henry Jekyll to an end" (ibid., p. 141). Who, in this case, is "I", since Jekyll is referred to in the third person? "I" may well be Hyde. Several lines above, Jekyll writes, "when I shall again and forever reindue that hated personality, I know how I shall sit shuddering and weeping in my chair" (ibid., p. 141). In this sentence, a transfer of the "I" is operating continually, perhaps making the reader sensitive to the pathos of Hyde as subject: the evil man who finally *attains his division, through his own anxiety.*

The three scenes

This examination of Jekyll's final letter does not resolve the enigmatic quality of his case; we have not yet mentioned an important event that figures in his statement. While Hyde is going from the hotel to Dr. Lanyon's home, where he hopes to find the drug that will turn him back into Jekyll, "a woman spoke to him, offering, I think, a box of lights. He smote her in the face, and she fled" (ibid., p. 135).

This scene constitutes the third version of what we have referred to as the primal scene, and the three, taken together, resemble Freud's (1919) analysis of the three phases of the fantasy in "A Child is Being Beaten". In Stevenson's tale, we would obtain the following:

> *Primal Scene (Scene I)*: a little girl is being beaten by Hyde, while a man is watching.
> *Scene II*: a man is being beaten by Hyde, while a woman is watching.
> *Scene III*: a woman is being beaten by Hyde, but who is watching?

Since this third scene had at least one witness – the one who reports it – we could say that Jekyll is watching. It happens that this witness is unsure of himself, and adds, concerning the matchbox, "I think". At the moment when this scene takes place, Jekyll seems already to have been partially absorbed into Hyde's personality, and is on the point of disappearing as a witness.[13] Yet the final witness, the tale's author, is Stevenson himself. We shall soon see how this hypothesis will be borne out.

In these three scenes, Hyde is in the position of the agent: the agent of castration, to introduce Freud's thesis, and the real father – who carries out the subject's castration – to present Lacan's, in his seminar, *The Other Side of Psychoanalysis* (Lacan, 1991, p. 128; also see Bruno, 2003b). This conclusion confirms, rather than contradicts, the argument that Hyde is a pure being of the drives. The fantasy, which is primarily sadistic, is located on Jekyll's side, in either an unconscious or a conscious form, and the bare drive, stripped of the fantasy, is found on Hyde's side. The murder of Sir Danvers Carew procures a sadistic jouissance for him (he "tast[ed] delight from every blow") (Stevenson, 1886, p. 127), but the jouissance that Stevenson attributes to him is certainly the result of a confusion connected to the author's own conception of the real father. The jouissance of the real father must always remain unknown: the very definition of this figure carries the logical implication that the jouissance that he is supposed to feel is the subject's own (see Stevenson's nightmare). Yet despite this reservation, Hyde is very much the agent of castration; he is an exception to the phallic law and is exempt from the passion of hatred for the man he kills. He is the object rather than the agent of hatred.

This leads us to question the figure of the father who is paired with Hyde: Utterson, who is decidedly a jack of all trades. He is a symbolic father, the one who conforms to the law in everything, and who, as a correlate, can explain everything, especially the turpitudes of the sons. The perfect son, quite consistently, turns out to be the perfect father. I shall not even enter into Stevenson's apparently rather complex relations with his own father, who supported his son, but had rather settled opinions on the path that he should follow: he suggested that, as a way of compromising between the careers of engineer and writer, his son should study law!

Jekyll refuses his division as subject and occupies the place of knowledge, delegating that of subject to Hyde. In doing so, Jekyll inscribes himself precisely in the capitalist discourse: his explicit hope is to disencumber himself of desire by constructing a relation in which the object-cause of desire would complete Hyde as subject. This completion would put an end to the subject's division, as well as to subjectivation itself. This subjectivation is to be found in the fact that Jekyll is never totally absent from Hyde. If he were, why would he want to become Jekyll again? *The splitting of the subject is therefore what resists the capitalist discourse*; it is what this discourse cannot tame. As for the solution in which Hyde would become the figure who commands, thereby incarnating the place of S_1 – the master signifier rather than the subject, $\$$ – this is precisely what Jekyll refuses with horror, for if it were to take place, it would involve accepting that Hyde is the agent of castration, which he does not want. Such an acceptance would, however, be the condition for moving back from the capitalist discourse to that of the master; S_1 would be found again in the place of the agent, and $\$$ in that of truth.

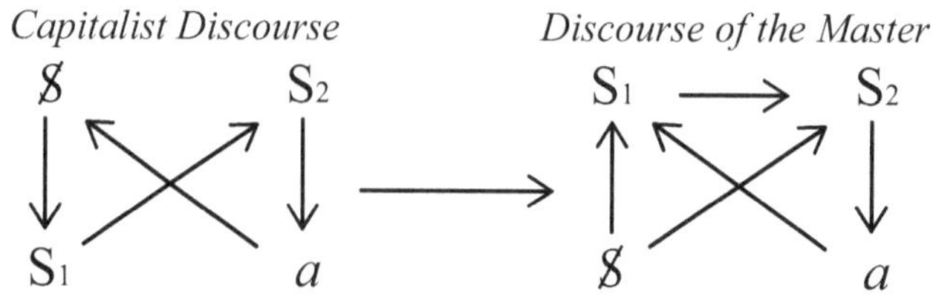

Through this return, the unconscious could reclaim its rights and an analysis could begin.

The last matter that Jekyll mentions is the possibility that Hyde will destroy his statement. Likewise, he notes that in setting down his pen, he puts an end to the life of Dr. Henry Jekyll. What is a tale if not the duration of its reading, during which the characters are alive? Can Hyde, in this fiction, exit from the fiction in which he was born, in order to prevent Jekyll from living in this fiction, and in consequence, deprive Stevenson of the status of being the author, and us of reading this masterwork? To whom is Stevenson alluding, in this highly discreet, shadowy passage, if not to his wife Fanny Osbourne, who, at an early moment, had suggested that the immoral first version of the *Strange Case* should be destroyed. And who better than his beloved cousin, Katherine de Mattos, could be the dedicatee of this first verse of the epigraph: "It's ill to loose the bands that God decreed to bind"?

Dark

Bertolt Brecht finished *Saint Joan of the Stockyards* in October 1931, between the great economic, social and financial crisis of 1929 and Adolf Hitler's assumption of power in 1933. A very short summary of the play could go like this: whereas in Friedrich von Schiller's 1801 play, *The Maid of Orleans*, Joan of Arc saves the king of France, in Brecht's play, Joan Dark saves Pierpont Mauler, a great capitalist. Mauler wants to canonise her, but she refuses, for by the end of the play she has understood that, in saving him, she has taken the wrong path.

The play (Brecht, 1938) is divided into twelve scenes of unequal length, some of which are then subdivided. The first ten scenes have titles that announce and summarise the action. Scenes 11 and 12 only note the setting. The title of the final scene announces the denouement: "Death and Canonization of St Joan of the Stockyards" (ibid., p. 303). To read this play, it is essential to follow the sequence in which it is presented, which can, without any misuse of terminology, be called dialectical. I shall treat not Joan Dark, but Pierpont Mauler, the "meat king" of Chicago (ibid., p. 202), as the main character. What sort of man must he be if he can arouse such love, devotion and credulity in a young woman who desires the good with an extraordinary intensity? I am using the term "dialectic" because the schema of thesis/antithesis/synthesis, when applied to Mauler, provides the architecture of the drama. Mauler is presented successively as bad and hypocritical, then, antithetically, as generous and sincere, and finally as a bad but generous person and a sincere hypocrite. That synthesis thus leaves us with an enigma: how can he be all of these simultaneously? The character of Joan would seem to be easier to grasp. Unlike another of Brecht's great female characters, Pelagea Vlassova from *The Mother* (1932), she does not attain a sense of class consciousness, except perhaps at the end, in a way that is undecidable. She is not a revolutionary, but her generosity and kindness are never questioned.

It could have been said that Joan's characterisation is consistent with the psychology of the German classical theatre of Schiller and Goethe, but an important characteristic distinguishes her from the characters of these dramatists. In her relation with Mauler, she is what Hyde is for Jekyll. There is, however, a reversal: for Mauler, Joan, rather than being evil, is pure goodness. Mauler must rid himself of his own goodness by locating it in someone else, thus rejecting his subjective division in the same way that Jekyll does. Joan is the excuse or even "alibi" – understood in its etymological sense as "elsewhere" – who enables Mauler to inhabit more easily the being that he achieves at the moment of synthesis: the generous villain and sincere hypocrite. Thus, there is, as in Stevenson's text, a game that involves both a pure being – now devoted to goodness – and a being composed of both good and evil. Mauler does not experience Jekyll's torment, and if he can finally be said to "kill" Joan in a way that constitutes her "suicide", he gets off rather lightly. In a certain way, the capitalist discourse certifies his ability to reach this end, which is also the end of the play.

Joan's case is more delicate but no less instructive: what blinds her and even leads her to betray the workers' cause, which she had believed that she was defending, is her reduction to being the incarnation of good, and thus of knowing nothing of evil. This could be Brecht's moral maxim: ignorance of evil is the mother of evils.

If this moral can be stated easily, the same cannot be said for its practical reason. Brecht's genius lies in his ability to add a dimension that, through its distance from the dimension of the two main characters, gives a depth to what is at stake in practical reason. This dimension is the fluctuations of the stock market, which directly determine Mauler's decisions, which always aim to valorise his capital. Here a remarkable dissymmetry appears: the value of Mauler's stocks is determined by a financial algorithm that is completely independent of his psyche. Joan's actions, however, are determined by a hollow dream: that her goodness could prove to unbelievers that evil does not exist. We shall not tarry at this point, since *Saint Joan of the Stockyards* is not an intimate, two-character play. Other figures populate it: capitalists, workers and the "Black Straw Hats", the fictionalised counterparts of the Salvation Army. These figures are not unified groups or masses. Each has his/her own individuality, which is itself interesting.

One of the questions dominating the play is whether the capitalist discourse – which *sets up* the dominance of the capitalist mode of production and its relations of production – reduces human action to the automatic functioning of a programme that is generated by iron laws. If this is the case, then the gap between the dimensions of good and evil would be abolished and what is at stake in practical reason would disappear. Perhaps, however, a particular human being, whatever the social conjuncture, can "feel the breath of another world", as Brecht (1938, p. 215) suggests, mockingly but sincerely, in the title of the third scene.

In this context, I prefer the term "practical reason" to "ethics", and this involves choosing Kant over Spinoza. Kant, by stating the concept of the categorical imperative – which is subtracted from the conditional character of contingency – may well have anticipated the age in which the generalisation of capitalist predation and the long-standing weakening of any effective religion have led to a world in which neither God nor human beings are feared. The result of this has been to connect the law to faith in capital, in a way that would perplex believers in Pierre-Simon Laplace's statistical determinism. To give only one example: should we attribute the success of the struggle to reduce the working day and to limit child labour – which Marx (1867) described admirably in the first volume of *Capital* – to the struggle of workers themselves or to an understanding, on the part of the political representatives of the capitalist class, of the threat posed by too quick a destruction of the productive forces? We could, of course, answer "both . . . and", or even connect the two with an ampersand, &, which could mark the sort of conflictual collaboration that is supposedly the condition of the progress of civilisation. Yet how can a strictly rhetorical solution be satisfying?

One of the problematic aspects of this situation is that the individual members of the capitalist class do not act in terms of collective logic; instead, they act under the strict condition that collective logic must not figure in their calculations. By "collective logic", I mean the awareness and understanding that the other person is also a subject. We tend to forget this, and this forgetting transforms the other subject into someone who is radically other: an alien figure rather than a counterpart. Is the best response to this situation the one that has already been tried in history: construct a "new man" – whatever meaning may be given to such a term – by completely destroying the existing/former man, perhaps even by killing him? Acting in this way, apart from any other consideration, may well involve a fetishistic belief in the determinism of filiation. Instead, if we do not believe that a capitalist can be touched by grace, we could always wait patiently for natural death to do its work. It is also interesting to note that the belief in the determinism of class membership and the belief in the determinism of filiation are consistent with one another. They both make collective logic impossible, debasing practical reason into a reason that justifies practice, whatever that practice may be.

This is why Brecht is interested in bringing out symptoms that can thwart the rejection of practical reason. Only such symptoms can confront the double dialectic of the stock market and the libido and confer upon this dialectic an irreducibility that could change history: these symptoms could prevent history from being nothing more than the history of human modelling clay. I shall now examine Brecht's text in order to analyse these symptoms.

First letter

In Chicago, the city of the stockyards, Pierpont Mauler receives a letter from his friends in New York.

Brecht, in the place of S_1, the writer who sets up the fiction, has a clear sympathy for Joan, thus revealing his proximity to Mauler, who is authentically touched by her, even if his emotions are also ways of taking advantage of her. In the letter from his friends, Mauler learns that "the meat market has been severely depressed" and that he should "drop the meat business" (Brecht, 1938, p. 203). He thus possesses knowledge, S_2 in the schema of the capitalist discourse. The object *a*, in turn, is by no means a false appearance: it is money, which can generate more money. He hides this letter from his partner, Cridle, but this does not mean that he is deliberately trying to deceive his associate. In this context, we can adopt a form of behaviourism that would be more extreme than the behaviourism of psychologists: when we observe, from the outside, the hiding of the letter, nothing enables us to deduce anything about Mauler's internal psychic processes. Perhaps he does not know what his hand is doing, and the stage directions throw no light on the situation. Whatever the case may be, everyone involved in the meat market – producers, retail traders, livestock farmers – is ruined by the shutting down of the two main factories. The producers and retail traders can no longer sell their commodities because of the crisis of overproduction and the reduced purchasing power of redundant workers. The farmers are ruined because Mauler is no longer buying cattle for his stockyards.

Joan Dark is a lieutenant in the Black Straw Hats and has very conformist and comforting views on divine jouissance and false earthly jouissance – the jouissance from which the workers have been alienated. Two characteristics, however, single her out: first, despite the warnings of her superiors and her colleagues, she *wants to know* – to know why the labourers are out of work. Second, she *recognises* Mauler, a fact that cannot be explained. She is said to be able to recognise him and does so; she picks him out of a group, even when he denies that he is Pierpont Mauler. What happens here is something like a Hegelian radiance: behind the bloody mask that Mauler has put on, and despite his disguising of his voice, Joan recognises a human being in him. The price of making oneself into the agent of capitalism – of devoting oneself body and soul to valorising capital – is dehumanisation. Mauler's sentimentality could thus be more than a way of deceiving others; it could also be a symptom of his refusal to cut himself off irreversibly from humanity. The problem with this reading of Mauler, which Brecht's text does not accentuate, is not the discreet suggestion of essentialism in its definition of what humanity is. Instead, such a reading misrecognises Mauler's undecidable ambiguity, which provides a structural principle that bears some resemblance to quantum mechanics. In the latter, we cannot simultaneously measure both the speed and the position of particles; there is an unpredictable element that cannot be eliminated. Likewise, at the level of practical reason, nothing can be said about Mauler. The same problematic can be found in *Galileo* (Brecht, 1938), where we cannot know whether the great scientist withdraws his work through cowardice or because remaining alive is a way of preserving the interests of science.

We shall now cross a barrier. Mauler, who has been unable – and has not even believed it possible – to corrupt Joan with money, has her descend into the depths, so that she can see how bad the poor are. Guided by Sullivan Slift, she meets a young worker, Mrs. Luckerniddle and Gloomb, all three of whom are members of the working class and, in various ways, behave reprehensibly. Mrs. Luckerniddle's husband has been killed in an industrial accident; he "fell into one of the rendering tanks . . . and he ended up with the leaf lard" (Brecht, 1931, p. 224). When the widow learns of this, she accepts twenty free meals as a bribe for remaining silent about the accident. Slift believes that such behaviour shows Joan the immorality of the poor, but she replies: "You have shown me not/The baseness of the poor but/*The poverty of the poor*" (ibid., pp. 229–230). This aphorism has become famous and we can infer that it has an implied counterpart, written in a sort of invisible ink, concerning Mauler: "You have shown me not/The immorality of the rich but/the wealth of the rich". Perhaps Mauler relies on Joan in order not to become a pure instrument of capital; in this, he would resemble Jekyll, who finally preferred to be divided, even at the cost of his death, rather than to be abandoned to pure evil. This is a subtle and problematic dance, for the comparison seems flawed: Jekyll, finally, does not want to come together with Hyde, whereas Mauler's relation to Joan is not defined in the same way. Mauler and Jekyll have in common, however, a refusal to be reduced to a kind of knowledge that would be unaware of itself. This tendency, indeed, can retroactively make Jekyll's reaction more comprehensible: what he refuses is not so much to be transformed into a figure who is dedicated to evil. Instead, everything suggests that if he were to lose control of the transformation, Hyde would end up being divided, just as Jekyll was. What Jekyll refuses is to be pure knowledge, an agent of the great linguistic computer and an element of the unconscious. As René Daumal (1938, p. 68) puts it, emphatically, in *A Night of Serious Drinking*, "I know everything, but I don't understand any of it".

This analysis provides us with a Freudian way out, which can honour practical reason without using the categorical imperative: the alternative is not between good and evil. Joan's good, as we shall see, is hardly better than Mauler's evil; as her name indicates, it is very "dark". Instead, the true debate takes place between Eros and Thanatos. The victory of Thanatos would reduce Jekyll and Mauler to being mere agents of knowledge, and they would thus be cut away from the true character of the drive, the site of the simultaneous intertwining and struggle between Eros and Thanatos.

Mauler's theorem

The second letter that Mauler receives threatens to pin him down, like a butterfly in a collector's glass case. It would make him nothing more than the place of knowledge: the knowledge of stock-market calculations. This letter comes, once again, from his New York friends (and we may start to wonder who is writing to these friends). It tells him to "buy meat" (Brecht, 1931, p. 246), and this is what Joan has also asked him to do, in order to save the manufacturers, the retail traders (who buy the canned meat) and the livestock farmers, and thus to rekindle the meat industry, which would enable the redundant workers to be rehired. We may suspect that the letter from New York does not use the same arguments. The members of congress have been corrupted and are ready to suppress trade barriers and open up the southern market. Buying the canned meat has thus become a good calculation.

Mauler first hesitates and then decides to buy, but in doing so, it is not clear whether he is following the letter's advice or Joan's pleading. In the decisive passage, he tells Slift, "Yes, yes, I did buy meat, but I didn't/Buy it because of the letter and its advice/(Which is all wrong anyway, pure theory)" (ibid., p. 245). Mauler seems to baulk at the prospect of being nothing more than an element of an analysis that has been made elsewhere. This does not mean, however, that he took his decision because of Joan. The secret of his decision lies in what can be called "Mauler's theorem":

> Somebody makes a mistake. Let's call it A.
> It's a mistake because his feelings got
> The better of him. Then he makes
> Another move. We'll call it B. B too
> Is wrong. But taken together A and B
> Two wrongs – will make a right
>
> (ibid., p. 248)

"A" is the decision to buy the cans of meat; "B" is what he is going to do: buy all the cattle, which he can sell at a very high price to the manufacturers, who are bound by contract to deliver the cans to him. Thus, he distances himself from the knowledge of his New York friends, which has become a sort of imperative coming from the superego, while also achieving a brilliant financial success.

The situation, however, does not improve for the workers, and Joan rebels. Mauler believes that he can calm her down by offering to donate money to the Black Straw Hats, but Joan does not place herself within the capitalist discourse. Breaking with it, she tells him, "Mr. Mauler, I don't understand what you've been saying/And I don't wish to understand" (ibid., p. 263). She thus leaves this discourse:

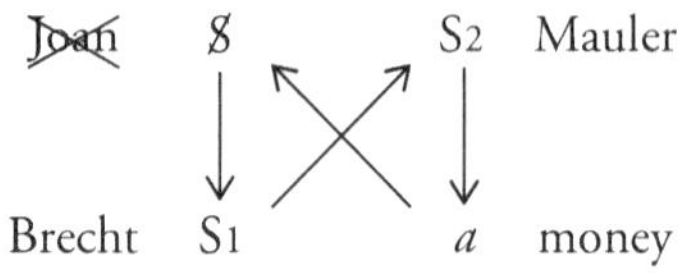

Joan's apostasy

Is this the end of their idyll? Not quite. In scene 9, Joan is now living in the stockyard area with Gloomb and Mrs Luckerniddle, the figures who were supposed to have shown her the fundamental corruption of the workers. She tells them a dream that she had had a week earlier. This dream should be left uninterpreted, except for its end, where she sees herself as a warrior, marching "With warlike steps and bleeding forehead" at the head of a multitude that is "wreaking immoderate destruction" and is "Perceptibly influencing the course of the stars" (ibid., p. 265, translation modified). Assuming a prophetic mode, she explains its meaning: all the poor will march on Chicago. In the dream, she has fulfilled her wish for a revolution, but this dream is not the prelude to a revolution, for no dream is prophetic, except when it is falsified fantasmatically. Instead, it is a prelude to her betrayal.

The revolutionary worker's movement has been preparing a general strike, which will be coordinated through letters that are being sent to worker-delegates at the main factories. Joan volunteers to carry one of these letters to the Graham factory, the area that is being watched the most carefully by the police. Despite an initial hesitation, the labour leaders decide to trust her, even if she has not renounced her belief that Mauler is a human being. They warn her, however, that if this letter is not transmitted, the strike will fail. Joan leaves on her mission to the stockyards, and then gives a very lucid speech about the system, denouncing its promotion of the belief that everyone can be a capitalist. Everyone is told, "Come up, then all/Of us will be on top", whereas in reality, "[t]his whole system's a see-saw": some can be on top only because many are on the bottom (ibid., p. 278). Yet there are already some clues – her irritation, her whims, her uncustomary injustice – that she is ready to crack up. When the reporters come to announce that Mauler has agreed to sell cattle to the manufacturers of canned meat, and that work can therefore begin again, Joan is in a hurry to believe them: "At least the righteous man among them/Has proved himself" (ibid., p. 280). She gives this speech at the very moment when the advancing army is using machine guns to subdue the crowd.

This is a religious moment, so a term from religion can be used to describe it: apostasy. Joan knows how the system works, but she does not understand the consequences. The weather is colder than it had been in her dream and her oneiric anticipation of the strike has rendered the actual strike null and void for her. She does not deliver the letter. When she explains her betrayal, she speaks of a refusal to betray: she refuses to rise up against the established order, without which she would feel lost. "The movement of the stars/Over his head would no longer be governed by/The old rule" (ibid., p. 283).

This nearly explicit reference to Galileo throws light on this moment, in which what is in question is the subject's relation to knowledge: the subject knows, without understanding the consequences of what she knows. In order for the subject to be able to understand the consequences of knowledge, this knowledge must have abolished the mirage of truth, and she needs this mirage in order to believe that she is innocent. It is not necessary that she feel guilty, for guilt and innocence are only two sides of the same coin, and this coin has the face of Adam stamped upon it. Instead, the subject must not refuse to understand what will happen if she does not grasp the implications of what she knows. As it happens, Joan does not want to know that if the letter is not transmitted to its addressee – despite her promise to do so – a chain will be broken. The result of this is that the worker-delegates will themselves end up in chains; Joan will see them pass in handcuffs before her eyes. What counts is not whether she is good or evil; instead, what is important is that she now refuses to know anything about the effects of her refusal to deliver the letter. She refuses this in the name of her "subjective truth", which is nothing other than a dignified name for her fantasy. The snow becomes the shroud that covers over this knowledge.

She then has a vision in which she sees herself as a criminal, who has "No bearings in/A world grown unfamiliar" (ibid., p. 283). There is something that she has not been able to confront by acting, because she still remains under the influence of an established order's truth, from which she could only have freed herself through crime. What she could not see is now returning to her in what we must not hesitate to call a visual hallucination. She has preferred a truth that conforms to her fantasy and now this vision makes a real present for her, a real that would otherwise have been buried forever under the snow, along with the knowledge by which the real signals to her. In the same way, a bit later, she begins to hear voices. Through the real of these voices, a knowledge that she had not wanted to hear breaks in: "O Truth, bright light, unseasonably darkened by a snowstorm!/Never more to be seen! Oh, what force in a snowstorm!" (ibid., p. 287). This "psychotisation" has a salvational value for her, showing the path that she will make her destiny, just like the real Joan of Arc.

Monopoly

Joan's development is symmetrical with Mauler's; while these events have been transpiring, he has not been wasting any time. He has acquired a monopoly on livestock and has made its price rise to dizzying heights. This may be why, once again, as he tells Slift, he begins to "feel sick" (ibid., p. 276). There is nothing new in this: it remains in the realm of the subjective truth that was criticised with Joan, and such truths can be used to justify both domestic and political tyranny. On the other hand, Mauler, having an idea of the repressive turn that the situation is going to take, has detectives look for Joan, so that he can protect her, but to no avail.

Now, once again, the action returns us to Joan's "seesaw"; we could well wonder whether there is any difference between its movement and that of the dialectic of desire. This seesaw swings back: the manufacturers of tinned meat, ruined by Mauler's manoeuvres, stop buying from him. The price of livestock collapses, and he goes bankrupt.

This is the situation at the start of scene 10: "Pierpont Mauler Humbles Himself and Is Exalted" (ibid., p. 288). Naturally, with this title's parody of Christian vocabulary, it is tempting to hear only its caustic connotation. This is especially tempting since this is the most violently anticapitalist and antireligious[14] part of the play. Through Mauler's cynical speech, it is "humanity" as it has been "dehumanized" by capitalism that triumphs (ibid., p. 298). Mauler's humiliation, however, does not last. Having taken refuge with the Black Straw Hats as one of the new poor, he is soon joined by the meatpackers and the livestock breeders. Graham, a meatpacker, then narrates to him the "battle" that ended with the collapse of the banking system itself (ibid., p. 292). Brecht makes this bravura speech worthy of the greatest epic narratives, from Homer to Corneille. For the third time, apparent defeat has become the instrument of a new victory.

A further letter now arrives from New York, and whether its advice is correct is of no importance, for it provides Mauler with the key that will lead to his promised "exalt[ation]": set up a single trust for which he will own half of the stock (ibid., p. 296). Everyone is enthusiastic about his solution.

A double desire

Let us return to Joan. The delegates of the workers have been imprisoned, and the general strike has been brought to a halt because Joan did not deliver the letter. When the reporters tell her this news, she faints. This is the denouement (scene 12): "Death and Canonization of St Joan of the Stockyards" (ibid., p. 303). Slift and Mauler are the first to understand how to use this champion of the working class, who was a rebel but not a revolutionary. They turn her into a media and religious figure who comes to symbolise the exorcising of evil, a banner around which both workers and capitalists can unite. Joan herself is dying of the cold, hunger and despair, but she is finally lucid: "Take care that when you leave the world/You have not merely been good but are leaving/A better world!" (ibid., p. 306). This is her critique of Mauler. She neither denies his aspirations towards the good nor accuses him of being a fraud; instead, *she reproaches him for what she also reproaches herself.* They had both believed that being good oneself is sufficient, just as it would be sufficient to be analysed oneself, without worrying about the effects of the system:

Those at the bottom are kept at the bottom
So that those at the top may stay on top.
And the baseness of those on top is beyond measure.
And even if they got better, it wouldn't
Help.

(ibid., pp. 306–307)

Mauler, as we would expect, lauds her good soul. Is this the final verdict on Joan's death? Now Brecht's play reaches its greatest brilliance: its maximal commitment is founded upon a point of undecidability, which only the reader's own commitment can settle. In his final speech, Mauler declares that:

A razor-sharp dichotomy
Cutting deep into my breast
Fashions two souls from my soul.
Though do-gooding suits me best
Meanwhile business interest
Also plays a certain role
Unconsciously.

(ibid., p. 310)

Before we reach the final chorus, spoken by everyone on stage, it should be emphasised that Brecht plainly yields, without any parody, to tragedy in its densest and most purified form, the model for which remains Greek. He does so in order to present a fundamental human contradiction, without either judging or resolving it. Everything that has preceded it certainly relativises this refusal of any judgement: Joan's distinction between good intentions and a concern with one's effects on the world remains a small and fragile movement towards a solution. Yet Brecht chooses the form of accepting the power of Mauler's message. The final speech of the chorus confirms this and it is clear that we cannot decide whether or not it expresses Brecht's point of view. Instead, an impersonal voice, the voice of no one, is speaking:

Humanity, two warring souls reside
Deep inside you.
No use trying to decide.
For you can't help having two.
With your other self contending
Cleaving, clawing, splitting, rending
Keep the good and keep the evil
Keep the god and keep the devil
In a conflict never-ending!

(ibid., pp. 310–311)

This is certainly a direct response to the end of Goethe's *Faust*. If, however, we follow the thread of analytic discourse, which I have tried neither to lose sight of nor to break, it is also a rejection of an imposture: the one that promises to suppress the splitting of the subject through the excess of a supply that would end up in extinguishing demand. Such an imposture could efface irreversibly the only trace that guides us along the invisible path of desire, to the point where, at the end of this course, desire can act without demand.

Notes

1 [*Translator's note*: See Freud (1937, p. 252, emphasis added):

> We often have the impression that with the wish for a penis and the masculine protest we have penetrated through all the psychological strata and have reached *bedrock*, and that thus our activities are at an end. This is probably true, since, for the psychical field, *the biological field does in fact play the part of the underlying bedrock*.]

2 Regarding the "new spirit" of the capitalist discourse, see Boltanski and Chiapello (1999).
3 This should lead us to revise, rather than completely abandon, Freud's economic model.
4 Here are the mathemes of the capitalist and the analytic discourses:

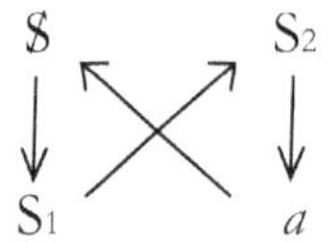

$$\frac{a}{S_2}\ \begin{matrix}\rightarrow\\ //\end{matrix}\ \frac{\$}{S_1}$$

5 To grasp what analytic discourse is able to achieve with psychotics, two factors must be noted: the paranoiac subject, at the cost of delusion, locates jouissance in the Other, within which the subject must find a place in order to find his bearings. Only the melancholic subject reaches the truth on this, in ruling that the jouissance of the Other is impossible to reach. This verdict, however, is precisely what s/he gets off on, at her/his own expense, for example by negativising the image of the body in the real.
6 In his essay "A Chapter on Dreams", Stevenson (1892, pp. 248–251) mentions the role of "brownies", who can be compared with molecules of the unconscious.
7 [*Translator's note*: In French this sentence concludes with a bilingual pun: "*Jekyll se suicide (kills je)*". The syllables of Jekyll's name are reversed, and what becomes the second syllable, "*je*" – French for "I" – receives the action of what is then the first syllable, "kill[s]". In this way, Jekyll's very name contains his suicide, once it is turned inside-out.]
8 It would be worthwhile to investigate the modes by which the subject can relate to the devil. Faust, the most eminent among them, signs a pact but succeeds in outwitting the devil. If we admit that Toussaint Turelure – a character in Paul Claudel's trilogy, which Lacan (2001b) discusses at length in his seminar on transference – serves as a figure of the devil, then Sygne de Coûfontaine makes a "pact" for which she would receive nothing in return. Finally, at the end of her life, she refuses a new pact that would distort the meaning of the first one. Christophe Haizmann, the painter whose story Freud (1923) reconstitutes in "A Seventeenth-Century Demonological Neurosis", *invents* a pact as an excuse for his inability to do without a nurturing, and perhaps even "nourishing" father. Such ethical choices, and they are not the only ones, mark out three major aspects of the subjectivity of our age. In the case of "Markheim", whether the figure involved is indeed the devil remains uncertain. The character who proposes the pact is, instead, the incarnation of temptation.
9 In this respect, Utterson resembles Sacher-Masoch, who was also a "Cainite".
10 Engels (1883) explored this tendency in the work of Alfred Russell Wallace, a first-rate English naturalist and scientist, who turned towards the study of miracles at the end of his life.

11 The gap between morality and ethics is a constant in Stevenson; for example, in "Markheim" (1887), the hero is a criminal in the world and pure in God.

12 As Lacan (1978b, p. 48) puts it, the capitalist discourse "works like a charm, like skids that have been fully greased, but that's just it: it goes too fast, it consumes itself [*ça se consomme*], and it does this so well that it uses itself up [*ça se consume*]".

13 Pierre Legendre (1989) discusses the case of a man who committed a crime while being filmed by a surveillance camera, and who remembered nothing when confronted with this recording.

14 This anticlericalism is not specific to revolutionary activists. Freud's (1928) discussion, in "Dostoevsky and Parricide", of repentance as a form of recidivism is similarly anticlerical.

2

FROM A TO Z

In the next three chapters, I examine the work of three philosophers (Louis Althusser, Gilles Deleuze and Slavoj Žižek) and one psychoanalyst (Félix Guattari). I have chosen them because they wanted, and were able, to take psychoanalysis into account, unlike other thinkers who believed that they could avoid it or adapt it in any manner they pleased. Even in criticising their ways of defining the problem of the relations between castration, subjective division and the symptom – definitions that would affect the aim both of an analysis and of psychoanalysis itself – I shall also be paying homage to their courage and perspicacity.

I do not want to summarise the results of my reading at the outset, except on one point, which is, as it were, the "guard rail" of this book: the symptom. Freud announced the splitting of the subject just before his London exile; it is as if the coming *Spaltung* between Vienna and London had led him to intuit it. The central question now is whether, without the division of the subject, a non-pathological doctrine of the symptom would even have been conceivable. In my opinion, this would not have been possible. The symptom – invented by Marx and given its foundation by Lacan – does not emerge unscathed by the major concepts of these four thinkers: Althusser's "bad subject", Deleuze and Guattari's "rhizome" and Žižek's "empty subject" are all modes of avoiding this constitutive division, although in Žižek, this question is very complex. This symptom is the corporeal event through which the body, at least once and in one place, subtracts itself from the Other's will-to-jouissance. By being spoken of, this body becomes a speaking body, and this event brings division into existence and makes it present: speech originates from the simultaneous splitting of the body by language and the splitting of language by the body. These four authors also sometimes mention castration, which I could define as an operation carried out by an agent – the real father – which enables the divided subject not to be drawn and quartered psychically, as is often the case when castration fails. Yet in doing so, castration privileges the phallus, thereby masking what could be called the innocence of splitting, since castration – whether or not it succeeds – links speaking to guilt. Consequently, an operation on the symptom proves necessary, through an experience that could occur in analysis, but also elsewhere. This operation will attempt to revitalise the symptom's relation to what it has always sought to do: create a diagonal of freedom between the Other's will-to-jouissance and the subject's own.

Althusser's comet

In 1966, the same year that the *Écrits* appeared, Louis Althusser (see 1966, pp. 33–37) circulated among his students a manuscript entitled "Three Notes on the Theory of Discourses". At that time, Althusser's interest in Lacan was intense, as he had already shown with his 1964 article, "Freud and Lacan" (Althusser, 1993, pp. 7–32) which had been published in *La nouvelle critique*, the journal of Communist party intellectuals. This article had already done much, in both France and Latin America, to rehabilitate the status of psychoanalysis as a revolutionary discipline. Whether or not this was a misunderstanding, its consequences have been unmistakable. Like Oscar Masotta, the Argentinian existentialist who was exiled in Spain, Althusser was one of Lacan's passers [*passeurs*].[1]

As the reader may know, the dramatist Heiner Müller (1982, p. 189) made a cruel and notorious observation: "The first event in Althusser's life was the murder of his wife". This assertion is not, however, immodest, and Louis Althusser would not necessarily have been shocked by it; in order that his status as subject not be dismissed, he had insisted on being judged for this murder in a criminal court. Perhaps, instead of saying "first event", it would be better to say, "first act". In any case, Müller justified his statement by noting that he was not interested in Althusser's theoretical work. Like any important dramatist, however, he was interested in discourse, an interest, indeed, that was striking. To take only one example, in Müller's (1980) *Quartet*, which was inspired by *Les liaisons dangereuses* (Choderlos de Laclos, 1782), the roles are reversed in the middle of the play. The Marquise de Merteuil becomes the Vicomte de Valmont and vice versa, a change that may be a response to Valmont's remark, made just before the reversal: "We should have our roles played by tigers" (Müller, 1980, p. 110). After this first change, Valmont becomes himself again, then turns into Merteuil again, and finally, upon becoming himself one last time, commits suicide in a supposedly "feminine" way by opening his veins with scissors. He then tells his former lover that he is dying because she has poisoned him.

This extraordinary use of the semblance tells us more about Lacan's concept of discourse than ten thousand pages of exegesis could. The theatre is the stage of discourse: it enables us to locate places and terms on it. References to the theatre take a priority in Lacan's teaching; he discussed at least one play by each of these authors: Sophocles, Aristophanes, Plautus, Shakespeare, Racine, Claudel and Genet (see León-Lopez, 1999).[2] And perhaps the subject of theatre is always the entrance into discourse, in that it is offered to human beings on condition that they can surmount the lethal jouissance of keeping themselves apart from the world. This entrance, however, can only take place in the gap between the places of production and truth in a discourse, a gap imposed by the barrier of jouissance.

To appreciate the theoretical impact of Althusser's "positions" on psychoanalysis, and in order not to get stuck in discussions of his disagreements with or misunderstandings of Lacan, I shall begin by isolating a central thread that appears in several texts: these include a speech that he gave after Lacan's dissolution of the *École freudienne de Paris*, his correspondence with René Diatkine and with Lacan, his 1973 text on transference and countertransference, and finally, the presentation intended for the Tbilissi conference and published without his consent.[3] All of these texts point to an enunciation that touches Althusser's experience as analysand directly; in this way, they are unlike some of his other works, which are more distant from this experience. These other works are also marked by the same symptomatic certainty that there is an absolute discontinuity between science and ideology (we know that one of the philosophical foundations of this distinction was Spinoza's third kind of knowledge).

Althusser's speech at the PLM Saint Jacques on 15 March 1980, given during an internal meeting of the *École freudienne de Paris* and published under the title of "In the Name of the Analysands . . ." (Althusser, 1993, pp. 125–144), was motivated by his disapproval of the way in which analysts tend to "drop" their analysands. This disapproval was both very old and very harsh; it may well have come to include Lacan after the latter's late-night visit to Althusser, following Lucien Sebag's suicide.[4] Perhaps this disapproval gives the speech its lucidity. In any case, although he was in a state of incontestable agitation, as Jacques-Alain Miller has noted (see ibid., p. 181, note 1), Althusser was able to ask a fundamental question: "But not one [analyst] asked whether in dissolving the Ecole and founding 'La Cause Freudienne', Lacan was not dragging them into a new Ecole" (ibid., p. 120). Nearly thirty years later, this remains an urgent question. In dissolving the *École freudienne de Paris*, was Lacan hoping to put an end to a school whose functioning was the reverse of what he had hoped for when he founded it? Was he, on the other hand, rejecting the very concept of a school, on the grounds that it was inappropriate to psychoanalysis? At the time, arguments drawing on supposedly "historical" explanations were made in order to show that the second option was indefensible, but that fact (which itself can be disputed) does not, in my opinion, render the question completely pointless today.

The other important aspect of Althusser's intrusion is also related to this question. He hoped to explain what he had noticed during the meeting of 15 March: most of the analysts who, in private, criticised, objected to or questioned Lacan's act nevertheless remained silent in public, and admitted to him that they were doing so out of fear. This situation can seem insignificant and commonplace; such incidents have been witnessed by anyone who has attended assemblies of analysts. All in all, it would be imprudent to prefer a psychotic "fearlessness" to neurotic "fear", according to a moral classification that could well be called "down to date". Yet Althusser did not attribute what he witnessed to moral conformity; instead, he developed an analysis of this collective silence that remains interesting:

> It is best to stop at this point, since the logic that demands that analyst-intellectuals – who are often very subtle and not racist and "Lacanian" adults, broadly speaking – assemble out of a need to be afraid of Lacan or of X . . . in order to be reassured, is a logic that far transcends analysts, since one can find its equivalent in a number of organizations – particularly workers' organizations (I mention them because I know them somewhat, but one could just as well invoke the Church or the army). In all of these, the need to be afraid can serve as a reason for belonging to a community of belief, thought and action; this reason assures you that you are indeed afraid and are right to be afraid, and at the same time reassures you against that fear and its reason, since you are no longer alone as a result of your belonging. This gives you the warmth – be it maternal or any other – of the active and protective group. . . . So, one falls back all the more on the group that satisfies this need for fear and protects against it.
>
> *(ibid., pp. 139–140, translation modified)*[5]

This speech, like the other texts in question, defends analysands against the hold of a transference that threatens to annihilate them. This position is implicit in his correspondence with Lacan. If Lacan did not immediately answer a long letter from Althusser – one in which the philosopher shows him the theoretical place that Lacan occupies for him – Althusser (ibid., p. 159) would immediately write a second letter that begins with the words: "Your silence has a great value for me. I expected it". This letter cannot hide his chagrin that the man whom Althusser considers to be a genius has not behaved as a mirror image: he has not addressed Althusser in the same terms in which the philosopher had addressed him. He parries this disappointment in a way that is very weak, attributing Lacan's lack of response precisely to his genius, while knowing that he has himself engineered this silence. The letter in which Althusser speaks of Lacan's failure to respond is dated Tuesday, December 10, less than a week after the preceding letter, which is dated Wednesday, 4 December.

A transferential misunderstanding, involving both love and hatred, is visible in this letter. Yet what is remarkable is a reversal, in which Althusser attributes to the analyst a fascination with the analysand or the "analysed". The letter, of course, testifies to the opposite: Althusser's fascination with Lacan. "The desire of the analyst. It sends us to the desire of the analyzed. Desire of a desire. Dual structure of fascination, whence so many interminable-unterminated analyses" (ibid., p. 163). This reversal is not, however, without value: the interminability of such treatments could well result from a desire of the analyst's, which would be nothing without the desire of the "analysed". This actually raises, in a negative form, the question of the analyst's relation to a knowledge of which s/he must become the symptom; without this, the analyst would be nothing more than the papyrus on which the scribe writes. This non-living analyst evoked in Althusser's remarks is nothing other than an avatar of the impasse about the real father. From this perspective, Althusser's arrow would not necessarily have missed its mark; unfortunately, however, his way of developing this point annuls its significance. Althusser imputes the establishment of the dual relation to the imaginary aspect of the analyst's desire, which can thereby be nothing without the desire of the analysed. It then becomes easy for Althusser to denounce the fact that this imaginary desire of the analyst is never called into question "in the analysis of the other imaginary, the one that the desire of the analysed attempts in vain to establish" (ibid., p. 166).

It should not be surprising that Althusser did not choose Lacan or one of his students as his analyst; René Diatkine was a member of the *Société psychanalytique de Paris*, and was thus, almost by definition, a champion of countertransference, which is precisely that which Althusser reproaches Lacan for being unaware of.

If we follow Lacan's critique of countertransference, it is certainly easy to dispense with this concept. Freud uses this term infrequently; it occurs only three times in his work, most interestingly in "Observations on Transference-Love", where his remarks prefigure Lacan's critique: "For the doctor, the phenomenon [of the patient's falling in love] signifies a valuable piece of enlightenment and a useful warning against any tendency to a counter-transference which may be present in his own mind" (Freud, 1915b, p. 160). Following Lacan, we can consider that an analyst operates as object rather than as subject, and thus does not act as an analysand. Thus, when Freud warns of the risk of countertransference, he is only warning doctors not to give up their position as analyst, which is a bare minimum. This single remark destroys Althusser's argument about the desire of the analyst.

The argument grows more interesting, however, if we consider it in terms of the analysand. Thus, in a text that was given the humorous title, "*Petites incongruités portatives*", before it was rewritten as "*Sur le transfert et le contre-transfert*", Althusser (1973) combats the opinion that the analysand's transference to the analyst is primary and that the analyst's transference to the analysand is secondary. He puts forward a thesis that, rather unexpectedly, undoes the symmetry of the analytic relation: countertransference is more important than transference. Although he does not provide a sufficient elucidation to this question, which he has had the merit of bringing out, he proposes what he calls the "primacy of *controlling* [*contrôle du*] countertransference" (ibid., p. 186, emphasis added). It is possible to understand this in various ways; I am of the opinion that Althusser could have benefitted from having an opportunity to explore, in the context of his own treatment, the different ways in which what he said could be understood. It could mean, first, that the process by which analysts are produced should be reconsidered; this could prevent the treatment from becoming an intersubjective relation. Second, and this anticipates what Althusser would call for in "In the Name of the Analysands", an analyst must neither act as a Pontius Pilate – which is also a minimum – nor use a power of intimidation, which the analysis bestows on him, and which – unless the analyst makes some slight avowal of his/her ability to be mistaken – can confer upon him/her an aura of infallibility. This sort of caricature can also be found among analysts, proving that it is indeed an effect of their production and not only of their infantile history. It happens that Althusser and Lacan agree about this point, despite their nearly total theoretical disagreement: they are both careful not to attribute to infantile history something that is the artificial effect of a certain conception of a psychoanalytic association, and, by extension, of the production of analysts.[6]

The section of *Writings on Psychoanalysis* entitled "The Tbilissi affair: 1976–1984" (Althusser, 1993, pp. 79–124) includes two texts that were written for a conference on psychoanalysis that was held in the Soviet Union. The first, which Althusser withdrew but which was later published without his permission, was written in the spring of 1976 and was entitled "The Discovery of Doctor Freud"; the second, written the following year, was called "On Marx and Freud". As is often the case with Althusser, the intended audience is crucial. Althusser thought that he was addressing a public of Marxist intellectuals, communist scientists from whom he would remove the blinkers that had led the Soviet Union to reject psychoanalysis. Discreetly, these two texts, which are neither pedagogic nor messianic, take on a status that differs from his other theoretical works; they seek to defend psychoanalysis from itself, thus enabling it to be integrated into dialectical materialism. For this reason, they do not mention Althusser's work on ideology – the ideological state apparatuses, the discourses, etc.

Instead of giving an exposition of the content of these two texts, I would like to explore Althusser's depiction of the relation between psychoanalysis and philosophy. First, in describing analytic treatment, he repeats his judgement about the relations between transference and countertransference. For Althusser (ibid., p. 89), countertransference is the analyst's introjective identification with the analysand, "which means that the analyst cannot manage to separate himself from the patient". Once again, one could subscribe to this view if the identification with the analysand were not interpreted in terms of the analyst's countertransference: if the analyst identifies with the analysand, the very position of analyst ceases to exist. Further, there is the unlimited series of the analyst's psychic states, which have no effect on the treatment if the analyst's place is maintained. Even further, there is the analyst's possible acting out,[7] which supposes that s/he identifies the analysand with an Other whose consistency s/he has not been able to reduce fully. Rather than being a countertransference, this is the transference of the non-analyst who exists *within* the analyst.

The second point, Althusser's understanding of repression, is even more determinant. "The second nucleus, revealed by the first [unconscious infantile sexuality], is the idea of a prodigious social *censorship* of those same unconscious sexual wishes" (ibid., p. 95). In this context, we may think of Wilhelm Reich or Jean-Jacques Rousseau's phantoms of an absolutely bad Other, but such references can only take on their full clinical significance if we examine why the fault is located in this way. The idea that repression is caused by parental – and beyond them, social – prohibitions is often wrongly attributed to Freud, but it is undermined by his second theory of anxiety, which he develops in *Inhibitions, Symptoms and Anxiety* (1926a). There he reverses his earlier thesis that the repressed portion of the libido is transformed into anxiety; now anxiety gives rise to repression. In this new argument, anxiety cannot be deduced from social censorship, which, instead, often resolves anxiety. Anxiety is a corporeal signal that there is a gap between a sort of virtual reality – to which language summons us – and trauma, which is constituted because we speak; the subject who takes the risk of speaking becomes an exception to this virtualisation. In other words, "social censorship" is the effect rather than the origin of this anxiety; it is nothing more than the groping attempt of civilisation to make anxiety bearable, because it cannot eradicate it absolutely.

Furthermore, although Althusser believes that the superego performs this social censorship, this is actually only its secondary function. Its primary function is to bring jouissance back into the place of the signifier, since in a primal logical time, the place of the signifier is the non-place, a sort of *nolle prosequi* [*non-lieu*] of jouissance. Yet when jouissance returns to this place, it does so at a price: it will now take the form of a fault or sin. This is the aporia of the superego: the more we follow its injunctions to jouissance, the greater the unconscious sense of guilt grows. As we know, the imperatives of the superego can cover a whole range of apparently contradictory imperatives, from "Thou shalt kill" to "Thou shalt not kill". In these two extreme cases, the subject obtains the scant jouissance permitted by the incompatibility between language and jouissance. Thus, the criminal would be equivalent to the saint, if a single difference did not make them antagonists: the place they give to the real other. I shall return to this question: the real other is neither the other whom I imagine nor the counterpart who is my equal; instead, it is a recognised alterity. In *State of Exception*, the second volume of *Homo Sacer*, Giorgio Agamben (1995, p. 36) forcefully brings out the homology between a state of exception as a "free and juridically empty space" and language, the empty space of speech, promoting a conception of law that could be related not only to the discourse of the master but also to that of the analyst. He does so by outlining the thesis of a kind of law in which the other could be the subject of something other than law.

Finally, Althusser's conception of the subject involves an obvious and irremediable disagreement with Lacan. For Lacan, who was following Freud's final statements about the dialectic between the recognition and disavowal of castration, the subject is split. Althusser considers Lacan's reading to be a misinterpretation; for him, there is neither a split subject nor a subject of the unconscious. He recognises only a single subject, which is constituted through an interpellation by Ideology; the consequence of this mode of constitution is the regular doubling of the subject by an entity that is its ideal specular counterpart: God. Thus, the only "subject" that can be named as such and would be immune to this ideological effect is the "bad subject", who is condemned to undergo a *passage à l'acte* in order to escape its vassalage to what, for Althusser, is the most terrifying figure of the Other: Ideology with a capital I.[8]

The other text, rewritten for the publication of the acts of the Tbilisi symposium, is entitled "On Marx and Freud". Even more directly than in the first, Althusser is addressing readers whom he supposes to be Marxists and is seeking to exonerate psychoanalysis by accentuating the homology between Freud and Marx's relation to science. He calls our attention, by the way, to the fact that both Freudian and Marxist science are "scissionist" – a term that he interprets, in a way that is not uninteresting, as resulting from the primacy of experience in both disciplines (Althusser, 1993, p. 109). Even if Althusser does not state this idea, it is difficult not to think that the conflictual character of these two sciences requires – if we want to be on the "right side" – that we choose the side of the analysands in one case and of the people in the other. He has almost crossed the Rubicon by making the analyst into an "enemy of the people". The reader, by a bit of forcing – and we know that caricature is the sincerest form of paying homage to truth – can glimpse that in psychoanalysis, there must be an opposition between the science of the analysand and that of the analyst.

I shall now return to the question of the subject, which is really what is at stake for Althusser. His violent criticism of the unified subject of psychology refers to Lacan's teaching, although he gets rid of its major consequence, the splitting of the subject. Thus, in developing the idea of a unitary subject that, like a fetish, would come to fill the absence of the subject of the unconscious, Althusser concludes that the subject of law must be considered as completed by the psychological subject, which is at least potentially conscious of itself (ibid., p. 115). Here again, we would expect Althusser to bring up the idea of a split subject, since, in Lacan, this splitting is based on the irreducibility of the unconscious. Furthermore, a bit later, Althusser seems to invite us to think that the subject is structurally divided between truth and what it is permitted to know; he mentions that "Every individual thus 'spontaneously' develops a reflex of 'defense' when confronting the unconscious, which is part of his own unconscious" (ibid., p. 120). Instead, however, there is a twist, in which Althusser forbids himself from taking the step that would allow him to accept this division:

> Every individual? This is not certain. It is not established that the defensive reflex is always equally active; experience shows, on the contrary, that there exist subjects in whom that resistance is – by virtue of their accommodation of their phantasmatic conflicts – sufficiently superseded to permit them to acknowledge the reality of the unconscious without triggering a reflex of defense or flight.
>
> *(ibid., p. 120)*

This is little more than a feeble dodge, in which an "exception" – which should be taken as a psychological consideration – only reinforces my judgement that Althusser uses the diktat of the "bad subject" to impose this lack of splitting upon the subject. There has been no act that would include the subject: an act that would take place between alienation and separation, between the subjection to language that divides the subject and the separation through which it is liberated. Therefore, the bad subject can only assert its truth by provoking its own destruction, and it does so by destroying an other who is too similar. I shall gladly group the texts that have just been examined under the heading of a "science of the analysand". In any case, these texts bear the same relation to texts less concerned with the analytic experience as the foundations of a house bear to its visible structure.

We shall now examine the works that constitute this visible structure. First, "Three Notes on the Theory of Discourses" (1966), which was written three years before Lacan gave his seminar *The Other Side of Psychoanalysis*. Here, Althusser distinguishes four discourses: scientific discourse, aesthetic discourse, ideological discourse and unconscious discourse. What he is seeking, above all, is to connect the unconscious and ideological discourses. Each of these discourses is characterised in two ways. First, there is the level of structure: ideological discourse has a specular structure, in which the human subject is reflected and doubled in the divine subject; the discourse of the unconscious has a metonymic structure, connected with the fact that a placeholder stands in for the subject-effect. Second, there are the elements of structure: "fantasies" for the unconscious discourse, and more diverse elements – from words to forms of conduct – for ideological discourse. What is relevant in this context is not the question of whether Althusser's construction is well founded, but its formalist character; like structuralism, this formalism is explicitly linked to a refusal to consider the question of the subject in any terms other than those of a subject-effect. The consequence is the "bad subject", which is not broken by being an effect. Yet Althusser allows this path to lead to a dead end, for he does not want to recognise that the "bad subject" is not bad, but instead is divided by its enunciation, which separates it from jouissance.

Therefore – and in this sense, Heiner Müller's diagnosis is correct – Althusser's theory of discourse is characteristic of what Lacan called the discourse of the university, which is one of the four configurations that are possible on the basis of the matrix that I have already indicated.

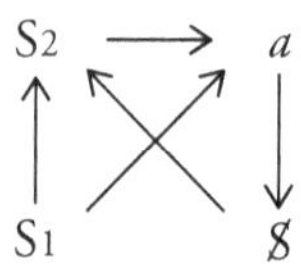

It may seem severe to apply this schema to Althusser's theory of discourses; it can even lead readers to accuse me of doing precisely what I am attacking: I am elevating Lacan to the level of some kind of knowledge that would have the status of a whole [*tout-savoir*]. Yet in this context, there is no difficulty, for Althusser's conception of science is clearly a form of this knowledge. The only difficulty is that Althusser does not hide that his teachers are Lacan and Marx.[9] What exonerates him from being a "knave" (Lacan, 1991, p. 61) and shows that his enunciation involved taking risks, or a forcing, is that his body opened the Pandora's box that contained language. Pandora was a woman, and if we take Hesiod's *Theogony* literally, this means that a woman was the first master. This origin was subsequently masked because people believed that they could correct this first lie,[10] since speech is itself a lie, by constructing a discourse that would separate the true from the false. On this site, first philosophy and then science have constructed their glory and unveiled their limits.

As a part of his implication in the discourse of the university, Althusser elaborated a theory of discourses, which involved a general theory – historical materialism – of which psychoanalysis would be a local theory. In this respect, all other things being unequal, his ambition was close to the ambition that underlies Lacan's four discourses. For readers who are familiar with Lacan's conception of discourse, any comparison of the two theories may seem inappropriate. Lacan understands "discourse" in a way that is very different from its common meaning as a form of speech; Althusser, on the other hand, used the word in its usual sense. His only specific originality is the proposition that "*every discourse produces a subjectivity-effect*", and thus each of the four forms of discourse (unconscious, ideological, aesthetic and scientific) "induces" a different subject-effect (Althusser, 1966, p. 48). Althusser sets up an opposition concerning unconscious and ideological discourse by claiming that the subject of the latter is "*present in person*", whereas the subject of the former "is *represented* . . . by *one* signifier which 'stands in' for it" (ibid., p. 49). This definition indicates a gap between Althusser and Lacan's formulations (we do not know whether this gap is deliberate or results from a confusion produced by a hasty reading). For Lacan, the signifier that represents the subject (S_1) is different from the signifier that serves as a stand-in (S_2), for the stand-in *is not representative*. As we have seen, ten years later, Althusser would repeat his refusal, which is already implicit here, of the splitting of the subject.

No one will be surprised that Althusser's theory gives precedence to the subject of ideological discourse. In "Ideology and Ideological State Apparatuses", Althusser (1970) develops this question much more fully and refers explicitly to this "bad subject", which becomes the exception to the state of ideological conformity produced by interpellation. Yet as early as 1966, the bases for this had already been established: "It is ideology", with a small "i", "that performs the function of designating the subject (in general) that is to occupy this function: to that end it must *interpellate it* as subject" (Althusser, 1966, p. 51).

These notes sought to relate ideological discourse to unconscious discourse. It would be better, however, to examine whether this problem is even relevant. Why is a theory of the relation between the unconscious and ideology necessary? On this point, I would be tempted to share the healthy simplicity of Freud, for whom no "social" effect is truly social, for it always depends on the individual's reactions. Social psychology is actually just psychology. Marx and Engels brought the term "ideology" to the forefront, but it was coined by Antoine Destutt de Tracy (1817), in his *Éléments d'idéologie*. For Destutt de Tracy, ideology is the science of ideas. In contrast, Marx and Engels, in *The German Ideology* (1932), perform a *coup de force*, emphasising that the function of ideology is to write a history that neglects the determinant role played by surplus-value in the various modes of production; ideology gives rise to a history that has been distorted into idealism and abstraction. Yet their observation goes beyond this, for they show that this ideology came into existence because those who produce and convey it have economic positions and interests that lead them to misunderstand the importance of surplus-value.

According to this account, however, Marx should himself have believed in the German ideology. If he did not, it was because, as subject, he chose another path. This remark may seem trivial, but we see its weight when applied to Wilhelm Reich's work. For Reich, a worker may choose to become a communist because of his/her class membership, and there is no need to make any psychological mechanism intervene. On the other hand, if a worker becomes a fascist, the existence of a pathological psychological mechanism must be postulated (for example, see Reich, 1933). If Reich's reasoning were applied to Marx, then Marx's invention of communism would be pathological. It would be better to conclude that there is no "natural" choice. Every ideological interpellation, to use Althusser's expression, is never anything but a plunging into a language that certainly has its own significations; only "half" of the subject, however, is ever interpellated in it.

If, therefore, the term "ideology" has any meaning, it is to designate false theories in the field of history. There are indeed false theories of history – the idea, for example, that society is an organism; such theories can degenerate into slogans, to the point of becoming ossified phrases. They are never "entities", demons that would magically instill an illusion or a false belief in someone. Ideology is never anything other than the product of a linguistic effect, one in which a theory becomes metaphorical. The subject, however, must always choose to accept this metaphorization. This invalidates neither Destutt de Tracy's project nor Marx's analysis; it does, however, invalidate the idea that *ideology is a collective unconscious*. Marxist Jungianism has still not been eradicated.

In his notes on discourse, Althusser finds himself on this slippery slope, and the best proof of this is that he makes the Other into both the entity of Ideology and a subject:

> The big Other, which speaks in the discourse of the unconscious, would then be, not the *subject* of the discourse of the ideological – God, the subject and so on – but the *discourse* of the ideological itself, established as the *subject* of the discourse of the unconscious, and established in the specific form of the discourse of the unconscious, that is, as an *effect* of this discourse.
>
> *(Althusser, 1966, p. 61)*

For Althusser, there is no subject of the unconscious; therefore, the Other, through an effect of the ideological discourse, comes to occupy this place as a false subject. Yet what need is there to bring in ideology if this subjectivation of the Other – this belief in the existence of an Other of the Other – can be sufficiently explained by the unconscious itself? The theory of fantasy does this. Why do we need to bring in ideology except because it has been posited as an entity against which the subject can do nothing? In other words, according to Althusser, to recognise oneself as subject is tantamount to accepting the consistency of the Other.

Althusser comes close, however, to what could have given him another solution when he says that ideological discourse serves in "the discourse of the unconscious . . . as a *symptom*" (ibid., p. 60, emphasis added). Such a solution, however, would have led him to abandon his initial conception of alienation, which had already been set in stone at the time of his 1964 article, "Freud and Lacan". For him, subjection is very much an alienation in the place of an Other who is a subject. In this sense, the mechanism that he describes is incompatible with what Lacan conceptualises with the term "alienation", where the Other is precisely not a subject. Lacan takes care to make an explicit statement about *what alienation is not*, and even if he is not aiming at Althusser, he hits him. Does alienation mean that the

> subject is condemned to seeing itself emerge, *in initio*, only in the field of the Other? Could it be that? Well, it isn't. Not at all – not at all – not at all.

> Alienation consists in this *vel*, which – if you do not object to the word *condemned*, I will use it – condemns the subject to appearing only in that division which, it seems to me, I have just articulated sufficiently by saying that, if it appears on one side as meaning, produced by the signifier, it appears on the other as *aphanisis*.
>
> *(Lacan, 1973d, p. 210)*

Polynices & Polynices

Anti-Oedipus (1972) and *A Thousand Plateaus* (1980), both of which were subtitled *Capitalism and Schizophrenia*, were written by a philosopher (Gilles Deleuze) and a psychoanalyst (Félix Guattari). The title of the first volume, *Anti-Oedipus*, announces its character very clearly, and its publication was an event. Yet the legacy of this book seems much less certain, and the schizoanalytic treatment that it promotes seems to have fizzled out, if, that is, there was ever much fizzle there.

By 1972, the *Écrits* had been available for six years. During 1971–1972, Lacan gave his seminar . . . *ou pire* (Lacan, 2011a) and a related series of lectures at Saint-Anne that has been partially published in English translation as *Talking to Brick Walls* (Lacan, 2011b). In them, he continued his investigation of what could be called phallic "imperialism" and the Oedipal "dictatorship", to choose two expressions that would not have displeased Deleuze and Guattari. Lacan was seeking to highlight the existence of a dephallicised jouissance that was specific to femininity – which does not mean that men are not involved in it – and which does not emerge through any acceptance of castration. If women are not wholly within the regime of the castration complex, the consequence is that Freud's impasse concerning femininity – the supposedly insurmountable persistence of penis envy – finds its exit not in a forcing but in a topographical displacement: the dead end remains a dead end, but numerous other roads remain available to anyone who wants to move about freely. Lacan's proposition seeks not to jettison the castration complex but to limit its scope to the definition of sexuation that it permits, and to undo its mad project of abolishing the dimension of the drives.

In writing the first volume of *Capitalism and Schizophrenia*, Deleuze and Guattari were not unaware of what Lacan was doing, but the reader of this book will not find a carefully argued confrontation with his work during that period. Paradoxically, *Anti-Oedipus*, despite its libertarian inspiration, presents itself as a closed system that is very difficult to enter into; it cultivates its own technical language and develops a reading-grid that is able to "decode" – a term that the authors are very fond of – all of the theoretical territory that is related, directly or indirectly, to human action. The entire book depends on an *organon* of dichotomies or differentiations. If we hope to be able to understand it and reconstruct its axioms, these dichotomies must be "tamed" and comprehended. The first of these is the distinction between "desiring-machines" and "bodies without organs". To say "we, desiring-machines" would be to go too far. Yet the prototype that the authors propose, following the principle of a machine that is never isolated but is always connected to another machine, is the breast-mouth couple: the breast-machine produces a flow and the mouth-machine cuts off that flow. The model is thus that of the montage of the drives, except that, unlike Lacan's, it is a *functional* montage.[11] Desire is thus defined as what does not cease to effect a coupling between a continuous flow and the removal or slicing off [*prélèvement*] of the flow: "desire causes the current to flow, flows itself in turn, and breaks the flows" (Deleuze & Guattari, 1972, p. 5).

As we shall see, this is where the vitiation of the Oedipus and castration complexes begins, for they reject the dissemination that is part of the regime of desiring-machines. This is shown with great acuteness in the chapter "1914: One or Several Wolves" in the second volume, *A Thousand Plateaus*. "[M]olecular multiplicities" are placed in opposition to what is supposed to be the phallic reign of unicity, which would set up a humiliating and defeated acceptance of the Oedipus complex (Deleuze & Guattari, 1980, p. 27). Their example comes from Salvador Dali, who stopped talking about "THE rhinoceros horn" – another overly opportune metaphor for phallic "unicity" – and begins comparing "goosebumps to a field of rhinoceros horns" (ibid., p. 27). Seen from this perspective, the ego itself is the opposite of a paranoiac corset: it is an undelimited zone of fluctuating and varied events.

Here the authors graft on what could be the book's most decisive thesis: the infantile Oedipus complex is an artefact forged by the paranoia of a father who imputes to his son the desire to kill him. Here is the key statement: "The paranoiac father Oedipalizes the son. Guilt is an idea projected by the father before it is an inner feeling experienced by the son. The first error of psychoanalysis is in acting as if things began with the child" (Deleuze & Guattari, 1972, p. 275).[12]

The concept of desiring-machines is paired with a second concept: that of the "body without organs". This expression was taken from Antonin Artaud's radio play, *To Have Done with the Judgement of God*:

> So it is man whom we must now make up our minds to emasculate.
> – How's that?
> How's that?
> No matter how one takes you, you are mad, ready for the straitjacket.
> – By placing him again, for the last time, on the autopsy table to remake his anatomy . . . .
> Man is sick because he is badly constructed.
> We must make up our minds to strip him in order to scrape off that animalcule that itches him mortally,
> god,
> and with god
> his organs.
> For you can tie me up if you wish,
> but there is nothing more useless than an organ.
> When you will have made him a body without organs,
> then you will have delivered him from all his automatic reactions and restored him to his true freedom.
>
> (Artaud, 1947b, pp. 570–571)

There are numerous readings of this poem, and they can be divided into two groups. On the one hand, through the body without organs, Artaud seems to be seeking to achieve a body without sexuality. Such readings argue that Artaud considers god (a term that is written here without capital letters) to be someone who gets off sexually on Artaud's body. It should be noted as lightly as possible that this single indication is sufficient to locate Artaud within paranoia, rather than schizophrenia. What is important, in this context, is not the general form of Artaud's subjection, which is absolutely secondary, but his relation to his symptom, to the singularity of his refusal to be "encaged" in the being of language. Artaud undoes what, through god, "machines" him as an object, one that has become the passive receptacle of an intrusive jouissance.

The second reading of the body without organs, which Deleuze supports explicitly in *The Logic of Sense*, is that it corresponds to a nonphallic, rhizomatic sexuality, which would be homologous to the heterogeneous objects of the drive. This reading is also irrefutable. Yet whichever interpretation one chooses, Artaud's "body without organs" is what is obtained by subtracting the body from the generative chain of the father and the mother; this would be done by "scraping off" the animalcule-god's organs. In other words, it would be done with the automatisms of its organism, which are like the after-effects or the side-effects of the infection of the body by god. In other words, it is necessary to begin with the colonising of the body into an organism in order then to exit from it; nothing indicates that there is any possibility of a primal bifurcation that would render such colonisation unnecessary. Having begun with the question of anti-Oedipus, we have now been led to question Deleuze and Guattari. Does their theory go beyond the Oedipus complex or fall short of it?

There is also a significant slippage in Deleuze and Guattari's use of the term "body without organs": they (1972, p. 32) speak of "a full body without organs", moving away from the letter of Artaud's work. This would be a body *before* the void and *before* lack, in a way that has serious consequences. It contradicts Artaud's proposition that the body is made of nothing, as he writes explicitly in his poem "And not like god": "the fact that what is nothingness is the body" (Artaud, 1947a, p. 264). What does this mean, if not that language is equivalent to this nothingness [*néantisation*], which, literally speaking, makes everybody. Therefore, for Artaud, "body without organs" and "full" are mutually exclusive notions. This is a complex question, for "nothing" is not "lack"; it is the reverse [*envers*] of full: "this wrong side out [*envers*] will be his [the body's] real place" (Artaud, 1947b, p. 570). We see thus that for Artaud, the body can only have a place as the underside of the full, the place that is imposed upon it by the animalcule-god.

This is the exact opposite of Deleuze and Guattari's thesis, which nevertheless makes this expression a major and unsurpassable reference. In their argument, lack, castration, etc. seem to be nothing more than paranoiac caprices. It would have been better, however – including and especially in terms of their determination to mark the limits of these terms – to examine how language itself made them necessary. It is therefore astonishing to see that, in taking nothingness into account, Artaud enables his "brothers" in castration – even those who are only neurotics – to find a sort of neighbourhood when faced with the walls of language. This wall obliges them to experience nothingness in order to inhabit their bodies.

The anti-Oedipal idea is entirely different: if the body is marked as zero, this is to signify the zero degree of numbering: the body precedes the One and is not the consequence of a nihilation [*néantisation*] by language. It is true that, in *A Thousand Plateaus*, Deleuze and Guattari devote a chapter to exploring how the body without organs or "BwO" is a "set of practices" (Deleuze & Guattari, 1980, p. 150). These practices mobilise "intensities" – "*pain waves*", "*refrigerator waves*" and other waves that belong to an order that is strictly impossible to interpret (ibid., p. 152). By thus treating the BwO "as the full egg before the extension of the organism and the organization of the organs" (ibid., p. 153), these practices have the aim of calculating the potential for intensity contained in this egg.

Fascinated by the facts of masochism, schizophrenic mutilation and melancholic negative hallucinations, Deleuze and Guattari do not overlook the question of the sombre side of the BwO: "So why these examples, why must we start there? Emptied bodies instead of full ones. What happened?" (ibid., p. 150). Yet the fact that they are writing after Freud does not lead them to wonder whether these specifically human facts may be related to the symbolic nihilation [*néantisation*] induced by language. Instead, moved by a passionate hatred for the symbolic, they prefer to mock the death drive. In this way, they miss precisely what limits the lethal hold of the symbolic: the symptom.

Seen from this perspective, the subject is a hanger-on, a parasite of the body without organs, and would therefore, oddly enough, have the status of Artaud's animalcule-god. The subject is a series of states, a host of metonymies that through their very "transitivity" (in the double sense of "transitive" and "transitional") make something present: the impossibility of any identification that would name and thus unify the subject. Since the body without organs is precisely the place where the desiring machines will take hold, it needs to be understood as fully as possible; we must not forget that these bodies do not efface the gap between the full body and the body-as-nothing. Artaud, indeed, was not satisfied with this volatile subject, for he never stopped using the body to forge an identity for the ego [*moi*]: "The self [*moi*] is not the body, it is the body that is the self [*moi*]" (Artaud, 1947a, p. 251).

The desiring-machines, to return to the other term of Deleuze and Guattari's opposition, are systems of cuts, which operate on a continuous material flow. Cut (or schiz) *vs.* flow: this is their minimal dialectical relation. Deleuze and Guattari are probably conceding the importance of language by having these machines include a code, which, however, is a code of "polyvocal" signs rather than a system of signifiers. This cacophonic code produces desire: it makes machines desire (Deleuze & Guattari, 1972, p. 38). This code also brings organs into existence, but in a way that does not connect each organ to a function; on the contrary, it makes the organ participate in negating its supposed function (an "anorectic mouth") (ibid., p. 38). This antifunctionalism is, however, more a sort of negative version of functionalism than a subversion of it, as it is in Lacan. There are three sorts of cuts: "breaks that are a slicing off (*coupures-prélèvements*)", which "have to do with continuous fluxes and are related to partial objects";"breaks that are a detachment (*coupures-détachements*)"; and the "residual break (*coupure-reste*) or residuum, which produces a subject alongside the machine, functioning as a part adjacent to the machine" (ibid., pp. 39, 40). These three operations – slicing off, detaching, residual breaking – are the components of the production of desire.

The body thus serves both to support the code and is a material reality that, paradoxically, is prior to the organism. The other material realities, however, which can become machines (the means of production) still remain undefined. A dialectic is taking shape (flux *vs.* breaks), one that is clearly opposed to the dialectic that the authors attribute to Oedipal psychoanalysis: in the latter, desire comes into existence as a lack of the object. According to Deleuze and Guattari, "Desire does not lack anything. . . . It is rather the *subject* that is missing in desire, or desire that lacks a fixed subject", because "there is no fixed subject unless there is repression" (ibid., p. 26). The objective being of desire is the real itself. The formulation "the *subject* . . . is missing to desire" would be extraordinary and absolutely true if it did not transform desire into an external entity, one for which the subject could lack respect, despite the fact that, in any case, no subject is without the filament – whether it be slender as a hair or solid as a tow rope – that connects it to the symptom. Indeed, the conclusions that the authors draw from their formulation confirm this reservation and reduce my initial enthusiasm: 1) "there is no particular form of" the real "that can be labelled 'psychic reality'"; 2) "the real is not the impossible", but the possible (ibid., p. 27, translation modified).

What, then, is the source of the lure or illusion that desire is correlated to lack? The answer is that, "We know very well where lack – and its subjective correlative come from, the fantasy. Lack [*manque*] is created, planned, and organized in and through social production" (ibid., p. 28). We can now understand at what level capitalism intervenes. As Lacan's thesis about the lack-in-jouissance [*manque-à-jouir*] that is produced by the capitalist discourse suggests, capitalism is, among all the modes of production, the one that pushes the manufacturing of lack to its height; this manufacturing becomes the very condition that enables capitalism to function. Desire as the effect of lack thus becomes the false capitalist version of desire, to which the authors can oppose schizophrenia, which, for them, preserves the true nature of desire. In doing so, they are referring not to the psychiatric entity that bears that name, but the essence of the process itself. The two authors do not fail, in a note, to signal the "two poles" of Lacan's theory of desire: an admirable one that is "related to the object small *a* as a desiring-machine", and another, which is more Oedipal and "which reintroduces a certain notion of lack" in relation to the Other (ibid., p. 27).

The "*capitalist machine*" "deterritorializ[es] . . . the socius" (ibid., pp. 33, 34); it abolishes particular social territories in a movement towards universalisation, but it is incapable of producing the code that would give a meaning to this universalisation. In this respect, we could add, capitalism is a-religious, despite a recurrent resistance on the part of religion, which tries to palliate this absence of meaning. Money neither makes sense nor creates meaning; Guizot's axiom "enrich yourselves!" does not provide any answer to the mystery of existence. There would thus be – note the use of the modal – a tendency towards schizophrenia within capitalism; this echoes Lacan's thesis about the foreclosure of castration by the capitalist discourse and could even provide an explanation of the difference between the foreclosures of the Name-of-the-Father and of castration. Nevertheless, the capitalist tendency towards deterritorialisation, the existence of which is incontestable, never ceases to approach its limit – schizophrenia – while also being prevented from reaching it, from "realising" it. Capitalism "continually seeks to avoid reaching its limit while simultaneously tending toward that limit" (ibid., p. 34).

We can thus see the principal thesis taking shape: capitalism, through its deterritorialisation, and by substituting money for codes, approaches schizophrenia asymptotically. It does not cease not to want to reach this limit. To prevent itself from doing so, it relies on the principle that contradicts schizophrenia: the Oedipus complex. Thus, the Oedipus complex is the means by which capitalism uses and literally perverts psychoanalysis. Castration – the theory that desire is caused by a lack – is the correlate of the Oedipus complex, and together they are able to constitute capitalism as a whole [*ensemble*], thereby strengthening its claim to universality, to the detriment of its dissociative, rhizomatic, affective action.

***

By promoting familialism, psychoanalysis places itself in the service of this project. The Oedipus complex serves to suppress [*réprimer*] desiring production; this socially manifest suppression conditions repression [*refoulement*] within the psyche. In the form of myth, the Oedipus complex reintroduces the meaning that is missing from capitalism. Even more importantly, this complex completes itself by bringing in the castration complex and a theory of the fantasy, thereby providing capitalism with what could be called a "therapeutic machine", one that validates and authorises the functioning that the authors have attacked. By the end of the book, nothing in Freud has been spared, and if Lacan emerges nearly unscathed from this beating, it is at the price of being emancipated, even against his will, from Freud's tutelage. It goes without saying that Reich remains in a state of grace. A question, however, arises: what is the nature of Deleuze and Guattari's critique of the familialism that they impute to Freud?

Their first reproach is that Freud constituted a general theory on the basis of what, at the beginning, was only one contingent connection among others, thereby transforming the Oedipus complex into a form of explanatory imperialism. They seek to demonstrate this forcing, for example, in their analysis of Freud's article "A Child is Being Beaten" (1919), dissecting the three moments of the fantasy for the girl.

They note cheerily that the father does not yet appear in the first phase and is no longer there in the third; his presence is only unequivocal in the second phase, about which, as Freud (1919, p. 185) notes explicitly, ". . . we may say of it in a certain sense that it has never had a real existence". Their criticism, however, seems more rhetorical than substantial; this is not because they question Freud's clinical observations and his reading, which are fragments drawn from analytic experience, and which are therefore difficult to cast doubt upon. It seems rhetorical, instead, because they are never interested in what Freud's actual thesis is; this is what they would need to criticise in order to damage his credibility. Freud emphasises that the source of fantasy's persistence and opacity is the subject's inability to *represent* the agent of castration, the real father. This then conditions the aporia involved in the subject's acceptance of castration, whether this subject is a girl or a boy: how can s/he accept what, structurally, corresponds to a necessary hole in what can be represented? Deleuze and Guattari are correct in attacking the ideologies of representation, but by imputing them to Freud, they accept the readings of the psychoanalysts of the IPA, readings that Lacan rejected. (It can be noted in passing that they are embracing, quite indulgently, the work of André Green.)[13] Likewise, they read the phallus in terms of representation, and this is why they reject this concept. They make it the representative representation, whereas, even already in Freud, it is the non-representative term par excellence. It is the condition of all representation, which is precisely what enables us to question the status of representation.

Their next, parallel step is no more convincing than this claim that Freud's treatment of fantasy is marked by Oedipal imperialism: they valorise the group-fantasy to the detriment of the "individual" fantasy. "The revolutionary pole of group fantasy" is extolled as being antagonistic to the "enormous inertia which the law communicates to institutions in an established order" (Deleuze & Guattari, 1972, pp. 62, 63). It is difficult to respect this slogan when we remember how much the inertia of groups – whatever their explicit political content may be – feeds the lies of institutions. Institutions impose their primacy upon the truth of the subject; more precisely, they pervert the subject's truth by accommodating it to their own worst tendencies. The fact that these words were written shortly after 1968 explains the authors' confidence in group fantasy.

Nevertheless, once my mood of initial rejection passed, I understood the importance of the central question that they are raising: are there individual fantasies or are there only group fantasies? For Deleuze and Guattari, these fantasies arise from two categories of groups: groups that are subjects and groups that have been subjected. The difference lies in whether or not they have been subjected to the imaginary structure of the Oedipus complex and castration. It can certainly be accepted, or at least not dismissed a priori, that an analysand's fantasies are actually group fantasies. Why not? Yet what is decisive in an analysis lies in the singularity of each subject's detachment of itself from the fantasy. The prototype of fantasy is the one in which the Other wants the subject to be castrated; the subject must find its own singular way of detaching itself from this fantasy. This detachment is a process that cannot be represented or take the form of an idea; to quote Freud's (1919, p. 185) exact words again, the second phase, which makes the fantasy hold together, "has never succeeded in becoming conscious".

As soon as we realise that castration is missing in what is called psychosis, the imperialism imputed to the Oedipus complex may well turn out to be fragile. We must remember that castration is the symbolic lack of an imaginary object (see Lacan, 1994, pp. 215–219) and consists in the fact that an empty place is left in the Other by the removal of an object; this empty place is filled by an image with which the subject identifies. If castration is to take place, this image must be negativised. In this configuration, the Other is neither the mother nor the father, who are only its supports. Instead, it is the "treasure trove of signifiers" (Lacan, 1960, p. 682): the mother tongue, inasmuch as it has not yet been constituted as a code. Nothing forces this negativisation to take place, but the consequences of its failure may be as intransigent as those of its "success".

Should castration then be thought of as a "whole" [*le tout*]? For psychoanalysis, the answer is that it absolutely must not be. At the very moment when Deleuze and Guattari were attacking castration, Lacan was showing that it cannot resolve all of what they call the game of the flux and the schiz, a game that, for him, is jouissance. Lacan does so by going beyond, rather than stopping short of castration. The absence of the category of jouissance from these books, moreover, is significant. Deleuze and Guattari are trying to construct a theory on the basis of real questions; however, if this category, along with the task of taking language into account, were to intrude into their theory, then it would be undone from within.

If the phallus is not all [*tout*], it is because structure is actually commanded by something else – by the symptom. The received and systematic opposition between the "schizophrenic" processes and the "Oedipal" matrix may not really be debatable, but the authors can be reproached for proceeding by means of an exclusive (rather than an inclusive) disjunction, a disjunction that they then attack for being part of the Oedipal regime. The Oedipus complex can certainly be considered, in terms of set theory, as an operation of mapping that "consists in establishing a constellation of one-to-one correspondences between the agents of social production, reproduction, and antiproduction, on the one hand, and the agents of the so-called natural reproduction of the family on the other" (Deleuze & Guattari, 1972, pp. 100–101, translation modified). Yet this idea that the father, the mother, the phallus and I are all mappings controlled by socio-economic formations, which then provide a false support for psychoanalysis, misses out on something important: this "mapping" can only be made because it corresponds to a logic whose foundation is located elsewhere than in it.

This foundation lies in each subject's relation to the "Other", a term that must be understood in its full ambiguity, as both the place of the signifier and the living support of this place. This relation includes a subversive set theory and topology; these are the respective fields, for example, of neurosis, perversion, psychosis. Bringing to light the logic of set theory – with its practice of establishing one-to-one correspondences – is not the result of a flaw in psychoanalysis. The flaw would not lie in a blindness to topology, but in the converse: in giving a preference to this topology without seeing the necessity of set theory. This would involve following an ideological choice that is as questionable as the familialist ideology that they impute to Freud.

⁂

I have presented Deleuze and Guattari's critique of Freud from the perspective provided by the forty years that have elapsed since the book appeared, and by highlighting its – possibly antagonistic – tension with Lacan. For these two authors, however, this critique constitutes the basis of schizoanalysis, which they present as a practical alternative to psychoanalysis, without defining it clearly. This form of analysis can be summarised in four theses:

1 "Every investment is social, and in any case, bears upon a sociohistorical field" (ibid., p. 343).[14]
2 "Within the social investments we will distinguish the unconscious libidinal investment of group or desire, and the preconscious investment of class or interest" (ibid., p. 343).
3 "Schizoanalysis posits the primacy of the libidinal investments of the social field over the familial investment" (ibid., p. 335).
4 The "final thesis ... is ... the distinction between the two poles of social libidinal investment: the paranoiac, reactionary and fascisizing pole, and the schizoid revolutionary pole" (ibid., p. 366).

These four theses are backed up by arguments, but the form in which they are stated suggests that schizoanalysis does not propose a new form of practice; instead, it concerns what could be called the "reading" – and not an interpretation – of this practice. The only modification that touches practice is the indication that transference should be "schizoprenized", rather than perverted (which is what Freudian psychoanalysis supposedly does) (ibid., p. 339). This modification follows from applying these four theses when responding to patients and is, moreover, not uninteresting. Lacan himself, after all, wonders about the limit of a "permitted" perversion in the transferential relation. Unlike Deleuze and Guattari, he does not consider that it is possible to eliminate this "turn toward the father" – *père-version* – from the beginning, since it is constitutive of transference. This "perversion" of transference can only be resolved by resolving this transference (which is the terminable analysis). We can see the practical gulf between these two positions. We have reason to wonder what the actual consequences of schizoanalysis would be, for it would impose its schizoid reading without taking into account the perverse dimension that conditions the very possibility of the message.

Hunting down the jouissance turned towards the father is hardly better than channelling this jouissance towards him. They are both ways of thumbing one's nose not only at the message of the symptom but also at the character of perversion. Perversion is a transgression that the father is required to bless; it transforms the structural lack of adequation in the relation between the subject and the Other into a symptom. Perversion only stops – as perversion, but not as symptom – when transgression is revealed as what posits the enactment of the law, if the subject takes such a transformation upon himself, without leaving this task to the father.

The four theses of schizoanalysis are disappointing because it is not clear how they are relevant: they do not mark out a clear border between the positions of psychoanalysis and schizoanalysis, except in the field of ideology. If we assume that the latter will have an effect on practice, it will be at a level – see the second thesis – that is not preconscious, but unconscious. The only relevant thesis would be the final one, through its very exaggeration: as a paranoiac, Artaud was a fascist, like Rousseau, Reich, Dali and so many others. Here, paradoxically, I agree with Deleuze and Guattari, in the sense that this "exaggeration" highlights the status of the symptom: it is the subject's life-and-death struggle against the form that subjects it. Thus, in my opinion, "schizophrenising" psychoanalysis means apprehending the symptom as what marks the nonexistence of the sexual relation (and thus not the nonexistence of the One, but the nonexistence of the whole). A paranoiac analysis, on the other hand, would suppress the symptom in order to force the sexual relation into existence. The difficulty with this formulation is that, whether one is paranoiac or not, nothing can abolish the symptom and make the sexual relation exist. This is the formula for atheism, or a reversal of Pascal's wager. If the God who would be able to understand us does not exist, then we should stop doing anything and everything at all – which is not the same as washing our hands of it all.

In fact, the key point of my own critique of Deleuze and Guattari is that, without their awareness, they fall short of explaining "structure", as Lacan, in his reading of Freud, understood this term. This weakness may well result from an ideological prejudice, which prevented them from understanding the full significance of the innovative intuitions that nevertheless fascinated them. For example, they constantly confuse desire and drive: they act as if Lacan had never differentiated them and shown how they create the division of the subject.

In "On Freud's 'Trieb' and the Psychoanalyst's Desire", Lacan (1964, p. 724) states:

> desire comes from the Other, and jouissance is located on the side of the Thing. Freud's second topography [the one that introduces the death drive, which Deleuze and Guattari reject] concerns the pluralizing quartering of the subject that results therefrom – yet another opportunity not to see what should strike us, which is that identifications are determined by desire there without satisfying the drive. That occurs because the drive divides the subject and desire.

Without wanting to start, or restart, the nonetheless necessary debate on the scientific status of psychoanalysis, let us note that Lacan's statement is a theorem that may well be as decisive as Galileo's law of falling bodies; treating it as an opinion, and even despising it as an opinion, can only result in the impasse that has been observed in schizoanalysis. In defence of schizoanalysis, it can be added that it has, at least, not become involved in the return to suggestion.

Freud does not place the father as an entity on one side and society on the other. If the traces of the father and the mother are not just flights of fancy, it is because they are the first social agents with which the *infans* deals. This *infans* should be understood as a sort of *homo non-psychologicus*; it wagers its life in the entry into language. Who would deny that the father and mother are products of society? Yet who would also deny that, because of the symptom, the mother and father are not merely social products, passive agents of a machine that works like clockwork? If desire then comes from the Other – from language as borne by someone who exists or has existed (this transcends the opposition between the living and the dead) – how do identifications, which try to ensure the hold of an intrinsically inaccessible Other, serve as suitable means of satisfying the drive that emerges, as irreducible, from language's failure [*échec*] not to miss [*rater*] representing the subject? This gap between identification and drive is manifested, on the side of the Other, by the confirmation that it cannot be absorbed; it remains irreducibly Other. On the subject's side, it is manifested by the symptom.

The same impasse can be envisioned in other ways; in analytic experience, what takes precedence is not the signified but the subject's relation to the bar that, in the algorithm for language, separates the signified from the signifier (Lacan reversed Saussure's treatment of the relation between the two). The father cannot be reduced to a signified, which would then have to be reduced to another signified, such as "desiring-machines" (Deleuze & Guattari, 1972, p. 297). Instead, the father is the index of the relation to this bar. In every case, this bar is structurally impossible to efface. It can, however, be written in two ways: as phallus, Φ, in cases in which the signified with which the subject identifies has been negativised, or as more or less discrete elementary phenomena – which can be highly variable and can go from hallucination to hypochondria – when this negativisation has not taken place.

⁂

The schizophrenic says, "The game has no rules": there is no semblance. The psychoanalyst must admit that this is right, yet must also say that the rule of the game is life itself, thus letting the schizophrenic know that s/he is rejecting this rule. Perhaps undertaking a reading of this book could turn a criticism of it into the same kind of dialogue. If we pair Deleuze and Guattari's arguments with Lacan's own contemporaneous teaching, the result could be a very severe judgement on them, and even a condemnation. Yet this condemnation is always a misdeal. Let us say instead that these talented "craftsmen" of language seem to have begun to dislike their tool; they seem superstitiously to attribute to it the malevolent power to use them, to "engineer them", in order to make them the henchmen of the despotism of the One.

Lacan claimed that "there is such a thing as One (*Y a d' l'Un*)" (see Lacan, 1975c, p. 5, note 19). There is no use in denying it, but it is necessary to sever the unity of this One. In relay racing, if athletes stop being united, this leads to defeat. In psychoanalysis, the situation is the opposite: not undoing this unity can also lead to defeat. This defeat, however, can be hidden by rhetoric, and there is, in this respect, a confusion concerning the status of the One. If the One is the interchangeable element, the *unit*, which would be the only basis for constructing a numerical order, Deleuze and Guattari's criticism would score a hit; they are correct in rejecting the identity of this One with itself and preferring a heterogeneous multiplicity. Yet Lacan's formulations about the One were attempts to confront a different clinical problem. The "One" that is posited is the name by which zero can be symbolised. The negativisation of the phallus is homologous to this fundamental logical operation, and the multiple can only be theorised on the basis of this. Yet, on the other hand, there is such a thing as the One of unicity, in the sense that nothing is identical to anything else: singularity founds heterogeneity, which is different from multiplicity: the latter can always be reduced to the denumerable.[15]

It can now be seen that Deleuze and Guattari's criticism aims at Freud but hits Marx, not by calling his discovery of surplus-value into question, but by observing that although he may have been a great painter, he was not a musician (or vice versa). In other words, in order to demarcate the field in which he was working, Marx was obliged to use a "clipping path", to borrow a term from photo editing. This means, however, that everything outside the field so defined is free for others to exploit as they see fit, as it were.

Let's therefore switch perspectives, erase all the preceding criticism from the canvas and take a new look at what Deleuze and Guattari try to introduce, in an avant-garde way, into the "contemporary psychoanalysis" of the new millennium, that is, at the malicious click of the mouse that is supposed to throw its stiff and starchy outlines into disarray. What is quite surprising is that their selective, and not always very charitable approach to psychoanalysis often ends up formulating criticisms that are not only homogeneous to Lacan's thoroughgoing criticism of post-Freudianism, but also bring out questions with far-reaching consequences. There is an urgent need to examine these questions in order to regenerate "post-Lacanian" psychoanalysis, thereby reawakening it from its monsterless nightmares. For example, "Surplus value of code is the primitive form of surplus value" (Deleuze & Guattari, 1972, p. 150). This statement refers to the work of the anthropologist Edmund Leach and concerns the conversion of "perishable wealth" – consumable goods – "into imperishable prestige through the medium" of "counter-prestations" (in the case of marriages) or spectacular activities (Leach, 1961, p. 89; as cited in Deleuze & Guattari, 1972, p. 150). Perhaps they are also thinking of Marcel Mauss' study of the potlatch and even of Georges Bataille's discussion of the economy of expense. Thus, Deleuze and Guattari meet up again with Lacan's thesis that surplus-jouissance precedes surplus-value.[16] The conversion they mention produces a jouissance-benefit – in this particular case, prestige. In this sense, this "surplus-value of code" is to be distinguished from Marx's surplus-value; the latter concerns the gap between exchange-values and does not consider entities, such as prestige, that cannot be integrated into the money-commodity-more money (M-C-M′) cycle. It thus becomes homologous to Lacan's surplus-jouissance. Just as *Marxlust* (see Lacan, 1970, p. 434) precedes the discovery of *Mehrwert*, so also capitalists, functioning in the place of surplus-jouissance, are never tempted to interrupt the cycle of M-C-M′ by going on strike themselves. They are never tempted to do so unless they have a political interest in this, one in which the M′ – the money increased by this cycle – would be threatened.

⁂

Deleuze and Guattari's reversal of the Oedipus complex and promotion of schizophrenia involves a caustic criticism of psychoanalysis. Despite the misunderstandings that I have brought out, their criticisms contain something that is quite accurate: their lauded multiplicity may well be the figure by which they seek to put an end to the One of unity, which continues to haunt psychoanalysts, despite their disavowals. This One of unity has appeared in many forms: from the one among others, which aims at a universalising (and Christian) homeostasis of narcissism (see Vasse, 1978), to the definition of the symptom as masking the nonexistence of the sexual relation (see Soler, 2002),[17] not to mention the paradoxical act of making the not-all [*pas-tout*] uniform. In all of these cases, contemporary psychoanalytic *doxas* seem to league together in a way that would retroactively show the truth of what these fierce critics of psychoanalysis say. All of these *doxas* militate in favour of a group-psychology that would take as its model the army, the church, the party or a business. People who promote them tolerate any criticism that does not draw conclusions from what it says; they channel the transference by means of "tour guides", whose job is to enable amused analysands to discover the great priests and priestesses of psychoanalysis.

An ambiguity, however, still remains. Inveighing against neurotics is a practice that can be found whenever the analytic discourse deviates into the discourse of the master. This can seem to contradict the observation that psychoanalysis has distanced itself from psychosis, which has been colonised by psychiatry. In reality, what is unbearable is to accept that the other gets off, because the imputation that this other is the Other still remains. It is the jouissance of the Other that is intolerable, because this Other wants me to be castrated. Analytic experience, however, shows that there is no jouissance of the Other, J(A̸), and if the other, with a small "o", gets off, this jouissance does not threaten me. Even if the fear that the Other wants to castrate me is unfounded, perhaps it still has to be eradicated as it testifies to a refusal of castration. The answer is that it should not at all be eradicated: if castration were to come from the Other, it would prohibit all jouissance, making me melancholic. This would not be the sort of castration that would be the condition for a different jouissance, a jouissance that would not be the pure and simple annihilation implied in the death drive. Far from being "ridiculous", the death drive is what enables us to explain how desire is what deactivates this drive by escaping from its legislation, through the symptom. The lack within desire is thus not a return to religion, but what is necessary to counter annihilation.

This leads us back to the question of the status of multiplicity, which turns out to have the same status in the deviations of post-Lacanian psychoanalysis that it has in schizoanalysis. The post-Lacanians evade multiplicity by seeking to obtain "ones" that can be fitted into a set, thus disguising the group's imaginary qualities as an institution. Schizoanalysis misses multiplicity in a different way: it hides the idea that the condition for a truly heterogeneous multiplicity is the fulfilment of each person's unicity. This is achieved – without taking this as a stopping point – through a transitory acceptance of the unity of one's symptomatic being. This being is equivalent to a division from one's being as a subject.

The last Hegelian

I

Slavoj Žižek can certainly not be reproached with what Deleuze and Guattari are guilty of: a deliberate misunderstanding of the message of psychoanalysis. In the introduction to *Subversions du sujet*, the French translation of his book *Tarrying with the Negative: Kant, Hegel and the Critique of Ideology*, he locates himself within it impeccably, arguing that psychoanalysis is a quest for the unconscious that unveils something other than the true personality: it reveals a "primal lie" located in each person's fantasy, "through which we try to veil the inconsistency of the symbolic order that we inhabit" (Žižek, 1993a, p. 13). Thus, he locates himself as anti-anti-Oedipus. Schizoanalysis tends to found itself on a truth that is to be discovered by schizophrenising the unconscious; it attempts to escape from the philosophical tradition of "critique", as inaugurated by Kant, and we need to pay close attention to the implications of this attempt.

Žižek, however, is not a Kantian. If he could be reduced to an epithet, it would be a "wild" Hegelian, or even a "wild and crazy" Hegelian. This does not mean that there is a flaw in the rationality and rigour of his understanding of Hegel. Instead, it is a way of paying homage to his ability to breathe life back into the primal pulsation of Hegel's questioning, which has been debased by the university's restoration projects. He starts with the question of the subject, giving Descartes, by his invention of the cogito, the credit for preparing the way for Kant's critical revolution. The first section of his book is significantly entitled, "The Void Named Subject". I have implicitly treated the problematisation of the void as inherent in the action of language: words produce the emptiness of the thing. Deleuze and Guattari positively mistrust the void, which is connected to the critical tradition. This tradition does not set up an ontological opposition between the void and fullness; instead, it examines the naming of the void, without always seeing this void as a consequence of language.

It is thus that Kant promotes the transcendental subject, the subject required as a thinking unit (and unity) that conditions the synthesis of empirical representations (although given in a priori forms) and nonempirical representations (see Kant, 1781, pp. 246–248). The unity of "I think" guarantees the object as object. As Žižek remarks very appropriately, this transcendental subject cannot reflect on itself, an impossibility that founds the distinction between phenomenon and noumenon: "*if I were given to myself phenomenally, as an object of experience, I would simultaneously have to be given to myself noumenally*" (Žižek, 1993b, p. 16).

In order to go beyond what seems to be critical philosophy's intangible point of equilibrium, Žižek's stratagem is to read Hegel as completing Kant, which first implies that the subject is "absolute negativity": it is, as negativity, the mark that the thing is not absorbed into the object (ibid., p. 23). There is thus always a remainder that the dialectic of subjective negativisation cannot eliminate; Žižek makes this remainder homologous to Lacan's object *a*. The second implication is that the subject "is the purely formal void which is left over after the substantial content has wholly 'passed over' into its predicates-determinations. . . [the] 'subject' is that very X, the empty form of a 'container' which remains after all its content was 'subjectivized'" (ibid., p. 21).

What is important in this context is not to judge the cogency of Žižek's reading of Hegel, and still less to criticise it because it contradicts Lacan's explicit statements. In a response to Jacques-Alain Miller in *The Four Fundamental Concepts of Psycho-Analysis*, Lacan (1973d, p. 215) confirmed unambiguously that he was "against Hegel". What does need to be considered is Žižek's theory of the subject: this theory is presented as deriving from Hegel, but it then becomes the paradigm of the theory of the subject as forged by psychoanalysis – by both Freud and Lacan – on the basis of analytic experience. Such experience would thereby realize *The Phenomenology of Spirit* in concrete form. Thus, to take up Žižek's major developments, self-consciousness "has to internalize this force of negativity and recognize in it its own essence, the very kernel of its own being" (Žižek, 1993b, p. 23).

Žižek thus starts with Hegel: negation "is the *universal will* which in its ultimate abstraction has nothing positive and therefore can give nothing in return for the sacrifice" (Hegel, 1807, p. 362; as cited in Žižek, ibid., p. 24). This is a crucial statement, for it indicates that there is some limit, some discretion, in the on-going dialectic: the point at which nothing can be given "in return for the sacrifice". He also asks, "what is 'subject' if not the infinite power of absolute negativity/mediation"? (Žižek, ibid., p. 23). This "that's not it" is very much that of Žižek's subject who knows – without always drawing conclusions from this knowledge – that s/he cannot be satisfied when the demand is satisfied; s/he cannot be satisfied with an Other who would believe that it could be completed by the subject's offer. It is a sort of seesaw that indicates the moment when a mental propaedeutics passes over into the experience of transference.[18] This seesaw is also a catapult, for it enables the question of the void to be displaced from the subject onto the Other; an imaginary askesis becomes a real separation. This is what Freud incontestably locates first in what he calls "maternal castration", where the subject is subtracted from being the Other's imaginary complement.

Of course, in taking this path, Žižek comes up against an obstacle: his own remainder, Marx. It is, however, with a certain joy that he sees Marx's true face: Marx's critique of Hegel's absolute idealism is his own self-criticism. For Hegel, the reconciliation is not the moment when "substance becomes subject"; this is Marx's illusion concerning what could be called the "dis-alienation" of the proletariat. "The dimension of subjectivity is inscribed into the very core of substance in the guise of an irreducible lack, which forever prevents it from achieving full self-identity" (ibid., p. 26). Ultimately, Žižek's reading of Hegel is congruent with Engels' (1886, p. 360) remark that in Hegel's philosophy, the system is conservative while the dialectic is revolutionary.

How do these formulations affect the status of the subject in psychoanalysis? What are the characteristics of this "subjective dimension", which is now the dimension of an irremediable lack? The conception of the subject as a lack, or rather – and this is not equivalent – as a void is very interesting. It is the kernel of the hysterical fantasy, which can be taken as the universal matrix of "subjectivity"; the very use of this latter word instead of "subject" is already significant. The hysteric fears the equivalence between the subject and "nothing", and in analytic experience, s/he resists the idea that the denouement of an analysis will confirm this presupposition; "I am nothing" would mean that in the place where s/he is seeking the truth of her/his being, there is only a void. However, this fantasy is congruent with a defence that enables her/him to avoid being an object on which the other gets off; if s/he is nothing, then s/he annuls any risk of this kind. In this context, we can recall Deleuze and Guattari's refusal to generate desire on the basis of lack. The religion of desire, which has often and correctly been attacked, may have more than one card up its sleeve, but it has only one card to play: hypostasising desire leads us to miss the drive, which is the other side of the same card. Desire is a lure, for behind the veil of Maya, there is nothing.

To return to Hegel, his conception of the subject as a pure negativity can only be evaluated if one remembers that it implies a subject as a dialectical process. The subject is thus, properly speaking, neither the nothing that would give consistency to the hysteric's fantasy, nor, in the field of Buddhist nirvana, the acceptance of nihilation [*néantisation*]. Žižek (1993b, p. 25) takes up the analysis of the subject's "internalization" of "revolutionary Terror", which concludes with a subject who is radically and "eternally split", since this internalisation can be read as the superego. Thus we return to the Kantian subject, which has now been raised to the level of the noumenon; Hegel's dialectisation of Kant then authorises the critical distance between Kant's two terms, "phenomenon" and "noumenon" to be reconceived as the real of the movement of reason (see Hegel, 1832). The other consequence is to give a new interpretation to the "negation of negation" (Žižek, 1993b, p. 25). This is not the always-renewed compensation for an always-repeated loss; it means, instead, that "what first appears as an external obstacle reveals itself to be an inherent hindrance, i.e., an outside force turns into an inner compulsion" (ibid., p. 25).

Two different judgements are possible here. On the one hand, Marx can be transformed into an authentic Hegelian idealist: he would thus embody a misunderstanding (in the sense of "it takes one to know one"), which is not without interest. By making the proletariat a "substanceless subjectivity" (ibid., p. 27), Marx is implicitly proposing a movement from prehistory to history, one that defines history in terms of the advent of a subjective substance, the new humanity. It could be objected that, through this *parousia*, the proletariat loses its symptom. To paraphrase Henri Michaux, "he who loses his madman loses his voice".[19] This would be an interpretation of Marx's impasse: he rejected the symptom, even if, according to Lacan's words of tribute, he also invented it.

On the other hand, the Hegelian subject, as Žižek rethinks it, bears a strange resemblance to "[t]he spirit which eternally denies", immortalised by Goethe (1808, p. 37) in the figure of Mephistopheles. More disquietingly, it even tends asymptotically towards Winston Smith, the main character in George Orwell's *1984*: this subject can only escape from guilt, which is maintained by the superego, by loving and submitting to the torturer. This is certainly not what Žižek says, but the way in which Hegel, the "most sublime hysteric", toadied to the autocratic Prussian state does not contradict this reference. Žižek's article "*Hegel avec Lacan*" also ends up touching on this same sort of allusion. By writing that "the subject, by definition, cannot master the effects of its discourse, since it is the Other who has this task" (Žižek, 1995, p. 108), he defines the subject as being trapped irremediably in the snares of religious discourse, a discourse in which the Other is indeed in control of this effect. Freud, in his article on Dostoevsky, had already criticised this figure of repentance.

This power accorded to the Other is confirmed again even more clearly if, returning this time to psychoanalysis, we pay attention to what Žižek says in a long parenthesis:

> And what is at stake in *la passe*, the concluding moment of the psychoanalytical process, is precisely the analysand's readiness to fully assume this radical self-externalization, i.e., "subjective destitution": *I am only what I am for the others*, which is why I have to renounce the fantasy-support of my being, my clinging to "my own private Idaho", to some hidden treasure in me, inaccessible to others'.
>
> *(1993b, p. 31, emphasis added)*

This definition of the subject reduces it to a sort of "mass-media" treatment of it, thereby producing what may be a radical and salutary rupture with any romantic emphasis on its ineffable qualities. Yet this definition also proposes that at the "end" of analysis – the equation of the pass and the end is already questionable – the "self" is externalised without any remainder; this externalisation promotes, in a way that affects his earlier argument, the figure of the analysed subject as a "surface" being, in terms of preprojective geometry, which cannot be topologised. Žižek is probably silently repeating a thesis by Jacques-Alain Miller, but as a result, like the latter, he misses what is essential.

The essential point is that subjective destitution removes a reflexive knowledge from the subject of the fantasy: a Schillerian knowledge in which the eye would see itself, the mouth would kiss itself, etc. This destitution also shows, at the level of the remainder that cannot be eliminated, that only the symptom knows; the pass must be judged from the standpoint of a mutation in the subject's relation to the symptom. This "inner garden" does not have to disappear. If we conceive of it in terms of the Hegelian dialectic – one that would *concern the symptom rather than the subject* – we could say that this garden becomes public, without ceasing to be a garden. Freud protects us from a conception of an analysed subject whose only narcissism would depend on the narcissism of others – unless we imagine, as "Catharists", a world that would be entirely free from narcissism, except from that of God. If we define the pass in this way, it would end up dissuading any candidate who is seeking anything other than an institutional promotion.

We can now understand how it is the symptom and not the subject that "emerges as the crack in the universal Substance" (ibid., p. 33). It may well be seductive to define the subject as the zero that commands the infinite series of ordinal numbers. God – why not believe this? – could well have created me as the zero that would serve as the basis of number. Indeed, Žižek himself deviates, without saying so, from this initial conception of the subject as void when he perspicaciously mentions the myth of a creation by a father who has passed from the status of the empty master signifier (S_1) to that of knowledge (S_2). When, as Žižek says, a father identifies with knowledge, he creates a monster: whether Frankenstein's monster or Roy Batty, the character played by Rutger Hauer in *Blade Runner*. Yet the father's movement – or rather, straddling of the position between S_1 and S_2 is the rule. This is why every human creature is a monster: a being that, by its symptom, sets itself up as a rebel against its creator, thus depriving the creator of his omnipotence and marking him as contingent.

The crucial step, however, has not yet been taken, since Žižek continues to think that this objection to the creator can only come from a monster; he therefore unveils what constitutes the "fundamental fantasy" of his critique, painting a portrait of the analyst as a cannibal. He writes about Hannibal Lecter, from Thomas Harris' novels:

> [Y]et even the utmost effort to imagine Lecter's cruelty fails to capture the true dimension of the act of the analyst: by bringing about *la traversée du fantasme* (the crossing of our fundamental fantasy), he literally "steals the kernel of our being," the *object small a*, the secret treasure, *agalma*, what we consider most precious in ourselves, denouncing it as a mere semblance. Lacan defines the *object small a* as the fantasmatic "stuff of the I," as that which confers on the $\$$, on the fissure in the symbolic order, on the ontological void that we call "subject," the ontological consistency of a "person," the semblance of a fullness of being – and it is precisely this "stuff" that the analyst pulverizes, "swallows".
>
> *(ibid., p. 48)*

This quotation may well be the one that makes Žižek's position most explicit. First, the subject is a void. Second, the object *a* is the stuff that gives the subject its status as an appearance of being. Third, this stuff can be devoured and destroyed. An allusion to the Eucharist follows, revealing the character of this ingestion. If the analyst is the one who devours, the analysand is the host, and thus the body of Christ, the substantiality of God. By devouring this, the analyst is identifying with the analysand. Fourth, the subject is annihilated.

Perhaps fortunately, this terrifying odyssey is based on a misinterpretation of subjective destitution. This destitution is *not* the subject's negativisation or its "realisation", as it were, of the Buddhist ideal of the void; it is also not, as has been noted, the hysterical fantasy. Instead, it is the destitution of the *subject-supposed-to-know*. This means that the analysed subject does not consent to submit to the Other; instead, by encountering the inconsistency of this Other – there is no Other of the Other – s/he discovers that there is an antinomy between the subject and knowledge. The name of this antinomy is the unconscious. Such a conclusion is not easy to theorise in Hegelian terms. The assertion that only the symptom knows is already apparent in Freud's conception of the symptom. The signifiers that are encrypted within it exist, concealed within this symptom. Freud's conception, however, lends itself to a misunderstanding: because the symptom has to be deciphered in order to be resolved, the idea that knowledge can thus be transferred to the subject seems self-evident. This idea is false, but opponents of psychoanalysis have not failed to use it against Freud by remarking that deciphering the symptom, and thus knowing what it means, does not make it disappear – which, indeed, is a proven fact.

What, then, does it mean to say that *the symptom knows*? Before discussing the answer, we need to examine the key that can unlock this question for us: the subject can only participate in this knowledge through identification. Such an identification with the symptom would be impossible as long as the subject attributes an unlimited knowledge to the Other of the Other: the figure who would say the true about the true, and who would be Hegel's absolute knowledge, which has no limit. Even if a materialist were to think that it would take the infinity of time to travel across such knowledge, this would still be a way of lending credence to the Other of the Other, whose final secret figure is nothing other than the subject itself (*agalma*). In such a situation, identifying with the symptom would be impossible, because identification would be directed entirely towards the Other of the Other, who would be considered to exist as subject. In this respect, the analysand would correspond strictly to Hegel, who closed his immense philosophy at the point just before the breakthrough of the pass.

In order for the removal of this misunderstanding not to give rise immediately to another, it needs to be made clear that only in the authentic misunderstanding that is involved in transference – which is the basis of all human experience – can we speak of an identification with the Other who would know itself. It should be noted that even if identification is conceived of in this way, it does not really occur in this way, since it takes place in relation to the real Other, the Other of a radical alterity, an Other that is not transparent to itself and is not reflexive. This alterity cannot be reduced to the One. In fact, it is when there is an identification with the symptom that identification can be thought of as making the real of alterity even more real (if this kind of comparative is meaningful here), especially since this alterity is dealt with, as symptom, by the subject him/herself. The subject thus acquires a relation to her/his own symptom that is absolutely homogeneous to the one that s/he could have to any other symptom – if s/he does not decide to desert, because there is no set pathway – her/his progression towards a saintliness that could be called secular.

In the identification with the symptom, it is therefore not the mechanism of identification that changes; instead, this identification is no longer controlled by the misunderstanding inherent in transference. In other words, transference is "resolved" [*résolu*], rather than "dissolved" [*dissous*], with the semantic dimension that could well get the upper hand [*prendre le dessus*]: I resolve even to love, or even to hate, if my cruelty is not sufficiently audacious for me to hold on to love.

***

This disagreement affects Žižek's way of reading Lacan's opposition between full and empty speech. This opposition is governed by the conception of the object *a*, if we take the word "conception" in the sense of procreation. In a discussion of the game of *Fort-Da*, which Freud (1920, pp. 14–16) recounts in *Beyond the Pleasure Principle*, Žižek, quite correctly, rejects the idea that the child engenders this object when he substitutes the bobbin for the mother; instead, Žižek (1993b, p. 91) makes it the "sacrificed part of the subject itself". He also argues that "*the object which compensates for the loss of the Mother-Thing is part of myself*" (ibid., p. 92). Here, once again, the fate of the subject is to be sacrificed primally by the loss of the thing and reduced to the void. Logically, this subject-void is the proof that the initial sacrifice was absolute, rather than partial. This thesis itself is enough to show the palpable distance between Žižek and Lacan. In Lacan, the subject exists only on the basis of its constitutive division. Although the unbarred S can be found in Lacan, for example in "Kant with Sade" (1963), where it becomes the figure for the pathological subject – the raw, suffering S – this is not at all the subject before division. Instead, this subject has been reconstructed on the basis of the model of the pre-critical philosophical subject; its only vocation is to assure the other subject, which conceives it, of its unswerving fidelity.

Concerning full speech, at a first level, Žižek's perspective converges with what Lacan says. Thus, when Žižek refers to Hegel's reading of the sacrifice of Christ, whose death on the cross is transformed into a triumph, he explains that:

> complete ground is the unity of formal and real ground: it is the real ground whose grounding relationship to the remaining content is again grounded in what? – *in itself* i.e., *in the totality of its relations to the grounded*. The ground grounds the grounded, but this grounding role must be itself grounded in the relationship of the ground to the grounded.
>
> *(ibid., p. 139)*

This formulation corresponds incontestably to one of Lacan's (1956a, p. 319) definitions of full speech: "[f]ull speech is defined by the fact that it is identical to what it speaks about."

Such a *parousia* of full speech inevitably evokes the *fiat lux*, the speech that makes the real emerge. It raises problems for Žižek, for it devalorises empty speech, the other term of the alternative. Žižek does not depreciate empty speech, for it corresponds precisely to the subject as void! Instead, he sets out an astute interpretation, which should not be rejected entirely: "for Lacan the exemplary case of empty speech is the password (*mot-de-passage*)" (Žižek, 1993b, p. 94). This argument is interesting because it excludes the statement [*énoncé*] considered in terms of its signification; what counts is only whether what the passand says corresponds to what the passer is expecting. This assertion is very close to the definition of the subject as reduced to the Other's statements about it, thus becoming the emblem of mass-media exposure and virtualisation. "I say what you expect" completes "I am what you say"![20]

This is not, of course, what Žižek means. In a way that is just as ingenious, empty speech, which has been revalorised as the crossing of a boundary, transforms the subject into a sort of temporary subject of the enunciation, an absolute enunciation; for the statement, "the enunciated context is totally indifferent" (ibid., p. 94), since it only has to be the "right" password. This absolute enunciation is the "name". The name subtracts the enunciator not only from the Other, but also from him/herself as subject; therefore, it becomes the linguistic matrix of the symptom, the negative fingerprint (see, for example, the negative hand stencils in the caves of Gargas). Nevertheless, it must be admitted that this plenitude of the enunciation, brought about by hollowing out any statement, does indeed suppose a statement that corresponds to what is expected by the passer, who is thus posited to be the Other.

This is the contrary of everything that Lacan expected of the pass. Žižek's proposition is more a sleight of hand [*tour de passe-passe*] than a part of the pass. On the contrary, in the experience of the pass, the only password would be one in which the statement cannot be annulled and would have nothing to do with the statement expected by the Other. This is the opposite of the way that Žižek completes his conception of the pass: only "empty speech", through its very void – through its distance from its stated content, which is perfectly indifferent – opens up the path to "full speech", a speech in which the subject can articulate its position as subject of the enunciation. It is thus that "only the spear that smote you/can heal your wound" (ibid., p. 92). Only through a complete acceptance of the void of "empty speech" can you hope to articulate your truth in "full speech". Amen.

The hitch, first, is that "the spear that smote you" will wound you just as much if it smites you again. The second smiting will only cure you if a different spear is used; this means that saying [*le dire*] founds doing [*le fait*], which is indeed what occurs in analytic experience. Late in his teaching, Lacan also explicitly criticised the opposition between full and empty speech. First, the expression, "empty speech" is a perfect designation of the sort of statement that, as it unfolds, moves further and further away from the kernel of being that it is seeking to grasp; it is like an awkward speaker who, the more he tries to correct a blunder, the worse he makes it. This is very different from the kind of speech that would be "identical to what it speaks about" (Lacan, 1956a, p. 319), a definition that contradicts the principle that the saying [*dire*] is ex-centric in relation to what is said [*dit*]. Lacan (1956b, p. 249), indeed, does not fail to add – in order to take into account an objection that he is tacitly opposed to – that "true speech" must include "the subject's realization of his history in its relation to a future". It must posit, in terms of topology, a point at infinity in which what is external to the circle can be integrated into it.

Lacan (1976–1977, 15 March 1977) comes to reject, explicitly, the binary opposition between empty and full speech. He does so by interposing a third structure, which is homologous to analytic interpretation and to poetic saying [*dire*]. From then on, full speech pertains to meaning (and direction) [*sens*], and, more specifically, to the *double* meaning that emerges in the founding or creative speech where God is the other side [*verso*] of the father and vice versa. Such speech is of the order of desire. Empty speech itself pertains to signification, and more precisely to empty signification; as such, it only has love at its disposal to create a message. Žižek's reference to the password is relevant at this level, but only at this level. Without even emphasising the erotic value of the term, we can note that passwords are frequently used by lovers as a private language that will be forgotten if they cease to love one another. Thus, "coffee" can mean "let's make love" and "sugar" a particular position. They can exchange these words in the presence of a third party, and the frisson involved in having a secret will be heightened by not revealing this secret in public.

***

The severity and even the acerbity of my criticism are ways of paying homage to Žižek's quickness of thought, which should inspire psychoanalysts. At the very least, readers do not find in his work the sort of parroting that, by its irrefutably learned quality, becomes even more ruinous for psychoanalysis. Despite Freud and Lacan's enormous efforts, psychoanalysis has not been exempted from attempts to make it say the opposite of what it says, or to remain at a sort of low-water mark, one where theoretical and clinical confusion will be expressed and transmitted with an impeccable scholarship. In Lacan's topology, a piece of string can go over *or* under something. In psychoanalytic language, a cat can be both black and white; black can be white and the feline theorist will always be able to fall on his/her feet.

My disagreement with Žižek concerns: 1) his precipitateness in making the subject equivalent to the void;[21] 2) the absence of a theory of the symptom. In an attempt at a sort of mathematical exhaustion, it would be possible to follow out the consequences of this "deviation" (Žižek would appreciate the political savour of this word, which is borrowed not from Stalin, but from Lacan). For example, when Žižek explains Hegel's return to the thing itself by defining it as the inclusion of the name in the definition of the object, he makes a convincing use of the logical distinction between description and name. Lacan also availed himself of this distinction in positioning himself in relation to both Bertrand Russell (1905) and Saul Kripke (1980) in his re-evaluation of the status of the Name-of-the-Father. This would have given Žižek the chance to exit from Hegel's *tout*ology – a sort of tautology of the whole – by establishing a distinction between the Name-of-the-Father and the symptom. The Name-of-the-Father participates in the whole and serves as the guarantee by the Other of the capacity of language to signify. The status of the symptom is different: if we take the common complaint, "I'd be willing to give up everything, *but not that*!", then the symptom would consist in the words "but not that", which are separate from "everything" or the "whole". It calls into question the guarantee coming from the Other. Yet, rather than pointlessly multiplying examples concerning the consequences of Žižek's deviation, it would be better to locate its source: the theoretical point where this deviation occurred. It seems to me that, in this theoretical edifice, the key to the vault is the conception of contradiction, as Žižek describes it:

> The last phrase in the quoted passage from Hegel's *Logic*[22] locates the contradiction clearly *inside "father" himself*: "contradiction" designates the antagonistic relationship between what I am "for the others" – my symbolic determination –and what I am "in myself" abstractedly from my relations to

> others. It is the contradiction between the void of the subject's pure "being-for-himself" and the signifying feature which represents him for the others, in Lacanian terms: between $\$$ and S_1.
>
> *(Žižek, 1993b, p. 131)*

To posit a contradiction between one of these constitutive terms (S_1) and the subject-void is to pass over the other constitutive term of the contradiction (S_2). With a slight adjustment to Bertrand Russell's (1902) analysis, this can be stated in terms of the paradox of the set of all the sets that do not contain themselves: as soon as this set is posited, the question of whether it contains itself arises.[23] The implication of signifiers $S_1 \rightarrow S_2$ is contradiction itself; this means that S_1, which forces its membership upon the set of sets that do not contain themselves, should not belong to this set. It also means that the other signifier (S_2), which does not claim to belong to it, could therefore belong to it. The result is that S_1 is indeed the master signifier; it signifies nothing other than its unwarranted membership in the set [*ensemble*] of all the sets that do not contain themselves (E). S_2, by not belonging to this set, concretises its being in the body at the level of the cut within the drive: the removal from this set of an object that *cannot* be a signifier. Here is the kernel of the impossible – of the real. If we want to develop this dialectic, we must remember that an articulation between S_1 and S_2 can only be conceived of and then made actual if the S_2 is preceded in this articulation by the empty set, which is the empty part of the subject: $S_1 \rightarrow (\emptyset, S_2)$. In other words, the S_2 would be preceded by the set that marks its absence in E, the place where it *should* be because it *is* not there.

For readers who began to read this book out of an interest in its section on the capitalist discourse, these considerations may seem off topic. Such readers may even be starting to wonder whether they could sue the publisher for false advertising. I may be able to offer them some slight apology by noting that the preceding considerations could throw a new light on the critique of political economy. Let us take, for example, Žižek's remark about John Maynard Keynes, who posited an equivalence between money and credit to which some Marxists have objected. "What Marx as well as strict monetarists commonly hold against Keynes is the conviction that sometimes, sooner or later, the moment will arrive when we actually shall have to 'settle accounts,' reimburse debts and thus place the system on its proper 'natural' foundations" (Žižek, 1993b, p. 81). If it is true that money is the form of signifier taken by exchange-value, and that the latter has been produced materially, it is also true that, in its temporal functioning, credit can anticipate money. In a sense, money can anticipate itself, according to the structural scheme of symbolic debt, without which no exchange between humans would be either possible or conceivable.

Does this observation force us to believe in the permanence of money? This permanence is related to the predicament of the younger generation: its members can only apprehend themselves as a distinct generation by recognising their symbolic debt to the preceding generation. The classic instance of such a debt can be found in the case of the Rat Man (Freud, 1909). This debt can cease to be a handicapping burden, shot through with the superego, once it has been detached from a desire of the Other that had nothing to do with its birth; it can only cease to be a burden if its existence is recognised. In other words, the virtual can have a real effect:

> As we know from Keynes onwards, the capitalist economy is "virtual" in a very precise sense: Keynes's favorite maxim was that in the long term we are all dead; the paradox of the capitalist economics is that our borrowing from the (virtual) future, i.e., our printing of money uncovered in "real" values, can bring about real effects (growth).
>
> *(Žižek, 1993b, p. 79)*

I agree with Žižek's treatment of Keynes's criticism of Marx. The significance of this criticism is not only economic but philosophical, for it includes the subject's relation to the symbolic as a component of reality. Such reality is not the real, and the problem is to construct a reality that would not close itself off from the real; this becomes quite a challenge once the real has been defined as what is impossible to symbolise. This is the unprecedented problem of psychoanalysis, and it has specific solutions that I shall not try to summarise here, since, throughout this book, I have been seeking to take them into account. Yet, in order not to stray too far from the Keynes-Marx dispute, I shall conclude that Keynes's theory is only valid if Marx's own theory remains true at the level of abstraction where it is situated; the limits of the virtual are not intrinsic to the virtual, as we see when financial bubbles burst, but depend on the risk of a return in the real.

This dichotomy between the virtual and the real has an echo: the dichotomy between the symbolic and the real dimensions of the desire of the Other. Žižek, in relation to the struggle to the death between the master and the slave, remarks that once the death in question is considered to be symbolic. then "the mere *possibility* of victory" becomes "sufficient" (ibid., p. 160). Starting from this and referring to Bentham's (1843) panopticon, Žižek (1993b, p. 160) argues that, at the level of fantasy, anxiety is produced much less by the certainty than by the possibility of being seen, and the "radical uncertainty" that accompanies this. He (ibid., p. 160) concludes that "This surplus of what is 'in the possibility more than a mere possibility' [i.e. anxiety] and which gets lost in its actualisation is *the real qua impossible*". This reading of Lacan's famous equation of the real with the impossible then enables him to paint a delightful portrait, caustic yet fair, of the master. He (ibid., p. 160) argues that "the way for a Master to strengthen his authority is precisely to present himself as 'human like the rest of us', full of little weaknesses, a person with whom it is quite possible to 'talk normally' when he is not compelled to give voice to Authority". Žižek's aim in this passage is perfect.

One question, however, remains: what is the value of this reading of the real? It is impeccable and is especially relevant in relation to anxiety as the affect of the real. It can be added that, for Lacan, fantasy is indeed the entry into the real, whereas the symptom is the entry into truth. Yet with the seminar on Joyce, *The Sinthome* (Lacan, 2005b), there is a reversal that leads us to redefine fantasy as the entry into the false, and the symptom as the entry into the real. It would be even more precise to say that the *real is the entry into the symptom.*

Let us consider the castration complex, which when it is put to the test, makes the real – the real that is immediately impossible – emerge as what is in fact being interrogated. It is impossible for the *infans* to become One with the maternal Other, and this impossibility involves *both sides* of this relation: the *first* or the *subject's side* and the *other side*. In Anneliese Schnurmann's (1947) case history of Little Sandy, which Lacan (1994) discusses in the fourth year of his seminar, there is an almost furtive, but utterly decisive remark: Sandy wants to be able to choose to detach herself from her mother, but does not accept that her mother stop being at her beck and call, or even at her mercy. This asymmetry refutes the idea that there is some kind of primordial fusion or primary narcissism. In the couple formed with the mother, the *infans* requires the possibility of detaching itself from the Other. In other words, the impossibility of making One (see Lacan, 1975c, p. 5) is there right away, on the *first side* and is a condition of the possibility of the subject's willingness to make One.

If we follow Freud, the entry into the castration complex – which, for girls, occurs before the Oedipus complex starts, and for boys, follows it – involves calling the *other side* into question. The maternal Other – despite what the subject tyrannically demands [*revendique*] – is not just ready and waiting to make One with the subject, even when the subject has an imaginary identification with φ, which is the element that is supposed to restore to the maternal Other the missing part whose absence is preventing her from making One. The fact that this is only an identification already indicates sufficiently that the subject does not lend itself as such to this reduction – or induction – of the Other to the One. By only *identifying with an image*, the subject preserves its ability to detach itself, and thus indicates the contingent character of "making One". Either make One or live: this is the subject's symptomatic dilemma.

Then castration, which logically concerns the *other side*, continues its neurotic, psychotic or perverse course. Castration is also at work on the *subject's side*, and what it produces there may well be the outcome that Freud considered satisfactory: the acknowledgement of maternal castration takes precedence over its disavowal; Lacan rethought this process in terms of the negativisation of the phallus, -φ. This outcome can never, however, become the sole and unique law of jouissance, since it concerns only the *other side*; meanwhile, the *first side*, the side of the *subject*, has already catalysed jouissance around the symptom. Although the process of castration – in whichever form it occurs – will always re-order this jouissance retroactively, this symptomatic process will never stop being – in the words of James Joyce – a "work in progress". It will always mount a structural resistance to any attempt to measure it. Therein, perhaps, lies Freud's error about the "oceanic feeling" in his exchange with Romain Rolland; he simply skipped over the White Goddess and focused instead on the Sun God, Aten.[24]

Let's return now to Žižek and his definition of the real as an excess – an excess of anxiety when something that is possible has not taken place but *can* take place. This *excess* could be an equivalent of the *symptom*. Yet as I have already insisted, Žižek not only does not speak of the symptom as such but eliminates it. The place where it could emerge has been blocked by the conception of the subject as void and the correlative conception of the analyst as the devourer of the *agalma*. There is thus a recurring confusion between the response of the real and a response of the Other; this confusion occurs because the excision of the symptom has removed the very backbone of the real. Thus, he writes that, "This 'answer' of the real on which we rely, this support in the big Other whose gesture of response 'subjectivizes' the abyss of the pure subject, is what Hegel has in mind when he speaks of the "cunning of reason" (Žižek, 1993b, p. 169). Likewise, in the passage from "*Hegel avec Lacan*" cited above, when Žižek, making an opportune distinction between discourse and its effect, adds that "the subject, by definition, cannot master the effects of its discourse, since it is the Other who has this task", he fails to grasp the character of the pass: the pass is precisely that by which the subject does not master the effect of his/her discourse but is also not released from its burden.

II

Thinkers who do not contradict themselves are nothing but censors.

By "contradiction", I do not mean changes of opinion that seek to adjust an unchanging grid to the vicissitudes of ideological correctness.[25] To contradict oneself is to try to correct one's aim, and Žižek's epistemic power is confirmed in a more recent book, *The Puppet and the Dwarf: The Perverse Core of Christianity* (2003), in which he does not avoid confronting the transcendent and making a certain number of changes in his reading of psychoanalysis. The puppet of the title is the phenomenal subject and the dwarf the noumenal subject. In questioning the truth of Buddhism and the three religions of the book, Žižek opens up disciplines that have become so closed off from one another that science cannot say anything about God or the saints without shutting itself up in positivism or drowning in spiritualism.

First, we find a healthy undoing of the attraction currently exercised by Buddhism, which, for many of our contemporaries, has become a seductive alternative to Christianity. Earlier, I qualified Žižek's position on the pass and the end of analysis as a kind of hysterical Buddhism: the subject is reduced to being only what others say of him/her, and this means being equal to the void, since I am not what others say about me. In *The Puppet and the Dwarf*, there is a related formulation: "I am what I do" (Lewis, 1966, p. 225; cited in Žižek, 2003, p. 22). Žižek rejects this statement, thereby showing the distance that he has taken towards a certain reading of his own thesis. The pleonastic character of this aphorism, which has an existentialist appearance, is not visible immediately. However, just as with the formula, "I am what others say about me", and now even more ironically, in this new context, the evacuation of any ethical dimension from "I am" and its reduction to a restrictive behaviourism leaves the subject void. Žižek (2003, p. 27) notes, with a cruel justice, that Lewis's definition makes "absolute discipline coincide with total spontaneity". The absence of any soul-searching characterises not only saints but also soldiers who obey criminal orders unhesitatingly. Generalising his criticism, Žižek shows that Buddhist doctrine is a great equaliser: if killing a fly is just as great a crime as genocide; if, as the *Bhagavad-Gita* says, "The self kills not and the self is not killed"; and if, more radically, birth and death are mere illusions, then what follows is a conclusion that must be rejected: the response of the Nazi executioners concerning the Jews whom they had murdered would be "you ought not to grieve" for them (ibid., pp. 30–31). Žižek also notes that the *Bhagavad-Gita* was Heinrich Himmler's favourite book and that the members of the Brazilian military dictatorship had adopted, behind their mask of conservative Catholicism, "an improvised Eastern mysticism as their unofficial religion" (ibid., p. 176).

This slight displacement enables Žižek to approach the question of castration from a new angle. Relying, as he often does, on the plot of a spy film, in this case Jeannot Szwarc's 1982 film *Enigma*, he argues that castration could well be based on "feigning [the] loss" of jouissance (ibid., p. 51).[26] Using the examples of obsessional rituals of sacrifice and of what he calls a "woman's sacrifice" in remaining in the shadow of her husband, Žižek argues that such pretences enable subjects to "dupe the Other" (ibid., p. 51): to make the Other believe that, through sacrifice, they are seeking, in exchange, to obtain what they are missing. The structure of the paradox is the following: 1) I possess the object that I was coveting in the Other; 2) I pretend that I do not possess it and let the Other see me looking for it; and 3) I make a sacrifice, which is intended to make the Other believe that I am not feigning and that what I am seeking is so precious that I consent to losing an object that is supposed to be important to me. Žižek (ibid., p. 52) can thus conclude, with good reason, that this "sacrifice is the most refined way of disavowing" castration; in feigning that he does not possess the object that would ensure jouissance, the subject reaches the incorrect conclusion that since he pretends not to have it, he really has it.

This misunderstanding, in which the subject, without knowing that he is doing so, makes himself the victim, is an exemplary illustration of the difference between castration – which enables us to pretend that we have abolished it – and division or splitting, which implies a loss that cannot be recovered. Splitting situates what has been lost outside the subject, for if what has been lost remains inside, it is not an object. It is necessary to understand, however, that what constitutes the passage from castration to splitting is not at all a movement from the relativity of lack to the absolute character of loss. Instead, it is the acceptance that castration is not whole [*n'est pas tout, ou n'est pas toute*], an acceptance that can easily be impeded because the belief that an Other is preventing our jouissance is profoundly comfortable to us. To return to the source, Freud's more or less contemporaneous discovery of both the bedrock of castration and *Spaltung* (splitting), does not contradict the pass, but, on the contrary, lays the ground for it. To accept one's subjective division is to accept that the bedrock is indeed a bedrock; this bedrock, however, does nothing more than to forbid access to a place where jouissance would be equivalent to dying.

On the basis of his shift in emphasis, Žižek's (ibid., p. 53) criticism of the "perverse solution that forms the very core of 'really existing Christianity'" becomes significant. He suggests that the border between Law and transgression could be better understood by defining "universal Law" as the "absolute transgression" (ibid., p. 36); in doing so, he both explains the failure of perversion and marks out its limit.

To posit the existence of the Law in order to be able to transgress it is to miss what is essential. The Law can only be born through a transgression, a transgression of what submitting to the sexual relation would impose on us: I would get off on the Other in the same way that I would let the Other get off on me. Sade's maxim[27] is only the dream of abolishing the symptom, which itself marks the nonexistence, not of the Other, but of the sexual relation.

This is also what authorises Žižek to toy with the idea of criticising Lacan's (1986, p. 319) overworked formula in *The Ethics of Psychoanalysis*: do not "give ground relative to one's desire".[28] In this case, I am very pleased to agree with Žižek. Jacques-Alain Miller and the Millerians have used this aphorism to justify a conception of the "reconquest" or "*reconquista*", in Schmitt's sense of the term, of the Freudian field (Miller, 1990; Schmitt, 1950, 1955). It can also, as Žižek (ibid., p. 54) suggests, be read in terms of Bataille's Sadean position that one should "think everything to a point that makes people tremble" (see Surya, 2002, p. 479; cited by Žižek, 2003, p. 54). This, however, is only one reading, one that Miller has neither promoted nor put forward; he has, however, made it possible through his own work of interpretation, a work that is the prisoner of his own determination to transform – under his aegis and according to his criteria – the psychoanalytic movement into a group that would resemble the army or the Church.

Unlike Bataille, for whom jouissance is the hypostasis of desire (see the five-issue journal *Acéphale*, partially translated in Bataille [1986]), the seminar on ethics posits that there is a point of disruption between desire and jouissance. I agree with Žižek, however, that Lacan's formulation has both a paradoxical dimension as an imperative, and risks giving rise to a religion of desire: a "dogmatics" of desire, to the detriment of its "dialectic". I would argue, instead, that what founds the ethical value of desire is cowardice: cowardice involves the moment when the subject gives up on his/her desire, a moment that is terrible because it makes guilt coalesce. Without such an experience of giving up, no subject would ever envision undergoing an analysis. To give up on one's desire is homologous to the gesture of a swimmer, just before a competition: s/he tastes the water. Without such a surrender, it would be impossible to accept the splitting of the subject.

For Lacan – as we can see from his next seminar, *The Transference* (2001b) – the ethical paradigm was not Antigone but Sygne de Coûfontaine, the protagonist of Paul Claudel's (1911) play, *The Hostage*. In a first period that lasts almost her entire life, she betrays her desire: both her love and the object of that love. Then, before dying, she refuses three times to *say* that she *has not* betrayed her desire. In her refusal *of* speech, she exiles herself from the lie that speech *is*; such a refusal goes beyond or falls short of any refusal that could take place *in* speech, and it leads to the birth of her granddaughter, Pensée. Although Paul Claudel was extraordinarily unpleasant, there was genius in him.

With this, some things fall back into order and give us a better sense of what is at stake in desire:

> the true problem is the mother who *enjoys* me (her child), and the true stake of the game is to escape this closure. The true anxiety is this being-caught

> in the Other's *jouissance*. . . . [I]nstead of the child mastering the game [of *Fort/Da*], and thus coping with the trauma of the mother's absence, we get the child trying to escape the suffocating embrace of his mother and construct an open space for desire.
>
> *(Žižek, 2003, p. 59)*

I have one reservation[29] concerning Žižek's rejection of Freud's explanation that the child was trying to confront the mother's absence; yet this distinction between jouissance and desire is the only one that enables us to construct a psychoanalytic, rather than psychological, conception of the symptom.[30] Likewise, I can only endorse his conception, in the pages that follow, of the difference between the desire and the jouissance of the Other, and his resulting definition of phallic jouissance as "*jouissance* under the condition of desire" (ibid., p. 61).

The next developments in *The Puppet and the Dwarf* are even better. As I mentioned at the beginning, in this book Žižek confronts the question of the transcendent. To paraphrase Baudelaire: "God is the sole being who has no need to exist to be perfect".[31] Žižek is Baudelairean in his analysis of Christianity, since he (ibid., p. 89) argues that the Christian identification with Christ is "ultimately [an] *identification with a failure* – and, consequently, since the object of identification is God, God Himself must be shown to fail". The statement could be completed with the words "to exist" in any other way than by the fall, which is the true beginning. The same logic is present in Žižek's apparently paradoxical analysis of the antagonistic relation between the death drive and the nirvana principle, the goal of which is death. The death drive, on the contrary, represents "the dimension of the 'undead', and of the spectral life which insists beyond (biological death)" (ibid., p. 93). I agree with the fundamental point of this remark, although the paradox could be presented differently: it is less a matter of a contradiction between Thanatos and nirvana than of a contradiction that is internal to the death drive's power of dissolution.

In a way that can now be understood clearly, because he gives a decisive importance to Lacan's repositioning of the castration complex in *Encore*, Žižek makes a probing comparison between the law in Judaism and Christianity. He does so by referring to Alain Badiou's book, *St. Paul: The Foundation of Universalism*, citing Eric Santner's formulation of the question Badiou directs to Paul: "Is all the subject within the figure of legal subjection?" (ibid., p. 116). As Žižek (ibid., p. 116), still quoting Santner, notes, for Lacan "there is *no direct path* from legal subjection to 'not all'; not all only opens up through a traversal of the *fantasy* of exception".[32] Through this proposition, he can claim that the Christian conception establishes a correlation between law and transgression (sin), thus obeying the "'masculine' logic of exception" (ibid., p. 116). Experiencing the law involves being tested by sin; this is why the law, which constitutes sin and reveals itself by means of sin, "has to appear to the subject as a foreign power crushing the subject" (ibid., p. 116).

At this point, it becomes difficult to grasp how Žižek situates the place of love in this conception of Christian law. He seems to adopt a double solution. On the one hand, "there is *too much* love" in the Christian law: the law only seems to impose itself from the outside if the subject experiences it as threatening "its attachment to the pathological *agalma* deep within itself" (ibid., p. 117). On the other hand, both Paul and some Lutheran theologians approach the opposition between law and divine love by de-emphasising the importance of the first and accentuating the second; love is reintroduced in a form that is divine and no longer human. Unless my understanding of Žižek is mistaken, it would thus be nonpathological. Certainly, as we have already stressed, there is an opposition between two conceptions of the fall; in the first, a "strange, perverse" God programmed it in order, next, through the offer of redemption, to glorify Himself; in the second, the "Fall is *identical* to redemption" (ibid., p. 118). In other words, if this second conception is correct, God would only be God by accepting – through the human being – not to be God. There is an even better way of formulating this, one that would present the underside of Baudelaire's statement about God: He would only exist as God by no longer being God. Yet why then should there be an opposition between "pathological" human love and divine love? It is certain that a thousand and one forms of love can be distinguished, in both the psychoanalytic and the literary "clinic", yet the true question about love may well be the following: isn't love what enables us to escape from the deadly attraction exercised by the conviction that there is a sexual relation (the dilution or contraction of two into One)? Doesn't love enable us to do this by *making up* [*suppléant*] for the nonexistence of this relation?

It is difficult not to sense that the ambiguity of Žižek's position concerning love is directly related to his mistrust of transference; as I have already suggested, this derives from the supposition that analysis (and the analyst as the operator of this aim) is determined to deprive the analysand of her/his "secret garden". Finally, even if Žižek's generous reading of Christianity is quite acceptable – except for theologians, who may find the kernel of atheism in it – why should it be ruled out that Christianity, and perhaps every religion, is perverse? Perhaps the only reason is that today, perversion, like psychosis, remains stained by a moralistic opprobrium that confuses our judgement.

It is difficult not to see that this discomfort about transference misses its mark: God is the target, but it is the analyst who is shot. This is apparent in the chapter entitled "Subtraction, Jewish and Christian", where Žižek develops a thesis whose premises are related to the attempt to exonerate Christianity from the charge of perversion (ibid., pp. 122–143). If Job is one of the most representative figures of Judaism, the figure of Jesus brings in another relation: a relation between God and the one who despairs of Him. With Jesus, the gap between the "desperate man" and God "is transposed onto God Himself, as His own radical splitting, or rather, self-abandonment" (ibid., p. 126). Jesus' despair, as caused by God's abandonment, is nothing other than the death of God the father, a death that "reveal[s] His utter impotence" (ibid., p. 126). Therefore, what Christianity would thus take upon itself would be a divine impotence, one, it is true, that has been surmounted (*Aufgehobt*) by the resurrection of God in the form of the Holy Spirit. Yet perhaps Job also had a premonition of this. Judaism, through the figure of Job, distances itself from any sense of resignation before God's "crushing" and incomprehensible injustice. Instead, there is a subtraction: Job realises that it is not he, "*but God Himself, who was actually on trial in Job's calamities*" (ibid., p. 127).

Try substituting the words "the analyst" for "God" here. Doing so would place this theory at the heart of Freud's account of the dissolution of transference, which is confirmed by an endnote, in which Žižek (ibid., p. 183) sees the murder of Moses not, like Freud, as the founding parricide, but as "the *humiliation* of the Pharaoh". Žižek then asks, "What if this humiliation of the father was the precondition for establishing Judaism as the first great religion . . . the religion of a group without a state identity?" (ibid., p. 183). Through this hypothesis, Žižek, discreetly but openly, casts doubt upon the religious foundations of the state of Israel.

This diversion of his course from an analysis of Judaism and Christianity to that of psychoanalysis becomes explicit when Žižek wonders whether "the revolutionary party and the psychoanalytic society" – a significant pairing – are not a new type of collective organisation: a community knit together not by a master-signifier, but by "fidelity to a Cause" (ibid., p. 130). This is a striking but vague remark. In the penultimate chapter of *Group Psychology and the Analysis of the Ego*, Freud (1921, p. 121) draws certain conclusions from his thesis that the community is founded by the father's murder – "on the basis of a shared guilt for parricide" – and that the dead father returns in the form of a master signifier: this thesis enables him to provide a relatively cruel definition of the human being. The latter is not a "herd" animal or *Herdentier* – an allusion to Wilfred Trotter's ideas about the "herd instinct" – but rather a "horde animal" (*Hordentier*). This means that Freud's analysis of the crowd or group (*Masse*) is based on the idea that the crowd (whether a natural one or an artificial one like the army or the Church, the community of believers) is a "revival of the primal horde" (Freud, 1921, p. 123). Because the crowd's identification involves substituting the object *a* for the ego-ideal – which explains horizontal identification – the "fidelity to a Cause", to use Žižek's terminology, is not at all opposed to the master-signifier. Instead, it is added to this signifier. In itself, such fidelity would seem insufficient without the presence of a leader (*Führer*). In this respect, one of Freud's valuable suggestions is to locate Nietzsche's *Ubermensch* not in the future but in the past: the primal father, "at the very beginning of the history of mankind, was the 'superman' whom Nietzsche only expected from the future" (ibid., p. 123).

Without going too far too quickly, it is already possible to locate the problem: if we seek to envision a mode of the collective that would be purified of any allegiance to a leader, this would give a place to the object that functions as a cause. Even if the object that Freud presented in his schema of group-identification and the formation of a mass is not the object *a*, it already occupies this place. If this object takes the place of the ego-ideal, it cannot establish a social bond that would be free from the discourse of the master.

What remains convincing in Žižek's analysis is his way of interpreting God. We have seen that God's impotence and incapacity enable him to exist: this is God as interpreted through the paternal metaphor. Yet this is not all: "The very notion of creation implies God's self-contraction: God had first to withdraw into Himself, constrain His omnipresence, in order first to create the nothing out of which He then created the universe" (Žižek, 1993b, p. 137). This interpretation identifies God with the power and potentiality of language, which annihilates the thing, but which is also consequently the source of the freedom to create. It might well be necessary to specify the connection between God-the-Father (the proper name, by which such a God limits the debasement of the thing to its virtualised state) and God-as-language, which – once the thing has been annihilated (the creation of nothingness) and taking into account the safety catch [*cran d'arrêt*] introduced by God-the-Father, since he cannot let there be *only* nothingness – turns God-the-Father's own power of invention back against him, leaving him speechless.[33] Lights! Camera! Action!

Notes

1 [*Translator's note*: For a discussion of the translation of "*passeur*" and the related term "*passant*", please see the translator's introduction.]

2 See Patricia León-Lopez (1999). It has been established that discourse, in Lacan's sense of the term, was dramatized in the theatre. It suffices to recall the extraordinary remark Eugene O'Neill supposedly made to his publisher: "I've finished the play – now I just have to write the dialogue", as well as Samuel Beckett's play *Quad*, an assemblage of stage directions without any dialogue.

3 [*Translator's note*: "*Positions*" is the title of a collection of essays published (in French) by Althusser (1976). It included "Ideology and Ideological State Apparatuses".]

4 [*Translator's note*: Lucien Sebag (1934–1965) was an anthropologist who had prepared for the *agrégation* teaching examination under Althusser and begun an analysis with Lacan. In his autobiography, *The Future Lasts Forever*, Althusser writes that a "panic-stricken" Lacan paid him a visit early one morning, immediately after Sebag's suicide, in order to explain to him the circumstances of what had taken place. Lacan had terminated Sebag's analysis when the latter had fallen in love with his daughter, Judith; he told Althusser that "It was impossible, for technical reasons" to continue seeing him. In an attempt to prevent the suicide, Lacan "had assured him that he would visit him at any hour of the day or night if he asked him to" (Althusser, 1992, p. 189).

Althusser (ibid., p. 189), for his part, notes that "I wanted to ask if he could not have had Sebag taken into hospital for his own safety", and adds that Lacan "would probably have told me that it was against the analytical 'rules'". Althusser also states that "I have often wondered what he would have done in my own case: if he would have left me unsupervised (I constantly wanted to kill myself) so as not to infringe in the slightest way on the 'rules' of analysis"].

5 Let us note that these words express either a fallacy or something quite subtle, since the object that the members of the group fear is itself a member of the group.

6 In the "Letter of Dissolution", Lacan (1980a, p. 130) wrote that one reason he had decided to put an end to the *École freudienne de Paris* was because it had become "an Institution, the effect of a consolidated group". If only he had lived long enough to be able to remind us of this warning!

7 [*Translator's note*: English in the original.]

8 [*Translator's note*: On the "bad subject", see Althusser (1970, pp. 268–269):

> Let me summarize what we have discovered about ideology in general.
>
> The duplicate mirror-structure of ideology ensures simultaneously:
>
> 1) the interpellation of "individuals" as subjects;
> 2) their subjection to the Subject;
> 3) the mutual recognition of subjects and Subject, the subjects' recognition of each other, and finally the subject's recognition of himself;
> 4) the absolute guarantee that everything really is so, and that on condition that the subjects recognize what they are and behave accordingly, everything will be all right: Amen–"*So be it*".

Result: caught in this quadruple system of interpellation as subjects, of subjection to the Subject, of universal recognition and of absolute guarantee, the subjects "work", they "work by themselves" in the vast majority of cases, with the exception of the "bad subjects" who on occasion provoke the intervention of one of the detachments of the (Repressive) State Apparatus. But the vast majority of (good) subjects work all right "all by themselves", i.e. by ideology (whose concrete forms are realized in the Ideological State Apparatuses). They are inserted into practices governed by the rituals of the ISAs. They "recognize" the existing state of affairs (*das Bestehende*), that "it really is true that it is so and not otherwise", and that they must be obedient to God, to their conscience, to the priest, to De Gaulle, to the boss, to the engineer, that thou shalt "love thy neighbor as thyself", etc. Their concrete, material behaviour is simply the inscription in life of the admirable words of the prayer: '*Amen – So be it*'.]

9 Lacan was sometimes very critical of the university discourse, noting its connection with "knavery" (Lacan, 1991, p. 61): it tends to lay claim, without justification, to propositions that belong to someone else.

10 [*Translator's note*: This can be related to the "hysterical *proton pseudos*" (Freud, 1950, pp. 352–357).]

11 For Lacan, the montage of the drive is not a matter of function. This is clear in the explicitly surrealist image he provides in *The Four Fundamental Concepts of Psycho-Analysis*: "[the] image would show the working of a dynamo connected up to a gas-tap, a peacock's feather emerges, and tickles the belly of a pretty woman, who is just lying there looking beautiful" (Lacan, 1973d, p. 169).

12 This idea is also developed in the first pages of *Anti-Oedipus* (Deleuze & Guattari, 1972).

13 The French mentality has, even among the most insightful of those who are plagued with it, a rather confounding ability: it always gets what is essential wrong at least once. For instance, Deleuze and Guattari take André Green, rather than Lacan, as the point of reference here. It is as if the authors were trying to inoculate themselves against the malady of submission by maintaining a certain distance towards the master, while praising one of his dissident students. The result of this kind of counterfeiting is always a tendency to recoil from thought; it is a way of opting for a cosmetically original position rather than the unimaginable one. If the latter were fully and irrevocably embraced, it would require one truly to leave the sheltering haven of the master.

14 [*Translator's note*: The translators of *Anti-Oedipus* use "investment" as a translation of the French word, "*investissement*", which is itself a rendering of the Freudian term, "*Besetzung*"; in the Standard Edition, this word became "cathexis". As James Strachey notes (1962, p. 63, note 2), "*Besetzung*" is "in ordinary use, and among many other senses, might have some such meaning as 'occupation' or 'filling'". The libido can thus be said to "occupy" a particular object, in a sense that is close to that of a military occupation. Strachey states that he coined the word "cathexis" on the basis of the Greek term "κατέχειν, catechein, to occupy" (ibid., p. 63, note 2). The French expression, "*investir un lieu*" can also be used to refer to an occupation – not necessarily military – of a particular place. The English words "invest" and "investment" possess similar resonances, which, however, struggle to make themselves heard above the overwhelming din of their financial meaning.]

15 For further discussion of these questions, see Alain Badiou's (1990) essential introduction in *Number and Numbers*.

16 [*Translator's note*: Lacan (1969, p. 18) writes: "Recently, in an ongoing course I am giving, I correlated this cause [the *a*-cause] and the function of surplus jouissance (*Mehrlust*, which is obviously homologous, but may not be analogous, to Marx's *Mehrwert*, since it is the cause rather than the effect of the market)".]

17 Soler (2002, p. 175) writes: "I will start again with the fundamental symptom. It fills in the yawning gap of the 'there is no [*il n'y a pas*]' – of the sexual non-relation – with the erection of a 'there is [*il y a*]'".

18 The "that's not it" of the obsessional – or of the hysteric in another form – touches on what is inconvenient for the subject and not on what is inconvenient for the Other.

19 [*Translator's note*: See Michaux (1997, p. 175): "He who hides his madman dies voiceless".]
20 This is not as close as it might seem to Lacan's (1973b, p. 491) concept of "*parêtre* [para-being]" in "*L'étourdit*". The *parêtre* concerns what allows the subject to devise a way to write the body and thereby become differentiated from its reduction to a being, something forced on the subject by the fact of being spoken by the Other. [*Translator's note*: Lacan's neologism "*parêtre*" is also a homophone of the French word "*paraître* [to seem]".]
21 A similar conception of the subject can be found in Millot's (2012, p. 94) discussion of Madame Guyon, the French mystic who was accused of being a Quietist: "the fundamental omission of oneself that is perhaps the place of the subject". The problem here probably concerns the distinction between the *moi* [generally translated as "ego"] as an instance of the imaginary and what Lacan himself called the "*Ego*", which plays a crucial role in Joyce's sinthome (Lacan, 2005b, p. 128).
22 [*Translator's note*: Žižek is referring to the following passage:

> Father is the other of son, and son the other of father, and each only *is* as this other of the other; at the same time, the one determination only is in relation to the other. . . . The father also has an existence of his own apart from the son-relationship; but then he is not father but simply man. . . . Opposites, therefore, contain contradiction in so far as they are, in the same respect, negatively related to one another.
> (Hegel, 1807, p. 441; cited by Žižek, 1993b, p. 131)]

23 [*Translator's note*: For more on Russell's paradox, see p. 132, note 18 below and the related discussion.]
24 [*Translator's note*: Concerning the "White Goddess", see Lacan's (1974a, p. 34, emphasis added) comment in "Spring awakening":

> How to know if, as Robert Graves puts it, the Father himself, the eternal father of us all, is not one Name among others of the *White Goddess*, the one that according to him gets lost in the night of time, because she is the Different one, the forever Other in her enjoyment – like those forms of the infinite whose enumeration we only start when we know that she is the one who will suspend us.]

25 From Bernard-Henri Lévy to Alain Finkielkraut, and without forgetting André Glucksmann: the extent to which what is "in" among these intellectuals involves the asphyxiation of their intellects is deplorable.
26 [*Translator's note*: Žižek (2003, p. 51) describes this film as follows:

> *Enigma* . . . tells the story of a dissident journalist-turned-spy who emigrates to the West, and is then recruited by the CIA and sent to East Germany to get hold of a scrambling/descrambling computer chip whose possession enables the owner to read all communications between KGB headquarters and its outposts. However, small clues tell the spy that there is something wrong with his mission: that is, that the East Germans and the Russians were informed of his arrival in advance – so what is going on? Is it that the Communists have a mole in CIA headquarters who informed them of this secret mission? As we learn toward the end of the film, the solution is much more ingenious: the CIA already possesses the scrambling chip, but, unfortunately, the Russians suspect this fact, so they have temporarily stopped using this computer network for their secret communications. The true aim of the operation was the CIA attempt to convince the Russians that they did not possess the chip: they sent an agent to get it and, at the same time, deliberately let the Russians know that there was an operation going on to get the chip; of course, the CIA is counting on the fact that the Russians will arrest the agent. The ultimate result will thus be that, by successfully preventing the mission, the Russians will be convinced that the Americans do not possess it, and that it is therefore safe to use this communication link. . . . The tragic aspect of the story, of course, is that the mission's failure is taken into account: the CIA wants the mission to fail, that is, the poor dissident agent is sacrificed in advance for the higher goal of convincing the opponent that one doesn't possess his

secret. The strategy here is to stage a search operation in order to convince the Other (the enemy) that one does not already possess what one is looking for – in short, one feigns a lack, a want, in order to conceal from the Other that one already possesses the *agalma*, the Other's innermost secret.]

27 [*Translator's note*: See Lacan (1963, p. 648):
Let us enunciate the [Sade's] maxim:

> "I have the right to enjoy your body," anyone can say to me, "and I will exercise this right without any limit to the capriciousness of the exactions I may wish to satiate with your body."
>
> Such is the rule to which everyone's will would be submitted, assuming a society were to forcibly implement the rule.]

28 Žižek (2003, p. 54) writes: "Far from being *the* seminar of Lacan, his *Ethics of Psychoanalysis* is, rather, the point of deadlock at which Lacan comes dangerously close to the standard version of the 'passion for the Real'".

29 This is not a minor reservation, for it involves the difficulty Žižek constantly has in differentiating between the real, the symbolic, and the imaginary without relying exclusively on binary relations between two of these three terms. See, for example, his discussion of the real and reality (Žižek, 2003, pp. 75–77); we note that language prohibits jouissance because it is also the condition of jouissance.

30 Psychiatry, psychology and many psychoanalysts hold that the purpose of therapy is to eliminate the symptom; they are like nudists, who are confused about the difference between skin and clothing.

31 [*Translator's note*: See Baudelaire (1897, p. 31): "God is the sole being who has no need to exist to reign".]

32 I (Bruno, 2003a, p. 19) have also stressed this point, in connection with the real father: "the function of the exception should be intrinsically correlated with its buttress of impossibility, at the risk of reintroducing suggestion". From this point of view, there is an (evangelical) risk of trying to make the ideal analysand into "one among others" (which is the title of a book by Denis Vasse [1978]). That would be to forget that the fantasy, before it is traversed, was constructed or put together, and that this putting-together cannot occur without such a reliance on the exception as impossible, including in psychosis, where the non-functioning of the real father leads the subject to embody the exception.

33 Again, see Artaud (1947a, p. 264): "nothingness [*le néant*] *is* the body".

PART II

The capitalist discourse

3

UMHA

In the preceding section, an examination of the splitting of the subject showed the true significance of the castration complex and how, when the capitalist discourse ends up sundering the subject, $\$$, from unconscious knowledge, S_2, it has deprived castration of its dialectic. In this kinetics, the more the subject drinks, the thirstier s/he becomes. This exhausting misunderstanding feeds on the capitalist axiom that it is not impossible for surplus-jouissance (*a*) to satiate the subject. Dr. Jekyll, in order to put an end to this vicious circle, commits suicide as Hyde. Joan Dark is led to her death by Pierpont Mauler, with the best of intentions, in order to preserve the criminal innocence of the unconscious. Mauler, despite his frequently displayed soul-searching, does not want to give up on this misunderstanding. What will become of him after Joan's death? Perhaps he will become both the wealthiest capitalist and a convert to a new form of Mariolatry.

The chapters on Althusser, Deleuze and Guattari and Žižek defined their theoretical relation to the splitting (*Spaltung*) of the subject. In Althusser, splitting is refused, which paves the way for the bad subject. Deleuze and Guattari give preeminence to one of the poles of this division – multiplicity – since this division can be located, in psychoanalysis, between the One and the Other. Finally, Žižek, connects the subject, as void, to the object *a*. What is striking about these three enterprises, retroactively, is that the last of them stands, without any doubt, in a very close relation to psychoanalysis. It is obvious that Žižek has read Lacan, including his late work, very closely. One problem, however, has not been resolved: the discourse of the philosopher is not that of the psychoanalyst. Lacan's verdict remains valid: we must separate ourselves from philosophical discourse in order not to become confused about what analytic discourse is.

Lacan's theory of discourse can be introduced in terms of the two themes of lysis and guise. "Lysis" marks the place of discourse: it belongs to the order of language, which dissolves the thing. A discourse can take place "without speech"; speech is not the only fate of language. Language can manifest itself in a graph, which implies writing and sets up logic. This is what we shall be dealing with here. The "guise" refers to the way in which a discourse is established, in order, on the one hand, to ward off the metonymic drifting that characterises speech in mania, and on the other hand, to inscribe the division of the subject within the constraints of the graph. Doesn't capitalist discourse, in exempting itself from this second characteristic, dictate a speech that is so over-encoded that the real is held at a distance, as if it were behind a glass? The imagery of the spectacle of war, for example, becomes so inflated that it covers over the real of what war actually is.

The arrows and the barrier

1) Instead of sketching an epistemological history of the category of discourse, I shall simply note that Lacan introduced his own discourses at the end of the 1960s, in his seminars *From an Other to the other* (1968–1969) and *The Other Side of Psychoanalysis* (1969–1970). Then, in "*Radiophonie*" (1970), he set down a first written account of this theory. The title of the seminar, *From an Other to the other*, already speaks volumes. It is telling that certain students of Lacan's have transcribed it incorrectly as "From an **o**ther to the **O**ther". This misunderstanding can easily be explained. The other is the alter ego of the dual relation, while the Other is polysemous; it is not only the "treasure trove of signifiers" (Lacan, 1960, p. 682)[1] and the place of truth implied by the existence of language; it is also the body that supports both of these, hence the expression "maternal Other". It can therefore seem orthodox to understand this title as retracing a genesis that leads from the imaginary register – the relation with the image of the other – to the entry into the symbolic order – the order of language. This is not at all, however, what Lacan was aiming at in this seminar. Starting with the Other, Lacan wonders how, through psychoanalysis, the other – other people in everyday life, the partner, the neighbour or the stranger, the friend or the enemy – can be recognised not as counterparts (this is the only kind of humanism authorised by the discourse of the master) but in terms of their irreducible alterity.[2] The date of this seminar is also telling. In his teaching, Lacan was always sensitive to historical circumstances, and this was his first seminar after May 1968.

2) If it can also be hoped that the reader will read Lacan, it cannot be expected that s/he has done so already. Therefore, it is necessary to give some idea, briefly and without any sugar coating, of what Lacan means by "discourse"; for him, this term does not, as it usually does, refer to all [*l'ensemble*] of speech, unless we want to define "all" as a mathematical set – which, unlike a class, can be empty, and empty precisely of speech.

In this sense, there is an opposition between discourse and speech, for in speech, the slippage of the signifier is more or less the rule. In a lecture given in May 1972, in which Lacan writes the matheme of the capitalist discourse (and to which we will return in what follows), this slippage is related to the fact that "there is no signifier whose signification would be assured" (Lacan, 1978b, p. 43). This signification "can always be a different one, and it even spends its time sliding as far in signification as you would like" (ibid., p. 43). Thus, discourse is, first of all, what enables us to ward off some of this slippage. If, for example, you are a man and go into a pharmacy to ask about medication for impotence and the pharmacist answers you by reciting one of La Fontaine's fables, you can conclude – precisely because you are in a pharmacy – that it is the pharmacist who is mad and not you. You would have good reason for concluding that she has taken you for a spectator, a French teacher, a theatre impresario or a casting director. A pharmacy is discourse: it enables you to specify places, relations and terms that have no need for actual speech in order to signify.

Of course, if this slight misadventure ever befalls you, you can also conclude that the pharmacist is not mad; she is simply joyous and mischievous, and her recitation suggests that poetry is better than chemistry at rearming Eros. To accomplish its function, discourse, as we are going to see, has a four-part structure. We shall also see, without too much pain, I hope, that for Lacan, the human being is at least as much a discoursing quadruped as a speaking biped.

3) Let us take leave of the pharmacist to go to a nonfictional example: Freud and the young woman whom we know, through his case history, as Dora.[3] In her encounter with "Professor" Freud, Dora commands him to produce knowledge about her case. Freud complies, giving a major interpretation that is mistaken, as he would recognise twenty-five years later. For the hysterical subject, this provides an inaugural proof that if the master *can* be mistaken once, he *must* always be wrong. Achilles will never reach the tortoise. Lacan subtracts the hysteric's Eleaticism from the pathology of neurosis and makes it one of the four discourses: one of three ways (for in this quartet, analytic discourse is set apart) of refusing to let the other be a subject. Either the other is a counterpart – and is therefore not an other – or s/he is not a subject. This unfairness is even more unanswerable because it claims to be its opposite, yet it is the fruit of an intellectual error: if the master, having been mistaken once, is always wrong, then the concept of error would lose all meaning. *Possibly being wrong* is not equivalent to *always being wrong*, just as potentiality is not the act. Positing that her/his partner mistakenly takes himself for a master, and failing to see that a *single* error does not disqualify him forever from being one, the hysterical subject – whether woman or man – parades her/himself as the only one who knows that s/he does *not* know. This is the hysteric's definition of the subject. Other people become thereby, at best, nothing more than sketches that are drawn on the mystic writing pad of her daydreams and then erased, victims of their belief that they are able to know. In the hysteric's defence, it should be added that in analytic discourse, believing that one is the only analysand may well be a necessary, although transitory lure. The example of Socrates leads us to think that an hysterical moment is required in every authentic philosophical enterprise.

This situation can be written as a matheme, a framework that imitates mathematical formalisation. Four places – the agent of the discourse, its other, its production and its truth – and four terms – the subject ($\$$), master-signifier (S_1), knowledge (S_2) and surplus-jouissance (a) – can be distinguished. We thus obtain a matrix:

Four Places

(1) agent	other (2)
(4) truth	production (3)

Later, Lacan would begin to refer to the place of the agent (at the top left) as that of the semblance [*semblant*].

4) This formalisation still needs to be explained, by showing the meaning of these places and especially of these terms. First, however, four preliminary remarks are necessary:

- In order to produce this schema, Lacan proceeded by trial and error, making successive approximations. The respective elaboration of places and terms ended up being articulated in this four-part structure; on its basis and because of the fixed character of the places, four – and only four – discourses can be constructed by rotating the terms.
- This matrix is antistructuralist. For structuralism, a system is defined as a set of elements whose places, definitions and relations obey a series of rules, by means of an empty place that makes the "play" of the set possible. Anything that is outside this system is not taken into consideration, so that each system is a universe, or a part of a universe. For Lacan, however, *there is no universe of discourse*. This lack leads to a presence: between the two lower places – where there would be a movement from production (3) to truth (4) – a barrier "of jouissance" appears. (Other Side, p. 108.) This is what Freud locates as trauma and Lacan as the real.[4]

5) Jouissance. Without understanding this category, it is impossible to grasp what discourse is for Lacan, since it is the barrier of jouissance that explains the gap between the place of production (at the lower right) and that of truth (at the lower left). Jouissance is fundamentally the fruit of Freud's second topography. Thanatos, the death drive, makes this "fifth element" manifest; all that can be said of it is that it results from both the advent of speech (of which language is a sediment) and its consequence: the representation of what cannot be represented. Death may be the only state in which "I" can *say itself* without becoming different from *what* it says, simply because the latter has been said. In this respect, jouissance would be what is unrepresentable in the subject, what would fail to come about through a representation by language. Lacan (1960, p. 694) lends a voice to jouissance, which states, voicelessly and from nowhere: "*I* am in the place from which 'the universe is a flaw in the purity of Non-Being' is vociferated".[5] Only Non-Being, which is strictly unthinkable, is pure, for death itself cannot prevent us from having been. The vocation of jouissance is to remind us that creation is negative.

Freud (1905, p. 182) grasped jouissance through its effects (repetition, masochism), but also invokes it with the dazzling example of a *mouth kissing itself*, or if we prefer

Lacan's (1973d, p. 179) paraphrase of this, a *kiss without a mouth*. And why not? Lacan promoted the category of jouissance to a major rank in psychoanalysis, but in doing so, he was following in Freud's footsteps. For example, in "The Economic Problem of Masochism", Freud (1924, p. 159) writes that "the Nirvana principle . . . would be entirely in the service of the death instincts". This statement deserves to be emphasised. As we have seen, jouissance has nothing in common with pleasure; the latter, with its twin, unpleasure, regulates conduct, inciting the subject to stay within certain limits. Jouissance only delights in what is outside the limit. Georges Bataille, whose work preceded Lacan's so discreetly, expressed its nature the best in *The Tears of Eros*, when he wrote "this book's meaning is the opening up of consciousness to the way in which the 'little death' and actual death are identical" (Bataille, 1961, p. 20, translation modified). This homology between orgasm and death-throes or agony (etymologically, "*a-gonon*", the end of a struggle) follows the path of Freud, who made the Nirvana principle the realisation of the zero degree of orgasm and jouissance. It also, however, tries to resolve this paradox, since in Freud, the height of orgasm leads to its end. Thus, just before no longer experiencing jouissance (death), a subject could encounter the height of jouissance. Bataille (ibid., p. 20) speaks of this moment of passage, of death, as one of "ultimate pain". Lacan's elaboration of the category of discourse enabled him not so much to resolve this paradox as to go beyond it. According to Lacan, discourse is what "makes do" with jouissance, unlike "discourse" understood in the more common sense of rhetoric, which wants to know nothing about it.

In his own way, Freud located the crux of the matter – or what might be called the sinews of war – in this jouissance-obstacle. This reference to "war" can be taken literally, for if there is a discourse that is specific to war, no real war can ever be reduced to conflict that is resolved by symbolic means. Even television, the magical instrument of derealisation, is unable to accomplish this.[6] When the nondiscursive breaks into discourse, this does not put an end to the civilising impact of the latter; instead, it incites us not to allow ourselves to be cradled and lulled to sleep by what the victors say (see Walter Benjamin): they claim that war disinfects us of evil. Jouissance is a barricade between two or more camps; it is an excess that, as soon as the first flesh has been made into the word, never ceases to complete the final butchery as quickly as possible.

6) If we retain just one characteristic of discourse, it should be this: a discourse is produced, but its truth is inaccessible. Truth is not a paltry matter. In Western philosophy, it is first and foremost, and always, a matter of the adequation between the idea and the thing. "There is a Swiss navy". Is this true or false? In examining this statement, we are at the level of what Freud discussed in terms of the judgement of existence.[7] The requirement that there be an adequation between the idea and the thing determines the programme of science, which can only, however, make a pronouncement when attempts at adequation fail. Scientific procedures can prove that a proposition is false, but that does not necessarily imply that what is not false is true; there is always a possibility that the claim that the non-false is true can itself be falsified (by proceeding to demonstrate the falseness of the proposition, whether through experiment or formal reasoning). Lacan works this problematic into psychoanalysis by playing on the equivocation between "phallus" and "*falsus*" ("false" in Latin). Thus, the phallic function says nothing other than "it is false that a man

is a woman". This function asserts that something is false, and it is only about what is false that such assertions can be made. Contrary to what our habits would lead us to believe, this does not debase the status of truth. Since truth can no longer be the faithful *copy* of the thing (the much-vaunted "reflection"),[8] it is always nothing other than what is *original* in speech; a lie thus only makes truth more radiant.

In this context, the statement, "I am lying" is no longer a paradox. We only have to admit that every enunciation, without exception, is true, and thus "I am lying" would also be true. Psychoanalysis is based on this principle, which justifies a form of association that is called "free": at the level of speech, every enunciation is true. One of the common mechanisms in the theatre is to have a particular character say, "I'm going", while the stage directions say that s/he does not move.[9] Even here, "I'm going" remains true. If the character were to say, "I'm staying", then s/he – or rather, her/his truth – would be different. Truth concerns the reality not of the action but of the character. The stage directions, which indicate that s/he remains, mark the entrance of a kind of knowledge that would put truth to the test. When the Holocaust denier Robert Faurisson argued that the Nazi extermination camps were really holiday camps, what he said was true in only one sense: it was a faithful part of his own self-portrait.

At the level of language rather than speech, however, the paradox is still able to create a contradiction. Logic constructs a language based on written letters or symbols that are abstracted from things and examines the question of truth at the level of propositions. If, for example, A – whatever A may be – is greater than B, and B – whatever B may be – is greater than C – whatever C may be – C cannot be greater than A. At the end of the nineteenth century, mathematical logicians began to be concerned with judgements about the existence not of things, but of formal propositions. In this respect, the major epistemic question of the twentieth century was whether the symbolic could be constituted as a universe that would exhaust the real. This task turned out to be impossible, and this impossibility is congruent with Lacan's conception of discourse.

7) This little journey into the province of truth gives us a better sense of what is meant by the incompatibility between the *production* and the *truth* of discourse. From the beginning, I have emphasised the lack of identity between discourse and speech. This nonidentity reappears here, throwing light on the status of truth in both of these: in speech, it is the substance of the enunciation, while in discourse, it is inaccessible. In order not to contravene this inaccessibility, analytic discourse situates knowledge as what effaces truth, while the latter is being renewed in and by speech. Knowledge serves as a border around the hole that has been made by the effacement of truth; this hole is both the condition for the constant regeneration of this truth and the index of its limit. How, however, can this effacement of the truth be reconciled with the proposition that "the symptom . . . represents the return of truth as such into the gap of a certain knowledge" (Lacan, 1966c, p. 194)? The answer is that if truth is supposed to be the "soul" of the symptom, then it cannot be spoken entirely. This is why its effacement is necessary in order to mark this final inaccessibility. Where truth, although present, cannot be said, a semblance – and a semblance is not just some random term – can be fashioned; it is an element of knowledge that takes the "blankness" of truth into account.[10]

8) Certain aspects of this conception of discourse resemble other, contemporaneous approaches to it. For example, Michel Foucault (1976, p. 123) defines discourse in a similar way: "discourse should be thought of neither as the collection of what is said nor as the way in which things are said. Discourse is the collection of constrained and constraining significations that are transmitted through social relations"; he thus emphasises that it is not the sum-total of speech, but a set of practices that regulate social interaction. Foucault does not, however, make the status of truth disappear. According to him, the task of discourse is, in effect, to "say the truth [*dire vrai*]" (Foucault, 1984, p. 678) and this task must be neither indifferent to constituted powers nor replaced by a prescription of what truth is. There is thus an "infinite labour" (ibid., p. 678), in which all members of the apparatuses of power must participate, not only as actors but as elements of this apparatus.

As I have said, Lacan does not trust discourse in this way; for him, the truth of a discourse can act without our ever being able to grasp it; perhaps, paradoxically, it can only be grasped when knowledge takes the place that constitutes it as a hole. Foucault, on the other hand, remains in the classical problematic of the Enlightenment. He is not blind, however, to the fact that, as he claims in "The Discourse on Language", a "profound logophobia" lurks under the flaunted logophilia of discourse (Foucault, 1971, p. 229). I shall not linger over the ways that he hopes to get rid of this logophobia, which are related to the aims of his archaeology, but his accent on a phobia that turns us away from thinking should be remembered, for it touches something important, and throws light on the ambivalence of his fascination with people who were often considered vile. He does not say that "abnormal" individuals should be distrusted just as much as coercive societies. There may be a difficulty, however, in supporting an individual's disobedience of a dominant discourse if this individual has been reduced to being nothing more than a product of this very discourse.

9) After this presentation of the matrix and the schemas of discourse, we can write the mathemes of the four discourses, in the order of succession that Lacan chose when he first presented them in *The Other Side of Psychoanalysis* (see Lacan, 1991, pp. 11–28):

U	**M**	**H**	**A**
University	*Master*	*Hysteric*	*Analyst*
$\frac{S_2}{S_1} \;\frac{\rightarrow}{//}\; \frac{a}{\$}$	$\frac{S_1}{\$} \;\frac{\rightarrow}{//}\; \frac{S_2}{a}$	$\frac{\$}{a} \;\frac{\rightarrow}{//}\; \frac{S_1}{S_2}$	$\frac{a}{S_2} \;\frac{\rightarrow}{//}\; \frac{\$}{S_1}$

A discourse can be defined through its differential relations with other discourses; this is the thesis that Lacan treats in the seventh question of "*Radiophonie*" (1970), written near the end of *The Other Side of Psychoanalysis*. There he examines the relation – or rather, the absence of relation – between the term that occupies the place of the production (on the lower right) and the one that occupies the place of truth (on the lower left). It should be recalled that this rupture results from the "barrier of jouissance".

If we concentrate only on the phenomenology of these four discourses, there is nothing original about them; this is even more true when we approach them through history. The Middle Ages saw the emergence of the discourse of the university. Abelard is an exemplary figure of the latter, for he sought to travel throughout the various regions of knowledge available in his age, in order to understand and map out their comprehensive organisation. He chose as partner a woman who was able to allow herself both to be his student and to be valued as object *a*; she could also, and perhaps especially, lend herself to an education that subjected her ($\$$). This subjection may well have operated through the magic of love, and this may endear this couple to us, but it also reveals that, without love, the discourse of the university cannot succeed in bringing together two elements that continue to remain distinct: teaching [*instruction*] and upbringing [*éducation*]. We know the exemplary end of the story: on the orders of a master, Héloïse's uncle, Abelard was castrated for having tried to instill in her a hunger for knowledge (see Clanchy, 1997). The striking parallel between the birth of the University and the invention of linear perspective, which enables a homogeneous space of knowledge to be conceived, can be mentioned in passing here.

To see the emergence of the *discourse of the master*, we do not need to go back to the Asiatic mode of production, which is too little known and too controversial as a concept. Slavery, serfdom and capitalism show us a relation of mastery over the other ($S_1 \rightarrow S_2$); this mastery is based on the exploitation of the other's knowledge (S_2) in order to produce, in the form of commodities or money, a value (*a*) that does not bring any satisfaction to the subject. The sequence is even purer with capitalism: the master has had to renounce enjoyment of his goods in order to begin the process of exploitation, but this process thereby implies that the producer (S_2) has become a consumer ($\$$). Without the modification that we shall soon encounter, the discourse of the master turns out not to be strong enough to protect us from an irremediable divorce between the subject ($\$$) and the value that has been produced (*a*).

The *discourse of the hysteric* may well be the one that is most easily readable. The history of this discourse presents us with a series of men: a series that goes from Akhenaten, the feminiser of culture, to Socrates – who is "taught" by a slave whom he transforms into a master – to the painter Christoph Haizman and Fyodor Dostoevsky, to whom Freud devoted articles, up to Hegel – "the most sublime hysteric", and ends up with scientists who define themselves by falsifying their teachers' theories. The hysteric as subject, however, entered psychoanalysis through a series of women, whose ancestors came from religious orders: the nun ($\$$) and her confessor (S_1). Behind them, in turn, are two shadowy counterparts, a couple that reveals what is really at work: the witch ($\$$) and her judge (S_1). The witch, the classical paradigm of the hysterical subject, is seeking a master, God, whom she can govern by proving that he is ignorant of the intimate mainspring of her desire. Human masters (confessors), who parade themselves as God's lieutenants, are left to choose between renouncing their beliefs or burning the woman who could make them doubt them. This relation also occurs in medicine, for example, in the couple formed by a hypnotist (S_1) and the woman who is subjected to his suggestions ($\$$);

thanks to Charcot, Freud encountered them in his youth. Let us note that in order to bring out what is at stake in analysis, Freud had to resort to a degraded form of it, one in which a two-person relation was transformed into a relation between a neurotic, on the one hand, and a "professional", on the other.[11]

Lacan (1968b, p. 7) criticised Didier Anzieu's (1959) thesis that Freud, in order to authorise himself as an analyst, had to undergo a "self-analysis". Lacan (1968b, p. 7) argues instead that Freud placed a "quack", Fliess, in the position of analyst: the position of someone (*a*) who aroused and sustained his desire to speak or write about the most intimate aspects of his questioning of himself as subject ($\not{S}$). Freud was thereby led to proffer his free associations – the master-signifiers of his life (S_1), to which no one else had access – to Fliess. What is important in this context is not whether this treasure was confided to good or bad hands; what is significant, instead, is that, when Freud discovered his colleague's lack of consistency and took his distance from him, he gave him a zero as an analyst. In other words, he did not name Fliess, retroactively, as an analyst. Yet this is what enabled Freud to name himself, in ordinal terms, as the first analyst.

This moment of naming constituted a decisive break. It would therefore be a mistake to reduce the forms of discourse by tracing their outlines onto historical figures, thereby reducing their polyvalence. The opposite movement is more appropriate: the emergence of analytic discourse should be considered as the one single historical moment. On its basis, the atoms and articulations of discourse can then be reassembled, by deconstructing their historical manifestations. This can be done by recognising the barrier between production and truth, a barrier instituted by jouissance. Such a recognition can occur, for example at the very moment that an analysand describes – with an exactitude that can be called absolute – the way in which he has been enclosed in the fantasy, an enclosure from which – he concludes – there is no exit. Perhaps what is needed would be to indicate that, with these words, he is speaking of himself as a statement [*énoncé*], and that his enunciation is not locked into it. This is not, however, enough. What encloses him is his adherence to his discourse, which has been transformed into a universe. As a consequence, he brings about his fantasy by speaking of it.

He needs then to stay quiet and allow – without being able to do anything about it – a meteor to appear; this meteor, in his speech, will come from two places at once, situated on both sides of the barrier: from S_1, according to the principle of free association, and from knowledge (S_2). The schema of the analytic discourse marks out two trajectories for the movement from knowledge (S_2) to the subject ($\not{S}$): one of them is direct and the other passes via *a*.

Lacan writes this process in the following way:

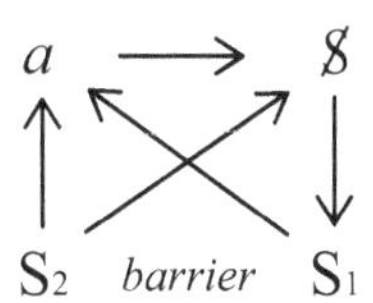

Discourse of the Analyst

Thus, there are four terms: $\$$, S_1, S_2, *a*. Yet before entering into the circular movement of discourse, we need to find a sort of governing principle that will enable us to grasp the meaning of each of these terms and to avoid, if possible, any misunderstanding that would be related to our regular semantic habits.

$\$$: the "barred" or "divided" subject. With this term, Lacan refers especially to Freud's final works, which argue that there is an intrinsic splitting (*Spaltung*) in every subject. a splitting between the recognition and the disavowal of the mother's castration.

S_1: the "master-signifier". This denotes the signifier that commands, or perhaps more precisely, the signifier of truth, which can be located easily in the slip of the tongue. In *The Psychopathology of Everyday Life*, for example, Freud (1901, p. 59) reports a slip of the tongue made by the President of the lower house of the Austrian Parliament, who, in opening a session, expressed publicly his secret wish: "I . . . herewith declare the sitting *closed*!". "Closed" is the master-signifier; it is the master, especially, of the subject who pronounces it.

S_2: "knowledge". In the preceding example, "closed" is a single signifier that represents the subject at the moment when it is said. Knowledge, on the other hand, is an articulation of signifiers. The unconscious is the knowledge that analytic treatment seeks to decipher; this deciphering occurs by interpreting not only the dream, but also the unconscious formations that manifest themselves in a subject's conduct and choices. Because all knowledge is constituted by the symbolic, which, as we have just seen, cannot absorb the real, knowledge must include a kernel that remains irreducibly unconscious. In order to forestall a confusion, I would like to emphasise that the reason that this kernel remains unconscious is not because something in it is ineffable or unsayable, or because since the real is supposed to be infinite, it would always overflow or be ahead of knowledge. This kernel is unconscious because a subject can only represent itself by excluding something from the representation: it must exclude the point from which it can be represented. The dream offers a metaphor of this point, if only by its multiplication of the figures who can represent the dreamer; yet this metaphor can only be interpreted if the subject, after awakening from the dream, gives up any hope of *knowing the point from which s/he is interpreting*. In this way, the subject is like a diver at the moment when s/he plunges from the diving board.

a: the "object little *a*". Lacan (1981a, p. 11) referred to this as his own invention. In Freud, the object is lacking and therefore becomes the basis of sexuality. This lack is not contingent, but structural, linked to the fact that the subject can only constitute itself as such – as divided – because it is born into a world in which it is spoken of. It is not only spoken of, however; it must also grasp itself through speech, in order to be able to speak (or not to speak) in turn. Lack is therefore to be situated as the result of a sampling or a removal of something from the basis upon and place from which the subject is spoken, which Lacan calls the Other. Once this object (breast, excrement, gaze, voice) has been removed from the Other, it cannot be restored to it; the condition for this withdrawal is the production of a subject. If this process were to be reversed, then the emergence of the subject would have to be annulled, and this is impossible. Lacan calls this "element" surplus-jouissance, or, in French, the *plus-de-jouir*, playing on the double meaning of the adverb *plus*, which denotes both the absence (no more) and the increasing (more) of jouissance. This means, first, that the object *a* cannot be integrated back into the Other; jouissance, in the sense of a mouth that would kiss itself, is impossible. Second, although that jouissance has not occurred, we can nevertheless get off; there is a supplement of jouissance or something that would take its place [*suppléance*]. Such jouissance is permitted as soon as the first, impossible, jouissance has been renounced. This algebra founds Lacan's theory of value, and we shall see how it enables Lacan to drive a wedge into the concept of surplus-value, in which Marx's genius is so clear.

It would not be superfluous to note how this inventory – in order to emphasise the extent to which the psychoanalytic terms, which are sometimes manipulated blindly – implies a syntax whose source lies in experience; the experience of analysis is impossible to model or simulate, and its framework must constantly be refounded through logic.

La Ronde

U

Following the order of the first sequence that Lacan presented, we shall begin with the discourse of the university. The barrier of jouissance is sketched on the bottom line:

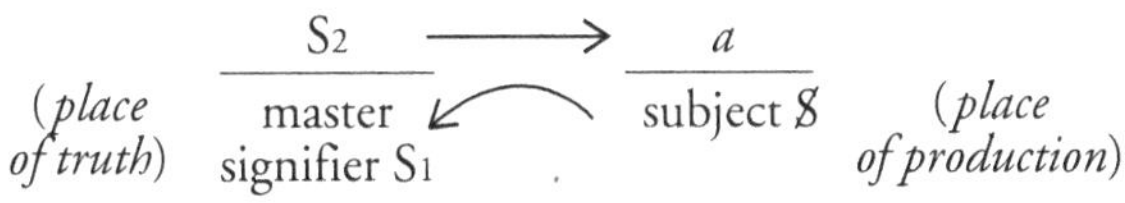

Lacan (1970, p. 445) comments on the curved arrow moving from right to left by noting that "the structure of each discourse necessitates an incapacity or impotence [*impuissance*] within it, which is to be differentiated as a disjunction – always the same – between its production and its truth". In the discourse of the university, this disjunction is "the gap that the subject rushes into, the subject that it [*qu'il*, the discourse] produces by having to suppose that knowledge has an author" (ibid., p. 445). In such a discourse, the subject is unable to articulate a master signifier that could guarantee truth; it is led to posit that knowledge (S_2) – which commands this discourse – has an author. The subject thus personalises the master-signifier and makes it the term from which knowledge originates. The author is a substitute for the absent commander.

A thesis is starting to take shape here: anyone who is unable to occupy the place that commands (S_1 in the discourse of the master) can hide behind knowledge. One of the consequences of this positioning is a misrecognition of the unconscious: a misunderstanding of the incompatibility between knowledge and the subject. The term "unconscious" does not mean "non-conscious"; it refers to the existence of a kind of knowledge that the subject cannot reach, a knowledge that, nevertheless, commands it. We shall see, however, how a subject can be guided by the knowledge contained in the symptom, and that the aim of analytic treatment is precisely to enable the subject to "have a knack [*savoir y faire*]" for being guided by the symptom (Lacan, 1976–1977, 16 November 1976).[12] The author is only a false master, who is supposed to suture S_2 to $\$$. Literary and artistic hacks are perfect illustrations of the consequences of this blunder.

In the discourse of the university, the subject is produced, and is precisely an effect. This irony should not lead us to turn up our noses at this discourse, any more than at any other discourse. What intensifies this irony is that, as we have seen, Lacan made this discourse the paradigm of the Soviet system, after it had been changed first by voluntarism and then by stagnation. In Lacan's own words:

> It is odd to observe that a doctrine such as Marx's whose articulation onto the function of struggle, the class struggle, which he instituted has not prevented it from giving birth to what for the moment is, indeed, the same problem that confronts us all, namely the persistence of a master's discourse. To be sure, the present one does not have the structure of the old, in the sense in which the old is installed in the place indicated under this big M [which designates the discourse of the master]. The present one is installed in the place on the left, the one capped by the U [which designates the discourse of the university]. I will tell you why. What occupies the place there, which we will provisionally call dominant [on the upper left], is the S_2, which is specified as being, not knowledge of everything [*savoir de tout*] – we've not got to that point yet, but knowledge taken as a whole. Understand that what is being affirmed is nothing other than knowledge, which in ordinary language is called the bureaucracy.
>
> *(Lacan, 1991, p. 31. translation modified)*

According to Lacan, the discourse of the university involves a "bending" of the discourse of the master. The "socialist" system still falls under the heading of this discourse of the master, which Lacan deplores. Next, in a certain way, the discourse of the university consolidates that of the master. It masks the fact that, beneath knowledge, the term that commands, there is S_1, a hidden master who claims to speak from the place of truth, whereas in the discourse of the master, the master only speaks in the name of a commandment that he takes upon himself, without claiming to do so in the name of truth. We can hang the portrait of Stalin onto S_1 and the acronym of the communist party of the Soviet Union ("CPSU" in the matheme that follows): this characterises the discourse of the university, which can be completed by the "new man" who will be produced (in the place of $\$$), and the mixture of material stimulus/ideological stimulus in the place of *a*:

$$\frac{\text{CPSU}}{\text{Portrait of Stalin}} \longrightarrow \frac{\text{Material Stimulus / Ideological Stimulus}}{\text{The New Man}}$$

The other problematic trait of the discourse of the university is that by placing knowledge in the position of the agent, free rein is given to the subject's temptation to make itself its own cause (*causa sui*), and thus the equal of God. We know that Saint Augustine tried to head off this slippery slope at the beginning of *On the Trinity*:

> those who suppose that God is of such power that he actually begets himself, are if anything even more wrong, since not only is God not like that, but neither is anything in the world of body or spirit. There is absolutely no thing whatsoever that brings itself into existence.
>
> (*Augustine of Hippo, 400 CE, pp. 65–66*)

This radical criticism of the idea of the *causa sui*, which reappears in almost identical terms in Nietzsche, enables Lacan (2005a, p. 64) to argue, in his comments on this text of Augustine in the single session of his seminar on the Names-of-the-Father, that there can only be a cause *after* the emergence of desire.

M

The discourse of the master is the twin of the discourse of the hysteric. This relation has remained the primal *Prägung*, or imprint, of psychoanalysis since Dora, after her short treatment, moved from the position of agent in the discourse of the hysteric to that of agent in the discourse of the master. Her swerve can be imputed to Freud's error in interpretation, which was not, however, the heart of the matter. Dora was satisfied by having found in Freud the prototype of the castrated master: the master who is always mistaken when he claims that he is able to reach the truth of the hysteric. She then wanted to act as master within the social bond, a movement that prefigures one of the outcomes of every institution, including the analytic institution.[13]

The discourses of the master and the hysteric form a couple, and it is in this coupling that the master experiences the failure of his knowledge; when the hysteric calls upon him to be a "real" man, he can only produce a knowledge that does not reach what causes this requirement. Correlatively, because he has not succeeded in being a man, he is not able to get a woman to be the "cause of his desire" (I am not saying "object"). Because this surplus-jouissance escapes him, the master turns to the slave – situated in S_2 – to produce it. Here again, however, the relation between the master-signifier and the slave's knowledge is marked by an impossibility: that of governing knowledge. Finally, it will only be possible to "circumscribe the real" of this impossibility on the basis of that lack-in-jouissance [*manque-à-jouir*]; in Dora, for example, this lack is presented in the $\$$ of the discourse of the hysteric at the "beginning", but is maintained "at the end" in the discourse of the master (on the lower left). To move from a specific example to the level of structure, we can say that the reason for this impossibility can be read in the matheme itself, on the lower line, where the terms on the left and the right are disjoined by the barrier of jouissance.

There is no relation [*rapport*] between the $\$$ and the *a*. It is as if the subject were at the Arctic Circle and the object *a* were in Antarctica, or vice versa. The subject is fundamentally a lack-in-jouissance, for it is separated from the object *a*, which does not fill it up. In the order of jouissance, the plus does not saturate the minus. Lacan says this in another way when he argues that there is no sexual relation: there is no sexual solution to the differentiation of sexed beings.

We can now write the matheme of the discourse of the master:

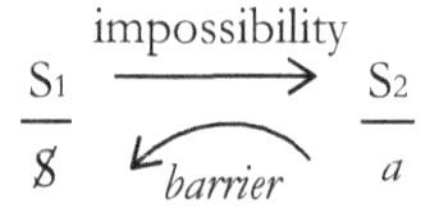

Discourse of the Master

This writing refers to the relation between the ancient master and slave.[14] The master (S_1) uses the slave's technical knowledge in order to produce (*a*). The transformation of labour-power into commodities would authorise Marx to name this "surplus-value", but generically, this is a surplus-jouissance; it is produced by the process in which the renunciation of jouissance turns out to be the only way of capitalising loss. Surplus-jouissance takes on its value in the master's inaugural abdication of a jouissance that has already been lost.[15] In analytic treatment, repetition can point to this process; it shows us how, through the repetition of a loss (a series of bungled actions), desire tries to give a renewed impetus to itself, to recreate a cause.

In *The Accursed Share*, Georges Bataille (1967), following Marcel Mauss, saw the pre-capitalist temptation towards an economy of expense; in the potlatch, this would give rise to an unrestrained jouissance that would be devoted entirely to glorifying the clan and its chief. An alternative to capitalism cannot, however, be anchored in a return to this economy, any more than astrology would enable us to go beyond scientism. Indeed, beyond such a dated example of the master-slave dialectic, what the discourse of the master founds is the discursive status of the unconscious. The term "master", like its French counterpart "*maître*", condenses two meanings that are distinct in Spanish: a slave-owner (*amo*) and an intellectual authority. For Lacan, this master is the allegorical and then historical figure of the signifier One. Within language, this signifier sets a limit to divisibility. Because it is a single and therefore not a differential signifier, it is only a virtual signifier. As Aesop says, *Hic Rhodus, hic salta*, Rhodes is here, here is where you jump. Until we consent to enter into the logic that will provide the key to the decisive homology between the unconscious and the discourse of the master, we can understand nothing about it.

To issue a first signifier is to take the risk of commanding; this brings with it the certainty that meaning will come about, for the first signifier can only be understood in the locus of knowledge, where it takes a place. The problem is that it can only take a place there at the price of being elided. This is how Lacan's formula, which has often been discussed at great length, "A signifier represents the subject for another signifier", is to be read. As soon as a signifier begins to represent the subject, rather than something that is not subjective, its status changes. It becomes the signifier that represents the subject as a statement [*énoncé*], and therefore cannot represent it as an enunciation – as the source of the statement. Thus, in the knowledge where it takes up a place, this S_1 is inscribed as what fails to represent the enunciation.[16] Without wanting to reassemble psychoanalytic theory as if it were a Meccano set, I shall note that its singular quality, in relation to science, is that it does not efface the constitutive gap between experience and structure, and this leads it to have to consent to a form that is frequently impassioned or rhapsodic. The function of the phallus is to condition the integration of the second signifier into the Other, thanks to the symbolic nihilation – the "elision" – of the first signifier, since S_1 and S_2 cannot coexist. The task of the analysand is to enable each lost S_1 to arise again, to put them back into circulation, through the paradoxical freedom to "say everything" or to speak in spite of everything; in the analytic discourse, each S_1 is produced in a place that is always disjoined from knowledge. Lacan writes this knowledge as S_2; it is a binary articulation of signifiers, in which one of the two signifiers can only figure in the empty place created by the elision of the first signifier.

What is the unconscious? *Before Freud*, it was seen as an anonymous network, one that did not have a locus. *After Lacan*, it has become the discourse of the master. This rather vertiginous leap leads to a corrosive revision of the *doxa*: psychoanalysis is not the midwife of the unconscious, and its job is not to highlight the value of the unconscious by revealing its secret riches. Psychoanalysis does not consist in substituting the unconscious for consciousness. If that were its mission, it would only be carrying out the project of the discourse of the master by enabling neurotics to transform themselves into masters.

The hysteric can do this easily, while the obsessional remains ambivalent about acceding to this status: can he want what he does not desire? The psychotic, finally, is not outside this movement, since, according to Lacan (1973a, p. 379), the "experience of the impossibility of pulverulent discourse" is "the Trojan horse by which the psychotic can enter the city of discourse as a master". In direct opposition to the avatars that reduce it to being an assistant to bureaucracy, psychoanalysis teaches the master that the unconscious is nothing more than a knowledge cut adrift, which no subject can master. A *subjectless knowledge*: this is the only definition that enables us to deliver the unconscious from the dimension of the psychic and its ideology of mastery. The unconscious is real. The discourse of the master teaches us that the unconscious commands us, but at the price of the subject's being elsewhere. This formulation may seem surprising and unorthodox, since it implicitly casts doubt on the phrase, "subject of the unconscious". This is quite precisely, however, what Lacan says (2006a, p. 385): the master "is strictly what we call the unconscious . . . namely what is unknown to the subject itself as such – an unknown from which the subject is absent and from which the subject is only represented elsewhere".

We can now reread the discourse of the master from this perspective. The passion for castration induced by the unconscious is the same passion that is refound in the renunciation of jouissance, a jouissance that has, in any case, been abolished. The master knows how to recuperate the best of this inaccessible jouissance through the magic object that transforms loss into surplus-jouissance. This, however, should be noticed: it is as master rather than as subject ($) that he benefits from surplus-jouissance. In other words, *a*, the surplus-jouissance produced by this discourse can only be satisfying when it excludes the symptom from reality; this is satisfying because the symptom signals a real that could shake up the fantasy. For these reasons, the discourse of the master is the reverse of analytic discourse. Fortunately for analytic discourse, the barrier of jouissance is preserved in the discourse of the master, thereby leaving us some hope.

H

In the discourse of the hysteric, the barrier of jouissance is located between S_2 and *a*: no knowledge produced by the master can grasp the truth of what makes the hysterical subject desire.

Freud's first clinical approach was centred on hysteria. Can hysteria, however, be equated with the discourse of the hysteric? A formula of Lacan's (1991, p. 129) – the "hysteric wants a master she can reign over" – invites us to do so. Yet if we consider that discourse marks out a mode of the social bond rather than of neurotic functioning, it would be better to emphasise that this social bond highlights desire, its just positioning – or just its positioning – in a way that concerns every subject, and not only hysterics; similarly, obsessional neurosis does not constitute a discourse but it does enable us to theorise the nature of thought. In this sense, the discourse of the hysteric is both valuable and irreplaceable, in large part because it locates desire in the place of the agent, as $, on the top left:

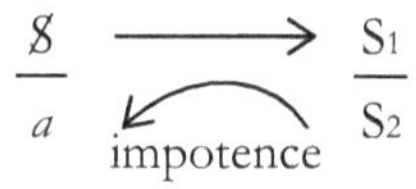

Discourse of the Hysteric

This discourse demonstrates and condemns the master's inability – and even impotence – when confronted with the task of producing a kind of knowledge about what causes the subject's desire. Thus, on the one hand, this discourse discredits the master, and on the other, it retroactively shows the necessity for the desiring subject of choosing a master in order to evict him from this position. This perpetual movement – based on the impotence or incapacity of knowledge (S_2) to do justice to the cause of desire (*a*) – maintains desire, but as unsatisfied. In castrating the master, the hysteric is also not sparing the father, thus suppressing the real agent who could lead her/him to consent to the mother's castration. This is one of the ambiguities of some currents of feminism, which may seek to promote the couple constituted by the hysterical subject and the castrated master as a general rule in culture. The emancipatory ideal is thus undermined by an economy of jouissance in which the sought-for partner is castrated (a class from which it would be false to exclude machos), which consequently leads to an impasse concerning that which cannot be castrated, something that every speaking being must come up against in order to gain access to the Archimedean point that would enable reality to be changed. *For each castrated master, there is a mother who remains untouchable.*

What is in question, to be still more precise, is desire, insofar as the subject makes itself the agent of discourse. It is therefore not enough to treat this desire as the best part of the social bond (this is the case even if desire, in Lacan, is Pauline, and can be deduced from the law). We saw this in our reading of Deleuze and Guattari's (1972, 1980) *Capitalism and Schizophrenia*. Even if desire is made schizophrenic, it is not certain that it can be cleansed of its tendency to become the subject's excuse: the subject can simply proclaim, "that's my choice", one in which any consideration of the other (person) would tend towards zero. Such a choice could manifest its vague hopes only in a dazzling but inconsequential display of the law of the heart or in that of the various cynical forms of the beautiful soul. Lacan took these two essential figures of subjectivity from Hegel (1807), who was himself inspired by Schiller's (1781) *The Robbers*; they cannot be reduced to a neurosis, but instead exemplify a subjective position. Certainly, in order not to be tempted to make this discourse moral by demoralising desire, we should note that if the hysterical subject was Freud's muse, she was also and remains the vestal virgin who worships truth; through the discourse of which she is the agent, she defends the truth of desire against the education/instruction of the master.[17] However, the best expression of this position is, rather, that the essence of desire can only be put to the test in wanting.

A

Last but not least, there is the discourse of the analyst. It is characterised by authorising a desire that is not a subject's desire but originates in a semblance of the object. This proposition of Lacan's is clearly as scandalous as Freud's attack on the equivalence between the psyche and consciousness and his daring thesis that there is an unconscious thinking. In this discourse, we encounter a non-subjective desire! Lacan's discovery begins and ends here.

It should be said at once that this desire without demand (see Lacan, 2001b, p. 370) is dissociated from the desire that manifests itself in the discourse of the hysteric, a desire that is attached pathetically to the subject; in the analytic treatment, this new desire has been transferred to the semblance of the object, which alone can be adapted to fit this unrepresentable object. Thus, a first conclusion already appears: by situating the subject of desire in the place of the other, the analytic discourse becomes the only discourse to apprehend the other – not the counterpart [*semblable*], but the other in its non-(veri)-similitude [*l'in-(vrai)-semblable*] – as a subject.

From the preceding discussion, the reader has probably been able to deduce the matheme of the analytic discourse:

$$\frac{a}{S_2} \; \underset{\swarrow}{\xrightarrow{\text{impossibility}}} \; \frac{\$}{S_1}$$

Discourse of the Analyst

Just as it is impossible for the master (S_1) to command knowledge (S_2), so it is also impossible for the analyst (*a*) to command the analysand ($\$$). This is a way of indicating the opposition between suggestion and psychoanalysis. During the treatment, however, transference covers over and masks this impossibility. An end, however, can be envisioned by remembering that although transference is a form of alienation, it also arouses, in the subject who trusts it, a desire for free association, which can be written as $\frac{\$}{S_1}$. Resolving transference conditions the conclusion of analysis; this comes within the grasp of the analysand as soon as s/he has experienced – an experience that requires patience – the inability of the signifier that has been produced (S_1) to represent her/him for the other signifier. Between what s/he says (S_1) and what s/he knows (S_2), there is a disjunction that interdicts jouissance. Accepting this disjunction implies consenting to a situation in which *the symptom, rather than the subject, knows*. One can wonder whether accepting the mother's castration would be equivalent to this new condition, and the answer would be that it both would and would not be. It would be, in the sense that this acceptance is a necessary condition for this change. It would also not be, for this acceptance does not make up for [*supplée*] what the Name-of-the-Father cannot accomplish: the movement beyond the phallic function. In saying this, I am encroaching on what I shall deal with in a more developed way in the final section of this book.

This disjunction and its consequences prove that there is an impossibility, and this condition characterises the relation written on the upper line: $a \rightarrow \$$. This same line will reappear in the capitalist discourse, where it will be marked as possible. Before this discourse can be presented in detail, however, it is necessary to examine the logical framework that Lacan borrowed from twentieth-century mathematical logic; this framework provides the key that will make the logical implication of $S_1 \rightarrow S_2$ intelligible.

Bertrand Russell occupies a central place among Lacan's references. If Russell left to Wittgenstein the sceptic's task of developing the idea of private language, his discovery of the paradox that bears his name remains historically significant, and not only because it eluded and even went against the work of Gottlob Frege (see Russell, 1902). Consider the catalogue of all catalogues that is supposed to list the catalogues that do not contain themselves. If this catalogue is on that list, there is a problem, because the catalogue is supposed to contain the list of all catalogues that do *not* contain themselves, which this catalogue now does, and this means that it violates the very definition of what a set is. Yet if the catalogue is *not* on the list, there is a problem as well, because it should, as a catalogue that does not contain itself, appear there.[18]

Russell formulated this contradiction in 1901, at roughly the same time that Freud's *Interpretation of Dreams* was published. It expresses the relation between language and speech perfectly, and highlights what Lacan (see 1973b, p. 483) called the "aspherical" character of this relation. The paradox allows us to define the master signifier, S_1, as the signifier that is a member of the set *even if it should not be*. If we remove the master signifier from the set, the latter will no longer contain itself, and therefore the master signifier should be a member of it. The S_2 is the second signifier, whose status is based in the fact that the first signifier has been excluded. This is what happens every time language is used in any way, even in baby talk, as we understand it. This logic controls how signifiers are differentiable from each other, and it runs counter to Saussure's idea about the two sides of a sheet of paper.[19] Of course, we could settle for saying that if there is only one signifier, nothing can be signified (everything is, say, a "strumpf") and that, for this reason, it is necessary to take the inherently differential or oppositional character of the signifier into account: "black" is not "white". However, that would be quite inadequate and would lead us to miss Lacan's essential point here.

The S_1 – the signifier called the "first" – is always an intruder in relation to the Other, that is, to the "treasure trove of signifiers" (Lacan, 1960, pp. 682, 684). That signifier belongs to language without belonging to language. What becomes of the second signifier – the signifier that, because it is not in the set, should be in it – in this case? It cannot be a member of the set, because if it were, it would become S_1. And here is the truly ingenious part of what Lacan does. What happens is that since this S_2 cannot be subsumed [*inscrit*] within language, it is subsumed [*inscrit*] within the body. It is written [*inscrit*] there as the signifying cut that is the Freudian part object: an object that has been removed from the body (breast, excrement, gaze, voice) and become separate from it. The halting movement, in which the master signifier is intrusively written [*inscrit*] into language while the second signifier is written [*inscrit*] into the body, sets up the disparity between the unconscious and the drive or, in the dichotomous terms of Freud's second topography, between the unconscious and the id. While the unconscious is a master who orders us around, the drive, literally, drives us – it steers [*conduit*] or sidetracks [*dérive*] us – for, as bound up with the living body, or better, with the way in which the symbolic is incorporated into the body, it produces and feeds jouissance insofar as the latter is condensed into the drive's objects. In this sense, the drive is the response to what, as far as jouissance is concerned, imposes itself as the consequence of Russell's paradox: *the locus of the signifier is the non-locus of jouissance*.

In *Jokes and Their Relation to the Unconscious*, a beggar who has borrowed money from a more prosperous acquaintance is surprised when his benefactor criticises him for using the money to order salmon mayonnaise at a restaurant: "I don't understand you . . . if I haven't any money I can't eat salmon mayonnaise, and if I have some money I mustn't eat salmon mayonnaise. Well, then, when am I to eat salmon mayonnaise?" (Freud, 1905, p. 50). An even better example would be Lacan's (1966f, p. 114) ironic remark that Marie-Antoinette made cake the object of psychoanalysis since it was "not to scarce bread, but to cake that the Queen sent her peoples in time of famine". Such is the object of psychoanalysis: something that is cut like a remnant [*reste*] from what has not been traced out between S_1 and S_2. This is a solution to Russell's paradox, but not one that Russell himself would have proposed, for he was stuck in the universe of propositional logic. In this solution, the signifier that should be in the symbolic because it is not there is, nevertheless, not lost; instead it operates from within the body, condensing jouissance on the inner and outer borders of the object of the drive.[20]

Incidentally, S_2 should be considered as both the second signifier and the link between the first and second signifiers. This linking is not achieved by adding the first and second signifier together, since that would involve sidestepping the problems raised by Russell's paradox. It is a linking that is *heterogeneous*, inasmuch as the signifier that represents the subject can only be in the set that includes the second signifier if, and only if, the second signifier is excluded from that set. This is how Lacan's time in the guild of structuralists came to a close.

Let's take a break.

I could have called this chapter "The Birth of Aphrodite and Athena". These myths provide two different ways of throwing cold water on the assertion that new life is generated when a man and a woman come together, and also, in a subtle way, on the belief that there is a sexual relation which can be written as "xRy".

This would be a good place to try to shed some light on how psychoanalysis creates another axiom, one that requires us to draw a distinction between being-though-generation [*l'être générationnel*] produced by mommy-daddy – a holophrase that is almost a hologram – and the being of the symptom [*l'être de symptôme*], that opposes the generational. We are going to see the consequences of this.

Notes

1 In this passage, Lacan (1960, p. 682) describes the Other is a "treasure trove" rather than a code. At the end of his teaching, starting with *Encore* (Lacan, 1975c), he examines the status of the Other's existence, which is not to be confused with its logical inconsistency. In his final work, the Other becomes the Other-than-the-Real, i.e. meaning. What are the consequences of this definition if "meaning is always religious" as Lacan (1980a, p. 130) wrote in the "Letter of Dissolution" of the *École freudienne de Paris*?

2 It is probably not mere chance that contemporary philosophers such as Agamben (2002) and Derrida (2000) have again taken up a question that seemed to have been fully worked out: what distinguishes humans from animals? It is worth recalling that Wittgenstein (1953, PPF i § 1) was asking this as well, at the very beginning of *Philosophy of Psychology – A Fragment*: "One can imagine an animal angry, fearful, sad, joyful, startled. But hopeful? And why not?"

3 Her real name was Ida Bauer.

4 The "real", however, is not synonymous with trauma. One could go so far as to say that by making the real a word, one effaces its semantic value as an "anti-word", since the real and meaning are mutually exclusive.

5 "Vociferate" means "to give a voice to" (from the Latin "*vox*" and "*ferre*").

6 We recall the great spectacle that was made of the first Gulf war.

7 [*Translator's note*: see Freud (1925, p. 237):

> The other sort of decision made by the function of judgement – as to the real existence of something of which there is a presentation (reality-testing) – is a concern of

the definitive reality-ego, which develops out of the initial pleasure-ego. It is now no longer a question of whether what has been perceived (a thing) shall be taken into the ego or not, but of whether something which is in the ego as a presentation can be rediscovered in perception (reality) as well. It is, we see, once more a question of external and internal.]

8 It has been shown that the translation of the Russian term used by Lenin in *Materialism and Empirio-criticism* as "*reflet* [reflection]" is incorrect.

9 [*Translator's note*: See, for example, *Waiting for Godot* (Beckett, 1954).]

10 Marx does not agree with this effacement of truth. For example, there is the truth of the proletariat, which he makes a subject – and, moreover, a collective one – without worrying that the "truth of the subject" might cover over an abuse of ethics.

11 Norifumi Suzuki's 1974 film *School of the Holy Beast* illustrates this debasement with all the cruelty that could be desired. The list of books dealing with the holy bond between the priest and the witch is too long to mention here. It has become common to note that a dash of the sacred adds spice to profane eroticism. Michelet's (1862) classic, *Satanism and Witchcraft*, can be mentioned, as can Michel Carmona's (1988) *Les diables de Loudun*, Robert Mandrou's (1979) collection *Possession et sorcellerie au XVIIe siècle*, and finally, the summa by Mario Praz (1933), *The Romantic Agony*.

12 Nerval's (1855) *Aurélia* enables us to distinguish between being an author (which anyone can become) and becoming a writer (which is not self-evident). On the basis of his symptom, which can be qualified, from the outside, as a psychotic episode, Nerval opens up a new relation to life, by means of an experience of writing that makes dreams, delusions and even hallucinations into a sort of compass. Thus, from the inside, he constructs a "reality", a term that is usually taken to be inimical to dreams, delusions and hallucinations, and highlights a dimension of reality that is ordinarily covered over.

13 Doesn't the substitution of initiation for psychoanalysis correspond, in terms of the extension of these words, to the substitution of institutions for associations? This is a very important and relevant question that is not unrelated to "article 52" passed by the French parliament in 2004. [*Translator's note*: This controversial amendment to France's public health code, which is sometimes referred to as the "Accoyer amendment" after the deputy who proposed it, set regulatory restrictions on the use of the term "psychotherapist" by clinicians practicing in France.] In any case, it is alarming when prominent psychoanalysts start writing that an analyst is trained *in* and *by* the institution, without mentioning that an analyst is produced, first of all, by his/her own treatment. It involves a sort of pre-Kantian determination to suppress, as it were, the resistance of the air so as better to clip the wings of the dove.

14 In the new French translation of Hegel's *Phenomenology of Spirit*, Jean-Pierre Lefebvre notes that the German term "*Knecht*" means "vassal". [*Translator's note*: The English translator of this work, A.V Miller, renders the same term as "Bondsman" (see Hegel, 1807, p. 111).]

15 The "calculation" involved in Pascal's wager is, in this respect, the strict computus of the discourse of the master. As Lacan (2006a, p. 396) notes: "Pascal was a master and, as everyone knows, a pioneer of capitalism". This assertion has the value of dissipating the misunderstanding that Pascal's wager prefigured analytic treatment. For example, see Michel Bousseyroux (2001, p. 31): "whoever wagers, like Pascal, from 'nothing to infinity', wagers only from 'dad' to worse, a wager that will not be disappointing". This contradicts what Lacan (2006a, p. 396) says about the wager: "Every time there is a wager about life, it is the master who is talking". In other words, this misunderstanding involves not seeing that the life that is at stake in the wager is never one's own; it is the slave's.

16 In one of his final seminars, Lacan (1976–1977, 10 May 1977) clarifies this as follows: "The S indexed as 1 does not represent the subject in relation to S indexed 2".

17 The discourse of the hysteric in particular, is the one in which the *double bind* of the master is revealed in its double meaning. Getting out of neurosis means getting out of this double meaning.

18 [*Translator's note*: Russell's paradox can be visualised as follows (Robinson & Groves, 2002, p. 28):

Let's imagine a catalogues of all catalogues. Is it, or is it not, a member of itself?

– If the catalogue "of all catalogues" includes itself as a member, then it is simply **one more** catalogue among **all** catalogues and is therefore **not** a catalogue of all catalogues.

– **OR, to put the same idea in another way** –

– It is simply one more **class** of catalogue among all other classes of catalogues...

– If this (or any) class of all classes **is** a member of itself – as a catalogue of all catalogues **is** a catalogue –then it should not be in this class which is reserved for though which are not members of themselves...

– however, if it **is not** a member of itself – as indeed a class of all classes cannot be a class of itself – as, e.g., a "group of men" is not a man – then it should be in this class and is therefore a member of itself.

Which is Russell's point: any set "X" (e.g., a catalogue of all catalogues) is a member of itself if, and only if, it is not a member of itself. This is self-contradictory.

]

19 [*Translator's note*: Saussure (1911, p. 132) uses the analogy of a sheet of paper to describe how thought and language cannot be separated from one another:

> A language might also be compared to a sheet of paper. Thought is one side of the sheet and sound the reverse side. Just as it is impossible to take a pair of scissors and cut one side of paper without at the same time cutting the other, so it is impossible in a language to isolate sound from thought, or thought from sound. To separate the two for theoretical purposes takes us into either pure psychology or pure phonetics, not linguistics.]

20 This logic involves the One and the Other. "Other" means that it is not identical to itself; if it were, it would not be Other. This places it in opposition to the "One", which is identical to itself. This "One" is the basis of repetition, i.e. of the fact that jouissance is always lost yet again and lost without ever having been attained. This one (Freud's unary trait) comes each time to mark each new failure with a notch. (This is the opposite of the notches made by prehistoric hunters to note their success in killing their prey.) This marking by the One can only take place because of the existence of language, the supposedly general murder of the thing. This justifies Lacan's qualification of the Other (the place from which language originates) as the empty set (Ø). With each failure to reach jouissance, the object *a* – surplus jouissance [*plus-de-jouir*] – emerges in the place of the empty set. The object *a* indicates both that there is no longer any jouissance [*la jouissance n'est plus*] and that, at the same time, because it has been reduced to nothing, it wants more [*elle en veuille plus*]. Something else needs to be written: the One of the extra signifier [*signifiant en plus*]; because it has not been proffered in new speech, it is not in the Other.

These actions give us some simple formulas: first 1 (1, Ø), then 1 (1, *a*). Within the parentheses (1, Ø) or (1, *a*), we must read S_2, knowledge, which is constituted not by adding together 1 + 1, but by the pairing of the two heterogeneous elements. It was to qualify these relations that Lacan, in one of his final seminars, made a clarification that I have already quoted: "The S indexed as 1 does not represent the subject in relation to S indexed as 2".

4

THE CAPITALIST EXEMPTION

A discourse without loss

1

Here is the matheme of the capitalist discourse:[1]

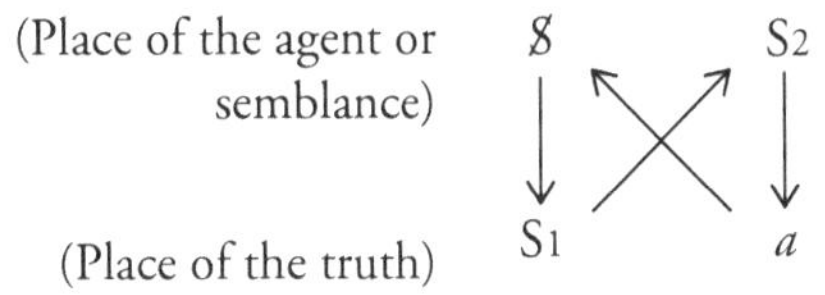

The matheme is constructed by inverting the terms found in the places of the semblance (or of the agent) and truth in the discourse of the master: $\$$ is now in the position of S_1 and vice versa. The direction of the arrow between $\$$ and S_1 remains unchanged, so that, in the capitalist discourse, it now moves from the top to the bottom. As a final modification, the arrow that had gone from *a* to S_1 moves from *a* to $\$$. The consequences of these changes require some comments.

Pleasure, like unpleasure, is a physiological reality. Jouissance is of a different order; if it does not exist without the body – the body as organism – it also does not exist without knowledge. In skipping the barrier of jouissance, it also skips an obstacle, the nature of which gives rise to a promise that can be kept only through annihilation. Jouissance is a "negative substance". This means that by speaking, I destroy myself as thing and that this self-virtualisation would provide me with jouissance if I were not, as a candidate for jouissance, annihilated by this very candidacy.[2] How can we get out of this infernal circle, even though those tormented by Satan (and this may well be Satan's hope) have the chance to participate in jouissance through his dark side? This dark side, in turn, is not as bad as vanity, abandonment or an emptiness of affect, to use the most common vocabulary. The central thread of this questioning has been woven in and out through the space/time of thought; the relief and even enthusiasm of the postwar period went hand in hand with a degradation, one that emerged through an emphasis on the absurd. Its herald was Albert Camus' (1951) *The Rebel*.

2

The Milan lecture, in May 1972, entitled, "On the Psychoanalytic Discourse", introduces the matheme of the capitalist discourse; through it, Lacan, brings out the impact of this use of language and suggests a way out of this nightmarish Möbius strip, provided that we are able to open this door. Perhaps an example – an unusual one for this context – may help us grasp what is at stake in this problem. In an analytic session, you go deliberately against Freud's advice not to look for information about how things "really" happened; you say to a female analysand, "You could ask your mother about this". During the next session, she tells you, "I couldn't ask my mother anything", and then adds, "It's like the time when my mother asked me, 'Whom do you prefer: your father or me?'" Nothing could stop her from hearing the analyst's words as coming from the Other of transference. The analyst's enunciation was reduced to the mother's, who, by her question, had closed the child up in a transferential cage: either you prefer me, or you don't really love me. If this analysand were to ask the mother anything, no matter how small, it would become the equivalent of the answer that she had not wanted to give at the time: I prefer you. As a result, she could only see her analyst as her mother's ally. The analyst, whom she had wanted to become her liberator, became her jailer.

This slippage was not as unfortunate as it may seem, since it helped the analysand to say something new about the closing-off of her relation with her mother. In the present context, it can provide us with the prototype of a way of leaving the capitalist discourse. In order to see how it can do so, we need to examine things more closely. The demand contained in the analyst's initial suggestion has a signification and can be understood "objectively" by approaching it simply in terms of its vocabulary and syntax. The analysand, however, apprehends it on a different plane; she hears it in a specific context, thus modifying its "objective" signification. As a result, following this suggestion would be the equivalent of accepting what she has always refused her mother: to enter into a transferential relation with her that would not be exclusive, but would take precedence over others. This then leads her to take a further step: she thinks that the analyst was asking her, indirectly, to treat her relation with him as more important than everything else. Let us say that *every signification is heard on a level that always affects the message: a meaning is produced that was not contained in the signification.* The "slippage" of the signifier means that the signifier is received on a plane that is always itself slippery. It is slippery because receiving a message involves not only its content and its emitter but also the relation between the receiver and the emitter, a relation called transference.

If we consider this fact in all its breadth, we can conclude, as Lacan notes, that a word can be made to say something very different from what it says. Someone who claims to be an atheist can be shown to believe in God, or psychoanalytic theory can be shown to say something that is the opposite of what one thinks it says, etc. Although in my anecdote, this slippage may seem to be a disadvantage – perhaps an unacceptable one – for the treatment, it is really quite the contrary. Through this misunderstanding, the subject can preserve, or rather bring into existence, the margin of indeterminacy that will enable her to grasp the forced choice of alienation and make it the symptomatic means of emancipating herself. For the neurotic, this will occur through the separation produced by the fantasy; for the psychotic, it will occur through the specific space that authorises him/her to have a delusion. True separation can be encountered, however, only once the fantasy has been dismantled and the delusion has been "stabilized in a . . . metaphor" (Lacan, 1959, p. 498).

These considerations take us to the heart of the questions posed by the capitalist discourse. Hollywood films such as *The Truman Show* or *Being John Malkovitch* portray people's efforts to escape from a virtualisation that seeks to programme them entirely. This virtualisation turns a stage or film set into reality, and thus reduces this fiction to being nothing more than the mapping (in the mathematical sense) of a linguistic function forged by an Other. The capitalist discourse seems capable of generating this sort of universe: "me, clone; you, hologram". In order to escape from this virtualisation, we must make the barrier of jouissance – which the capitalist discourse has rendered inoperative – function again. In psychoanalytic terms, the capitalist discourse dissolves the drive into the unconscious. From Jean Baudrillard to the multimedia artist Tony Oursler, the theme of the cunning triumph of virtualisation has now been fully sketched out. This may also be what the psychoanalyst Jean-Claude Maleval (2003) is evoking with his expression "foreclosure of reference". I myself especially like the French children's show, *Bonne nuit les petits* [Good Night, Little Ones], in which Oscar, the nephew of Nounours, the Teddy bear, turns himself off with a remote control; this shows us that virtualisation can only succeed through the initiative of the agent who is also its object.

Let us look at this problem from a different perspective, that of Orwell's *Nineteen Eighty-Four* (1949). Winston Smith, imputing to Big Brother a determination to make him submit to a sacrificial castration, comes to love Big Brother. Love seems to emerge alchemically from an annihilation to which one consents. This is not a baseless notion, provided that we see that this transformation of the emotion does away with Big Brother, since Big Brother is nothing other than the great persecutor as such.[3]

As we have seen, the unrestrained slippage of the signifier is connected with the fluctuations of all signification. This slippage must also be examined in relation to meaning. Lacan reminds us that S_1, the One of the signifier, rotates through each of the places in the discourse: those of the semblance, the other, the production and the truth. Because it can be translated from one discourse to another, a meaning can be born. This thesis is found explicitly in "*L'étourdit*": "This touches on the fact that meaning is never produced except through the translation from one discourse to another" (Lacan, 1973b, p. 480). Meaning, as distinct from signification, implies that the signifier can be translated. There is meaning only to the extent that there exists something that is outside a purely denotative language; this "outside" is speech itself, inasmuch as it supposes a subject.

Several questions can be raised here. Was Lacan correct in using the term "discourse" to describe the functioning of capitalism? A first error must be eliminated here: a discourse is not a set of words. The expression "capitalist discourse" designates the social bond that stems from the domination of the capitalist mode of production. The term "discourse" has, as it were, been substituted for that of "relations of production" and throws light on certain aspects of these relations. A more difficult objection can also, however, be raised: the disjunction that is internal to jouissance – and which can be found in all of the four discourses – is absent from the capitalist discourse.

Does this absence discredit the use of the term "discourse" in its Lacanian sense? In order not to answer this question too hurriedly, I will simply remark that the barrier of jouissance is not really the condition *sine qua non* of discourse. The necessary condition of discourse, as Lacan reminds us in this lecture, is the semblance: there is no discourse that is not of the semblance.[4] The unchecked slippage of the signifier has a positive aspect: it enables us to exit from the aporia of jouissance. It runs the risk, however, of becoming so uncontrolled that it would destroy the bond assured by the function of language. The semblance prevents this from taking place. The semblance [*semblant*], or its French homophone, *sens blanc* [blank meaning],[5] also takes the side of this slippage; it does so in opposition to language, which claims to make complete and absolute sense of everything. Instead, the semblance permits our exchanges to have an acceptable level of misunderstanding. The objective of theatre is to make this semblance implode, or rather to reveal the conditions that allow it to function, conditions that would otherwise remain unperceived. It happens that, in the capitalist discourse, $\$$ occupies the place of the semblance. If the absence of the barrier of jouissance has a major consequence for this subject, the very fact that it occupies the place of the semblance has a stabilising effect: the semblance enables the capitalist discourse to ward off the inordinate slippage of the signified.

The semblance is what, despite both this slipping and the complete impossibility of jouissance, enables language, through discourse, to create a bond and ensure a regulation and circulation of jouissance; it is able, in principle, to distance us from the spectres of mania or of a *passage à l'acte*, both of which are ways of putting an end to this bond. The price of such regulation is the conventionality and artificiality of our linguistic exchanges, which make the search for the truth of meaning into a bargain; we get it at a cut rate.

In this context, I would like to introduce another unusual but, I hope, revealing example, one that concerns the pharmacist from the preceding chapter. The capitalist subject believes that this figure can reveal what s/he desires, but surprisingly, the pharmacist becomes important here by refusing to sell a product. Through this trick, the capitalist discourse demonstrates its "superior" grasp of desire. It does not satisfy need, for which it substitutes desire. The proletarian would like to have public housing, but instead is offered a villa, thereby placing the subject as consumer in command. From then on, the subject's desire – as consumer and customer – becomes the effect of the reformulation – or interpretation – of the demand by the other, the pharmacist, who is located in S_2. In the matheme of the capitalist discourse, this circuit goes from $\$$ to S_2, by way of S_1, and thus via a master signifier. This principle of authority is concealed (since it is *under* the subject), but it is always necessary in order to certify the kind of knowledge that is in question. In experimental psychology, its trace can be found in the Stockholm syndrome as well as in those chilling experiments that show how submission to authority can turn almost anyone into a torturer. In the matheme, the rising diagonal of the vector that goes from S_1 to S_2 points to this power, which can be found anywhere at any moment. Throughout history, only the discourse of science forged by Descartes' *dubito, sum* has been able to make it totter or tremble, without abolishing it.

The arrow, $a \rightarrow \$$ is found in both the capitalist and the analytic discourses, but it functions in them in completely opposed ways.[6] In the analytic discourse, it is marked by an impossibility. In the capitalist discourse, however, surplus-jouissance (a) is supposed to saturate the lack-in-jouissance ($\$$). Whereas the capitalist discourse promotes the submission of knowledge to a masked authority, the discourse of the analyst writes a permanent disjunction between the master signifier and knowledge, a disjunction that could only be removed if jouissance were to fill up the place of the signifier.[7] Finally, it should be remembered that in the analytic discourse (as in the other three original discourses), one place – truth – has a special status. In the four discourses, you can start out from this place, but you cannot reach it, since the two arrows *move away* from it. This inaccessibility of truth in discourse does not mean that it does not exist. Truth exists and speaks, but you cannot speak it. The capitalist discourse, on the other hand, is constructed in order to *miss* the inaccessibility of truth. Not only is the place of truth accessible, but it must also be passed through in order to reach knowledge. *Truth, in the capitalist discourse, has the same status as it does in astrology; it cannot be falsified.*

The capacity of the mathemes to generate such readings and consequences may be surprising, and this is especially true of the capitalist discourse, which has a somewhat improvised quality. Lacan himself emphasised that these mathemes only "imitated" mathematics, and he sought later, in topology, to find a way of making judgements that would not be subjected to the caprices of language. It is also true, however, that the choice of a (mathematised) writing is, in itself, a choice in favour of science.[8] Writing, with its terms, its signs, its punctuation and its rules for placement in space, imposes orientations and leads to conclusions that limit, a priori, the slippage of the signifier, on the condition that we resist any imaginary instrumentalisation of writing, which, in the end, would involve magic. This is why it is false to say that psychoanalysis, as Karl Popper (1974, pp. 254–255) claimed, is unfalsifiable (an objection that Freud had already perceived). If psychoanalysis is problematic, it is because it is *always* falsifiable, right up until the moment when it ends. Indeed, it could be said that the end of an analysis is the end of the jouissance that comes from falsifying analysis: will [*volonté*] then becomes the safety catch [*cran*] of desire, something that, in the same step, the will understands to be both indestructible and discontinuous. It would not be too extreme to say that the analytic discourse is constructed on the principle of the inaugural and irremediable loss of jouissance, and that the nostalgia for falsifiability is only the ghost of this loss. The capitalist discourse presents itself as a discourse that has no loss and no entropy.

In this discourse S_2 is the slave-servant whose knowledge can be activated. The relation $S_1 \rightarrow S_2$ – the diagonal arrow that goes from the bottom left to the top right – can be transposed onto the capitalist/worker couple, since what intervenes in production is the *savoir-faire* of the labour force: the highly variable degree of the worker's skill, which goes from the status of being semi-skilled to that of engineer.

The S_1 does not possess knowledge; it derives its capacity to command from financial power. The worker obeys and produces surplus-value, which Marx discovered. We know that for Marx, whom no one challenges on this point, capitalism is characterised by the fact that labour-power has become a commodity, just like wheat or iron. Thus, with capitalism, surplus-jouissance (*a*) takes the form of surplus-value. Surplus-jouissance also calls to mind Freud's *Lustgewinn*, the "yield of pleasure", and already in Freud (1905a, p. 28), this yield makes up for the structural failure of jouissance, as is demonstrated by the fact that humour produces a *Lustgewinn*. *Mehrwert*, then, is the extra value produced by the salaried worker, throughout the working day, after having first reproduced the value or his/her labour-power. In order to reproduce her/his capacity to work (education, food, lodging), a worker needs to create a value of, let's say, four daily hours of labour. If s/he works eight hours, however, the difference – eight minus four – constitutes the *Mehrwert*.

In this sense, capitalism precedes and conditions psychoanalysis in shaping jouissance by means of value. This value is exchange-value, not the use-value that must be renounced in order to make the primitive accumulation of capital possible. Something makes our ears prick up here: it is the "surplus", the *Gewinn* (yield), rather than the *Lust* (pleasure). Lacan retroactively introduces into Marx's discovery of surplus-value the element that explains the power of the capitalist discourse. Without substituting surplus-jouissance for surplus-value, it becomes impossible to explain the gap between the "real" economy – which follows the principle of surplus-value – and the economy that functions through globalised finance. Surplus-value only constitutes the motive force of the capitalist mode of production as long as it enables there to be jouissance; if it did not do so, no one would care about it.

Yet who gets off here? A Marxist could retort that the proletarian sells his/her labour-power simply in order to survive: people eat to live rather than live to eat. "The jouissance that you're talking about", this Marxist might say, concerns the capitalist. This objection cannot simply be brushed off, for it comes from the real of the class struggle. However, the "cunning" of the capitalist discourse involves interesting the proletarian in jouissance, and in order to do so, it transforms the proletarian into a consumer, a capitalist subject: the $\$$ is in the place of the agent. Thus, money no longer serves as an instrument of measurement or as the universal equivalent; instead, it is only valuable to the extent that it engenders itself or seems to engender itself, in a parthenogenesis that excludes the productive process.

Marx, according to Lacan (2011b, p. 90), completed the capitalist discourse by giving it "its subject, the proletariat. Thanks to this, the discourse of capitalism has flourished in every nation-state that has taken a Marxist form". This rather daring judgment rectifies his assessment two years earlier, in *The Other Side of Psychoanalysis*, that the Soviet system functioned through the discourse of the university: knowledge, taken as a unified whole, was its agent, and the "new man" was supposed to be produced by it (Lacan, 1991, p. 206). In my opinion, this earlier judgment is correct, but the subsequent collapse of this system gives weight to the later thesis. Concerning this collapse, it would be comic, but fair, to argue that with the dissolution of the Soviet Union, the capitalist discourse experienced its first real defeat. Why not say that the Soviet system constituted the supreme stage of capitalism, for its axioms did not challenge the functioning of the capitalist discourse? The appropriation of surplus-value did not stop. It was distributed differently, and apparently – or, in any case, according to the ideology – S_1 and S_2, the capitalist and the worker, were no longer in an antagonistic relation: the former tried to get people to work too much, and the latter to diminish the amount of labour. Otherwise, the slogan, "we are all capitalists" sapped the Soviet system like the "old mole" (Marx, 1852, p. 185). Since the system was never able to acknowledge that this was its slogan, jouissance tended to get a lot of bad publicity; the proletarians had to renounce it in order to have a better future, while the bureaucracy transformed itself into a bureaucracy of jouissance.

In all this, there are strategies for obtaining jouissance, which can be distinguished in terms of the way in which we conceive of two couples within the discourse: $\$ – S_2$ and $\$ – S_1$. The first of these couples presents us with the two guises of the proletarian: $\$$ is the proletarian whose desire yields to surplus-jouissance (work more to get off more)[9]; S_2 is the worker as producer (work less in order to be less exploited). The other couple shows us the two positions taken by the capitalist. The capitalist is also sundered between the figure who appropriates surplus-value and commands the process, and the subject who consumes. Once this relation has been established, it cannot be revoked. The worker, in S_2, can go on strike, but the capitalist, in S_1, cannot. The capitalist philanthropist or patron of the arts will never go so far as to question the capitalist discourse itself. On the other hand, the capitalist can put him/herself in the ascetic position of subject, without thereby modifying the process. If the proletarian withdraws, as far as possible, from the position of subject of consumption, this will not have much of an effect. It is obvious, finally, that within the framework of the capitalist discourse, if the proletarian consumes more – a change that would go against the grain of the capitalist mode of production – this never puts a stop to the production of wealth.

From this, we must conclude that only the strike, a work stoppage, can constitute the symptom. We must also conclude that highlighting the contradictions between $\$$ and S_2, and between $\$$ and S_1 reveals not a splitting but a sundering. The key to this discourse is the recognition that the necessity of surplus-jouissance is based on the status of jouissance as a "hole that must be filled" (Lacan, 1970, p. 434).

Marx fills this hole through surplus-value. This is why Lacan (1970, p. 434) says that *Mehrwert* [surplus-value] is *Marxlust*, Marx's surplus-jouissance". Surplus-value is the cause of desire, which the capitalist economy makes into its fundamental principle: the principle of extensive production. Capitalist production – the cycle M – C – M′ (Money – Commodity – Money + Money) – implies that consumption must always increase, but this production would come to a sudden stop if consumption actually procured jouissance. Consumption would then halt, production would slow down, and this cycle would end. If this has not occurred, it is because this economy, through a *reversal* that Marx did not foresee, produces a lack-in-jouissance. *The more I consume, the greater the gap between jouissance and consumption becomes.* Thus, there is a struggle involving the distribution of this surplus-value, which "only leads those who are exploited to compete on the basic principle of exploitation, in order to harbour their indisputable participation in the thirst of lack-in-jouissance" (Lacan, 1970, p. 435). Vilfredo Pareto, one of the theorists of neoclassical economics, forged an exquisite expression: the "ophelimity" of a glass of water. Pareto made an incontestable observation: a drinker takes less pleasure in a third glass of water than in the first. He then deduced a law from it: the value of the water decreases in proportion to its consumption. The opposite law, however, governs the capitalist economy, in which we do more than simply drink without being thirsty. Beyond even the drunk who can't say no, in the capitalist economy, "The more I drink, the thirstier I get".

The choreography of love

As we have just seen, in the capitalist discourse, the accessibility of truth goes hand in hand with a suppression of the disjunction between the places of truth and production (on the bottom left and right). This suppression exonerates the capitalist discourse from a requirement that was believed to constitute all discourses.

The other structural characteristic that we have examined is the creation of a vector, $a \rightarrow \$$, which does not exist in the discourse of the master, from which the capitalist discourse derives. This arrow is also not found in the discourse of the hysteric, and although it does appear in the discourse of the analyst, it is marked explicitly as impossible. Only in the discourse of the university, which has a special kinship with the capitalist discourse, does this arrow function.

Within this framework, we can now approach another aspect of the capitalist discourse. As Lacan stated:

> What differentiates the discourse of capitalism is *Verwerfung*, the fact of rejecting, outside all the fields of the symbolic. This brings with it the consequence I have already said it has. What does it reject? Well, castration. Any order, any discourse that aligns itself with capitalism, sweeps to one side what we may simply call, my fine friends, matters of love. You see, it's a mere nothing.

> This was precisely why, two centuries after this slippage, which after all we may call a Calvinist slippage, castration finally made its irruptive entrance in the form of the analytic discourse.
>
> *(Lacan, 2011b, pp. 90–91)*

The heart of this statement is its connection between the setting aside of "matters of love" and the foreclosure of castration. Before we approach it directly, a few remarks can place it in perspective.

First, according to Lacan, love is what makes up for the nonexistence of the sexual relation (where the mere addition of man + woman would give one access to a jouissance that is primary and absolute). There is no sexual relation because of castration, and the acceptance of this nonexistence can authorise a sexual encounter that is contingent (see Lacan, 1975c, p. 145). The foreclosure of castration, on the contrary, has a very different consequence: it makes the sexual relation possible (which can then be indicated by the arrow, $a \rightarrow \$$, which can be read as "a woman fulfils a man"). In consequence, love, as something that makes up for this impossibility, becomes obsolete. The mechanics of sex would then become the physics of love, and there would be no need to differentiate between sex and love; a manual of sexology would be the same as the map of Tendre (see Lacan, 1957b, p. 339).

What is more subtle and difficult is an equivalence that Lacan posits in "*L'étourdit*": "Death [*la mort*] is love [*l'amour*]" (Lacan, 1973b, p. 475). This reminds us of the romance of Iseult and Tristan, in which death does indeed signal love. Either there is love or there is death. Or again, if love, which makes up for the nonexistence of the sexual relation, is an inaccessible outcome, death will do quite nicely. Only death will be able to make up for the situation in which castration has left us. Let us note, to strengthen this reading, that Lacan attributes this equivalence between love and death to Freud. What appears more directly in Freud's work, however, is the equivalence between death and jouissance. If, for Freud, jouissance is impossible for the living being, and is always lost (whatever the status of primary jouissance may be), the sole virtue of love, as distinct from desire, is that it brings with it the promise of something that can make up for this loss. Its narcissistic structure lends itself to this, especially given the lethal foundation of narcissism, and to realise this specularity of love can be deadly.

The foreclosure of castration, the other term involved, is distinct from that of the Name-of-the-Father, which serves as the basis of the distinction between psychosis and neurosis. He uses the arrow, $a \rightarrow \$$ to indicate a subject that, in an asymptotic accountancy, is completed by its surplus-jouissance. At the limit of this accountancy, we can hope to reach an unbarred subject: the "new man", who will soon be joined by the most valuable capital, woman. The cycle Money – Commodity – more Money – which Marx had so impeccably taken apart – is homologous to the Easter computus; by virtue of money, capitalism *virtualises all living things through money creation*. In such an economy, even the cost of death would count for something, and, in contrast to Freud's interpretation, the world would be loveless, with the exception of a religious love for that highly abstract Other, the capitalist system.

What is in question here is the status of death. On the side of psychoanalysis, this is the for-nothing that makes it equivalent to the for-nothing of love, thwarting any full accountancy of the real (what would it cost to buy the universe and who would want to buy it?). On the side of capitalism, death would be transformed into a substance through its commodification, based on an unlimited linguistic virtualisation. The real would be equal to reality and the sexual relation would be necessary; it would be the law by which the world works. This world would be nothing more than the reflection of the sexual relation.

As a result, when Lacan speaks of how castration irrupts back in through the analytic discourse, we should take him at his word: castration, as revealing the *absense* of the sexual relation, only becomes *for itself* with Freud. It had already been indicated, more or less, through the Oedipus complex, which was not, however, enough to permit the *Bejahung* (the yes to . . .) of castration, even if this consent is already present with language.

With the coming of capitalism, everything concerning the action of castration is foreclosed from discourse, starting with "matters of love": this could cause difficulty for the Oedipus complex itself. To mention sexual criminality, which, in changing forms, has always constituted *something of* the scandal of mores, there are two ways of struggling against it: reintroducing castration or transforming the Oedipus complex into a law. The effectiveness of the second solution is limited; only an acceptance of castration can enable the subject to accept such a law. In counting on law, one ends up forging a pseudo-castration, which would be complete and total. This pseudo-castration would only feed the misunderstanding of sexual difference, since it would reduce the feminine to a binary negative term in relation to the masculine.

The foreclosure of castration does not mean the manufacturing of psychotics, for it also concerns neurotics, pushing *both of them* to seek through power – either as masters or as those who benefit from the latter's position – a way to keep castration foreclosed. Can the hysteric and the obsessional neurotic be said to foreclose castration? In his case history of the Wolf Man, Freud (1918) threw light on this foreclosure in a way that can accommodate neurosis (see Sauret, 2009).[10] This suggests that castration cannot be brought wholly and totally into the field of the symbolic. The capitalist discourse transforms this partial restriction into a general rule. It must be emphasised that a misunderstanding of castration is a structural, and not an accidental, part of the castration complex. Such a misinterpretation is inevitable when femininity is not apprehended as being *beyond* castration. Being beyond it means that castration is necessary, but not sufficient.

Now let us examine the context. Lacan (2011b, p. 77) quotes a poem by Paul Fort: "*If all the lasses in the world were to join hands . . . they could make a ring around the world*". Lacan does not content himself with pointing out that the lasses themselves never dreamed of this. Unlike boys, they do not need to make a circle: a circle, for example, of officers or even a Freudian circle. Boys go around in circles because they are afraid of finding themselves alone with one girl. For this reason, it is up to the girl to separate the boy from his circle, from his "*Masse*". Nothing is missing from this choreography of love, not even the fact that before she succeeds in taking a boy out of his circle, a girl will go around with another girl, whom she will then leave on the sidelines, as soon as she has succeeded in kidnapping a boy.

If girls tend to go "two by two", this has its foundation in what Lacan (1962, p. 619) refers to as a jouissance that is "enveloped in its own contiguity". In this respect, feminine homosexuality could be particularised as a relation of Other to Other, and not of same to same. This is the case with the relation between Lol V. Stein and Tatiana, in Marguerite Duras' (1964) novel, *The Ravishing of Lol Stein* (also see Lacan, 1965). Tatiana is the secret side of the other woman, the one who is supposed to know how to make men desire, and who thereby finds herself transformed into a potential companion in jouissance. Could the Female Homosexual's beloved, indeed, be interpreted as a woman who might have been desired by the father?

What can be said of these "matters of love" when they are approached from the feminine side? First, they are different from Freud's conception of Eros, as he presents it in *Civilization and Its Discontents*: "Eros and Ananke have become the parents of human civilization too. The first result of civilization was that even a fairly large number of people were now able to live together in a community" (Freud, 1930, p. 97). Here, Eros proceeds by means of *Vereinigung*, a "making one" or unification with which we are quite familiar. Unification contributes to civilisation, by constituting circles that become larger and larger, going from the clan to humanity.

In Freud's words:

> Since civilization obeys an internal erotic impulsion which causes human beings to unite in a closely-knit group, it can only achieve this aim through an ever-increasing reinforcement of the sense of guilt. What began in relation to the father is completed in relation to the group. If civilization is a necessary course of development from the family to humanity as a whole, then – as a result of . . . the eternal struggle between the trends of love and death – there is inextricably bound up with it an increase in the sense of guilt.
>
> *(ibid., p. 133)*

According to Lacan, love does the opposite: it dissolves the circle by removing an element from it. He thus envisions "matters of love" as a *disunification* and situates love more on the side of Thanatos than of Eros. The mythography of Eros is not at all unilateral.

Claude Lévi-Strauss deserves recognition for having emphasised the positive character of the Oedipal prohibition in *The Elementary Structures of Kinship*:

> If these modalities can be subsumed under the general term of exogamy . . . this is conditional upon the apperception, behind the superficially negative expression of the rule of exogamy, of the final principle which, through the prohibition of marriage within prohibited degrees, tends to ensure the total and continuous circulation of the group's most important assets, its wives and its daughters.
>
> *(Lévi-Strauss, 1969, p. 479)*

Lévi-Strauss thereby covers over matters of love in his own way. He reduces women to values or assets and neglects exoandry, in which men leave their group and join their wives' group. As soon as women are considered as subjects, rather than as goods, this kinship structure takes priority over the others. This angle itself justifies feminism.

The feminine requirement of a minus-one (which may serve as the basis of its monandry) and of an "*Homoinzun*"[11] who will be her own, rather than being a boy like all the others, is not symmetrical with masculine exogamy. We will understand this distinction better if we remember that in order to bear leaving the circle, a man needs to transform *a* woman – the one who has chosen him – into *Woman*, quite simply by locating the Name-of-the-Father in her. This is a law: in order for a man – in this case, a neurotic man – to be able to attach himself to a woman, he must discern a paternal signifier in her. This is how he deals with the trauma of the encounter with the Other sex.[12] In psychosis, this transformation of a woman into *Woman* cannot be effected through the Name-of-the-Father as operator and therefore implies that man himself must become Woman, "the woman that men are missing" (Lacan, 1959, p. 472); without this woman, they are doomed to remain in the circle (as the psychotic will not fail to denounce). For a woman, it should be emphasised that she awakens the man by separating him from the group. This dissymmetry between masculine exogamy and a woman's choice of a man is a part of the dissymmetry between what is generally attributed to man – the fantasy of the *Vereinigung* – and what a woman reveals: love is an election, a choice that implies a dissolution.

We know the extent to which, for Freud, the question of understanding femininity was both decisive and insoluble. He considered anatomical and psychological determinations to be insufficient and concluded with an observation that – although it does not give us a positive definition of what a woman is – does provide a differential assessment: a woman differs from a man because she is not a woman from the moment of her birth but becomes one. Man as *being* is opposed to woman as *becoming*. This is Freud's final lesson.[13] We can wonder why Freud, who had written about the choice of love-objects, did not try to define women through their mode of choosing such objects. In any case, this is what Lacan did.

It can even be claimed that in the sexuation table in *Encore*, Lacan provides a matheme for this mode of choice: the wall – erected by language – between the sexes can be crossed over from left to right – from the phallic side to the side that is not-all – by following an arrow: $\$ \to a$ (Lacan, 1975c, p. 78). Lacan's comments on this arrow leave us in no doubt about how he schematises mens' choice of a love-object: "He is unable to attain his sexual partner, who is the Other, except inasmuch as his partner is the cause of his desire" (ibid., p. 80). After this, if we had the idea – and may God protect us from this – that there is a symmetry between the sexes (which would suppress their differences), we would expect a woman's love-choice to be written as $a \to \$$; this could be the matheme for the masculine cliché of woman as seducer. This is not at all, however, what Lacan writes. Through her choice of sexual partner, a woman inscribes herself in the phallic function: ~~Woman~~ $\to \Phi$. Yet, on the other hand, she has a relation with the Other, not through the intermediary of the *a*, but as radically barred. It does not seem risky to me to read the arrow, ~~Woman~~ → $S(\not{A})$ as indicating the feminine choice in love: it dissolves the set by extracting an element from it. Beyond this, it should be noted that the capitalist discourse defines the vector, $a \rightarrow \not{S}$, as the possible; the movement that would have gone from the not-whole to castration is reduced to something like a supermarket of love and desire, offered up for the subject's consumption. Thus, the capitalist discourse forecloses castration and, when all is said and done, also calls sexual difference into question. The capitalist discourse is Jungian.

This consideration opens up a path for understanding how sweeping aside matters of love can be related to castration in the capitalist discourse. In his "Guiding Remarks for a Convention on Female Sexuality", Lacan (1962) recognises the anti-entropic effects of feminine homosexuality, as they can be observed, for example, in the Précieuses. He also notes, in passing, that the Précieuses differed from the Cathars, who in sundering good absolutely from evil, anticipated the capitalist paradise, or – and this may be the same thing – fuelled a millenarianism the effects of which are not always cheering.

The Précieuses organised themselves in salons at the beginning of the seventeenth century and there is no doubt that they took the initiative in choosing a love-object. According to the classical analyses, such as Paul Bénichou's (1948), men who were admitted into the salon had been taken from the group of knights. This is a fair, if cavalier view. Knights were gradually disappearing, thanks in part to the Précieuses (and had, of course, been given their deathblow by Cervantes, who had mocked the knight errant's desire to preserve chivalry singlehandedly). In the salon, such knights were taught how to speak, rather than to kill or rape. It may well have been this "borrowing" of men that offended Molière, but this does not discredit the Précieuses' mode of choosing love-objects. They are a perfect example of the civilising work of women, which Freud had glimpsed: the dissolving of the group of men and the constructing of a community that acted through *dissemination*.

The Amazons, the other example that comes to mind, raise thornier questions. They are known through Greek mythology, beginning with Homer. Historians have said less about them, since their historical prototypes remain unknown, and it is uncertain whether they really existed. One journalist-historian, Lyn Webster Wilde (2000), in *On the Trail of the Women Warriors*, hypothesises that they had been displaced from the southern to the northern edge of the Black Sea and beyond, towards Ukraine, where numerous tombs of female warriors have been found. In this connection, I find it interesting that the oldest tomb, dating from around 1200 BCE, of a female warrior to have been discovered was in Colchis, in present-day Georgia, the home of Medea. She was accused of killing her two sons, just as certain Greek authors had accused the Amazons of infanticide. Whether or not this is the case, there is one constant in this mytheme: the women chose the men whom they had defeated in battle, after which there was a celebration, the Feast of Roses, where each woman married the man whom she had conquered. The best-known of the Amazons is Penthesilia, their queen, who fell in love with Achilles at the siege of Troy and would have done anything to defeat him and take him away from the circle of the Greeks. If, according, of course, to ancient Greek authors, this circle represented the progress of civilisation, then it is interesting that it was a barbarian who introduced matters of love into civilisation. This is the paradox in which Thanatos civilises Eros, the paradox that Giorgio Agamben (1995) seeks to account for in his stimulating work, *Homo Sacer*. In the myth, it is Penthesilia who is defeated and dies; Achilles, defeated in his turn by his love for her, embraces her, a rather sensational case of male necrophilia.

Heinrich von Kleist's play, *Penthesilia*, reverses this situation by having Penthesilia kill Achilles. Once he is dead, she eats him raw, having the honesty to do so herself, instead of giving this task to her dogs, as Artemis had done with Actaeon.

> How many a maid will say, her arms wrapped round
> Her lover's neck: I love you, oh so much
> That if I could, I'd eat you up right here;
> And later, taken by her word, the fool!
> She's had enough and now she's sick of him.
> You see, my love, that never was my way.
> Look: when *my* arms were wrapped around your neck,
> I did what I had spoken, word for word:
> I was not quite so mad as it might seem.
>
> (Kleist, 1808, p. 146)

In such a context, it can be said that "A kiss, a bite,/The two should rhyme" (ibid., p. 145).

The radical character of these actions provides a dazzling insight into the mysterious cannibalistic primary identification discussed by Freud (Freud, 1940a, p. 103). These women, in the throes of disgust, and whom Penthesilia judges correctly to be mad, are not exempt from a condition that we find in bulimia: bulimics eat the father again and again, because they have not dared really to eat him, as Penthesilia does. We know that in psychosis, this "remake" of primary identification can take the form of psychotic ingestion.

A moment ago, I mentioned Agamben's *Homo Sacer*, which is as important a reference now as Michel Foucault's *The Birth of the Clinic* (1963) was in the 1960s. This book discovers and analyses a logical paradox that can only be solved topologically.

Homo Sacer refers to a very specific Roman law formulated in Festus:

> The sacred man is the one whom the people have judged on account of a crime. It is not permitted to sacrifice this man, yet he who kills him will not be condemned for homicide; in the first tribunitian law, in fact, it is noted that "if someone kills the one who is sacred according to the plebiscite, it will not be considered homicide". This is why it is customary for a bad or impure man to be called sacred.
>
> *(Agamben, 1995, p. 71)*

Agamben thus brings out a contradiction: death is a judicial punishment on the condition that it not take the form of a judicial punishment. In logical terms, an element is subtracted from a set in such a way that it becomes impossible to reintegrate it into any set at all. This logic is the same as what presides over a woman's choice of a man as love-object. Once Achilles has been chosen by Penthesilia, he can no longer be the Greek whom he had once been.[14]

Notes

1 This way of writing the discourses comes from *Television* (Lacan, 1974b, p. 13); it differs from the version found in "*Radiophonie*" (Lacan, 1970, pp. 447–448) in the use of the crossed arrows. The specific matheme of the capitalist discourse can be found in *Lacan in Italia* (Lacan, 1978b, p. 40).

2 The definitive form of this thesis may perhaps be found in Lacan's (1981b, p. 20) opening statement at the 1980 seminar in Caracas: "It follows that the best thing *la langue* can do is to demonstrate how it is in the service of the death instinct".

3 George Orwell, who worked as part of the British secret services after spending the Spanish Civil War in the International Brigades, was not unambiguous in his choice of political camp.

4 [*Translator's note*: In renaming the "agent" of discourse as the "semblance", Lacan was, in part, emphasising the close relation between this semblance – an "appearance" or "seeming" – and truth. As he argues in *D'un discours qui ne serait pas du semblant* (Lacan, 2006b, p. 26) "Truth is not the contrary of the semblance. Truth is the dimension . . . that is strictly correlative to that of the semblance". In discourse, truth is not accessible directly, but something of it can *appear* or manifest itself through the vector that moves from it to the semblance.]

5 [*Translator's note*: See *R.S.I.* (Lacan, 1974–1975, 11 March 1975):

> The Real is "blank meaning" [*sens blanc*], that is, the blank meaning by which the body serves as a semblance [*fait semblant*; could also be read as "the body pretends"]. A semblance in which all discourse coalesces [*se fonde*], starting with the discourse of the master, which turns the phallus into signifier index 1 (S_1).]

6 Serge Lesourd (2006) emphasizes the rising diagonal of $a \rightarrow \$$ and relates it to the matheme for perversion ($a \lozenge \$$), thus connecting capitalism with the epiphany of a subject who is capable of experiencing "jouissance without any constraints". Without discussing directly this identification of the two mathemes, I would note that in the matheme of perversion, the $\lozenge$ of alienation/separation is placed between a and $\$$, rather than an arrow that is oriented in a single direction. It should also be recalled that, according to Lacan (2013, p. 569), perversion involves a logical protest that goes against normalizing identifications. I thank Marie-Jean Sauret for bringing this passage to my attention. [*Translator's note*: The injunction to experience "jouissance without any restraints" was a slogan popular in May 1968.]

7 In this respect, moreover, the discourse of the master, as the discourse of the unconscious, shows us the impossibility of commanding knowledge, whose real aspect is grasped by the analytic discourse.

8 This writing can, moreover, be independent of any transcription of the spoken word, as can be seen in the use of the little arrows in quantum physics (see Feynman, 1985).

9 [*Translator's note*: This is a play on Nicolas Sarkozy's campaign slogan during the presidential campaign of 2007: "Work more to earn more".]

10 It should, of course, be noted that certain analysts consider the Wolf Man to be psychotic.

11 [*Translator's note*: "*Hommoinzun*" is a play on "*au moins un* [at least one]", which introduces a reference to "*homme* [man]".]

12 In "Medusa's Head", Freud (1940, p. 274) describes what he calls the "apotropaic" function: an image of castration, as terrifying as it may be, is better than the unthinkable confrontation with a hole that has no boundaries, which would be an absolute absence.

13 [*Translator's note*: See Freud's late article "Female Sexuality":

> The sexual life of the woman is regularly split up into two phases, the first of which is of a masculine character, whilst only the second is specifically feminine. Thus in female development, there is a process of transition from the one phase to the other, to which there is nothing analogous in males.
>
> *(Freud, 1931, p. 228)]*

14 In psychoanalysis, there is the example of an element that serves as exception to the set: this is the real father, who as agent of castration, re-imposes the primacy of the living being over language.

PART III

On the symptom

5

THE SENSE OF SYMPTOMS

If the symptom raises decisive questions, this is not only because it brings Marx and Freud together, while also separating them; this concept also does the same for psychoanalysts. I shall argue that the symptom is a primal marker of the sexual nonrelation – the constitutive failure of sexuality – which gives sexuality its libidinal colour. Other psychoanalysts however, see it as masking the nonexistence of this relation. In my opinion, this view is contaminated by a psychiatric conception of the symptom, which emphasises the discourse of the master over the analytic discourse. At the moment of its birth, the baby is already spoken of, and this linguistic bedrock makes it exist, while also – in a contradictory way – annihilating it as a thing, just as a word is supposed to replace what it designates. The inaugural emergence of the symptom manifests the irreducibility of the "thing" that has been brought into existence. "I don't want the Other to get off on me" means that I do not want to be reduced to what I am in the Other's speech. Even before the mirror stage has conferred an imaginary status upon it, "I" is defined by its alterity to the figure whom the Other is speaking about. This is the symptom, and it can take the form, for example, of an early refusal of the mother's milk.

A second debate is also occurring among psychoanalysts. Some of them – relying on Lacan's (2005b) development of the concept of sinthome in his seminar on Joyce, which I shall examine below – treat the Name-of-the-Father as a particular case of the symptom. Others, among whom I count myself, take the distinction between the Name-of-the-Father and the symptom to be essential, holding that each of these terms implies an antagonistic relation between subject and Other. The Name-of-the-Father ensures a phallic signification by which the One sets a limit to the Other. This Other is a boundless alterity that can take the form of a manic use of language, in which a stable meaning cannot be pinned down successfully. What Lacan calls the sinthome is the product of an identification with the symptom, an art of making do with the symptom (this is how Joyce transforms "imposed words" into "epiphanies" [see ibid., p. 75]). The sinthome can certainly "make up for" [*sup-plée à*] (ibid., p. 710) the absence of the Name-of-the-Father (at least in Joyce), but this making-up [*suppléance*], which tames the violence of the signifier, *is not* the sinthome's primary function.

Its primary function is to provide an alternative to what presents itself as an action that claims to be taken *in the name of the Other*; this is what occurs when the Name-of-the-Father has been established or made up for. The does not imply that the sinthome serves as the basis of an action taken *in the name of the subject*, but rather that it *ek-sists* in relation to both the subject and the Other, a position that some call "grace" and others the "muse".

From Marx to Freud

The symptom has a meaning or sense (*Sinn*). This formula can be reversed: every meaning-event is a symptom. This reversal can prevent the symptom from being reduced to its pathological dimension. *The real and meaning are incompatible, and the symptom, through an inconceivable circuit, knots them together.* In his lecture "The Sense of Symptoms", Freud (1916–17, p. 257) begins by saying that "the fact that symptoms have a sense and are related to the patient's experience" (and if they do not, then they are not symptoms) was discovered neither by Breuer nor by himself. Instead, Pierre Janet, and before him, the "great psychiatrist Leuret" had believed that symptoms have a sense: Janet claimed this for neurotics and Leuret for the "delusional ideas of the insane" (ibid., p. 257). Delusion has a very particular status, which requires symptom and fantasy to be disentangled from one another. Delusion could be defined as a fantasy in which access to the agent of castration – the real father – has been closed off, because there is no symbolic key. When Lacan says that the Name-of-the-Father is this key, we must first ask what a name is. It may well be the specific word that replaces the concrete father, but it is also something that starts out as real, before any signification has been deduced from it. It follows that delusion is not solely or even principally an unconscious formation, whose meaning could be brought out by *translating* it into ordinary language. Instead, it is the very armature of the relation with the Other, inasmuch as the will-to-jouissance would be located primally in the Other that is, first of all, language. As soon as the subject – in what can be called a "theft" – takes the will-to-jouissance away from the Other, this will define the truly Promethean process of the subject.

This theft divides both the subject and the Other: the partitioning-off of the Other by which the subject accomplishes the translation of will continuously implies that the subject must also excise a piece of him/herself. This will become the currency exchanged for the piece s/he excises from the Other. For example, a child with autism who could only "borrow" an object from me if he left me with an equivalent object. The infernal circle of the melancholic subject involves identifying with this object itself; the object is the means by which this will is translated, and the subject becomes lost in an identification with it. The only way in which s/he can limit her/his identification is by discovering a symptom that testifies to the incompleteness of this identification. It should be noted that, for Freud, this discovery implies the recognition of the unconscious. Nevertheless, this discovery can only take place when one is in the throes of the symptom, a moment when its meaning is successful.

This is decisive, for the gap between a symptom and its meaning, which Freud names the unconscious, means that the real can only be defined as outside meaning. This suggests that jouissance, the specifically human relation to being that language both opens up for us and encloses us within, is never "whole". As a principle, jouissance cannot bring about an adequation between the idea and the thing, which was and remains the dream or fantasy of the University: from Plato to Spinoza, from Spinoza to Heidegger. Marx belongs to this sequence: by not analysing the jouissance in the symptom, he opened up the path to an interpretation made by the discourse of the university. This was the notorious conception of the reflection. Even breaking the mirror will not enable this unexamined jouissance to materialise.

What is the status of the symptom? In the *Introductory Lectures on Psychoanalysis*, Freud chooses to take his examples from obsessional neurosis, which does not involve a conversion from the psychic to the somatic. He defines the obsessional symptom as a constraint of both action and thought, in which the neurotic finds himself "obliged against his will to brood and speculate", in ways that make no sense for him (ibid., p. 258). Although such constraints can be displaced, it is "quite impossible for him to omit" or suppress them (ibid., p. 258). Freud gives two examples, the first of which is more successful in making the symptom intelligible.

In this clinical sequence,[1] it should be noted that, for a reason that Freud tells us that he is holding back, the obsessional symptom does not disappear, even if the patient herself interprets it. In the interpretation, the part of the symptom involving "desire" or a "wish" appears clearly: the symptom enacts the wish that the wedding night had been successful, whereas her husband had, in fact, been impotent. She wished to "make her husband superior to his past mishap" (Freud, 1916–1917, p. 263). The "defensive" element of the symptom is more obscure, however, although we are told that she has been separated from her husband, without learning the reasons for this separation. Freud thus emphasises an Oedipal wish, although we could see in it a wish for sexual jouissance, which was not achieved because of the husband's impotence.

The defensive side could involve a refusal to be indebted to her husband for this jouissance. Symptoms differ radically from dreams, in which wish-fulfilment is sufficient: through the "figuration"[2] in the dream, jouissance passes into the unconscious. The page has been turned. The symptom operates at a different level, for it must also, and especially, satisfy desire. For it to do so, wish-fulfilment must not *become a debt that reinforces the subject's subjection to the Other*. In both of Freud's examples, there is something that points to this requirement: interpretations only have an effect because the patients have made them themselves, rather than obeying Freud's suggestions. This requirement does not apply only to transference within analysis; it occurs in every relation with the Other. For example, the Rat Man's great obsessional fear does not go away through some element in his interpretative associations that would serve as a sort of mathematical integral; instead, it disappears when he remembers a sacrilegious thought that involved his father and his lady (specifically that they should go off together and have children) (see Freud, 1909, p. 218). This leads us to think that the resolution of the symptom does not involve its pure and simple disappearance: it is resolved when the wish that had been its motive is authorised to be fulfilled. This authorisation occurs at the same time as a separation between the subject and the Other: a separation not from the desire of the Other – which cannot be accomplished – but from its jouissance.

Once again, the reader may find that these considerations are unrelated to class struggle and capitalism. S/he would be wrong, however, for maintaining that the homeostasis of the capitalist mode of production depends upon an economy of jouissance, one that neither the dictatorship of the proletariat nor the Cultural Revolution were able to undo. Capitalism succeeded, in different ways, in defeating the two great Marxist revolutions of the twentieth century, the Soviet and the Chinese. We can even wonder whether the personalities of Stalin and Mao, even more than the often sombre policies of the capitalist world, were the Trojan horses that enabled the capitalist discourse to be extended. Through Freud, Lacan – even before he discovered or cobbled together his capitalist discourse – had a theory of the symptom at his disposal. This served as the Archimedean lever by which he could begin to explore Marx's blind spot, even before history had made it dazzlingly obvious.

In the introduction, I mentioned that Lacan paid homage to Marx as the inventor of the symptom. This homage is an interpretation that involves Marx's relation to Hegel. At each dialectical moment, Hegel's teleological cunning of reason operates by introducing a negative aspect into the *Aufhebung* of knowledge: this aspect is truth. Marx, as early as his *Critique of Hegel's Philosophy of Right* (1843), responds to this method by making a materialist assertion: "it isn't like that at all". Knowledge can never achieve a definitive incorporation of truth (see Askofaré, 1989).

Lacan, who defines the symptom as "the return of truth as such into the gap of a certain knowledge" (Lacan, 1966c, p. 194), credited Marx with a critique of absolute idealism, one that invented a relation between knowledge and truth. The symptom thus becomes an irruption of truth. On the one hand, anything that shows that surplus-value has been extorted is fundamentally a symptom; this distinguishes it from ideology, in which the real appears in a deceptive form, masking, perpetuating and hiding exploitation. Ideology presents the proletarian's sale of his labour-power to the capitalist as part of a contract that has been entered into freely, one in which the capitalist pays for labour-power at its correct value. This "mapping" of the symptom to exploitation highlights one way of characterising the symptom: a facade (the fair payment for labour-power) hides its status as symptom. In this way, the symptom emerges in what is out of place, staining this facade. It thus stands in an ambiguous relation with truth, for it is also true that labour-power is paid for at its correct value. Yet to refuse to go any further than this "truth" is to refuse to constitute as a symptom anything that calls it into question – for example, a strike. Lacan is attentive on this point, since he alludes admiringly to Marx's (1867, pp. 301, 300) reference, in *Capital*, to the capitalist's "laughter". In his 1968–1969 seminar, Lacan (2006a, p. 65) states that Marx's mention of this laughter unveils "the essence of surplus value".

In Marx's text, this laughter is related to the fact that the capitalist buys labour-power at its value, in terms of the socially necessary labour time needed to train and maintain the worker. The capitalist thus becomes the owner of the use-value of labour-power; were it not for the symptom, which acts as a sort of killjoy, no one would find fault with his "right" to use this now alienated power however he likes. As Marx emphasises:

> the daily sustenance of labour-power costs only half a day's labour, while on the other hand the very same labour-power can remain effective, can work, during a whole day, and consequently the value which its use during the day creates is double to what the capitalist pays for that use; this circumstance is a piece of good luck for the buyer, but by no means an injustice towards the seller.
>
> *(Marx, 1867, p. 301)*

This luck may make the capitalist laugh, but this laughter also lays bare his cynicism: he delights in cheating the proletarian by buying labour-power in this way. The worker cannot contest the correctness and legality of the exchange, but through the symptom, legality becomes the place of a conflict. Without the capitalist's knowledge, this laughter becomes a symptom for the proletarian: "Why would he be laughing if he hasn't played a trick on me – a trick that I can't do anything about?" This is the proletarian's question.

It would therefore not be going too far to consider the discovery of surplus-value as equivalent to the discovery of the symptom. The theory of surplus-value establishes the necessity of the symptom and conditions its possible resolution; it enables us to discover a truth – exploitation – that is truer than the truth of free contracts. "A truth that is truer than truth" could be one definition of the real. In this context, what is important is independent of economic calculations, which tell us, for example, that buying labour-power for one day only costs the equivalent of a half-day of work. The important point, instead, is that the symptom shows the emptiness of arguments arising from the protestant work ethic: "Why don't you become a capitalist too?" Such arguments collide with the fact that, for the proletarian, selling one's labour-power is a forced choice. Only through such a choice would the proletarian enter into a relation of production founded on exploitation.

How then can s/he get out of it? Can workers exit from it only when the development of the productive forces has rendered exploitation no longer necessary? Can the worker escape from it without waiting for this to happen, by modifying her/his economy of jouissance: by taking leave of the iron law that governs the cycle of the capitalist discourse? Can s/he do this not only through her/his status as exploited worker, but also by questioning her/his status as consumer? Concerning this alternative, Marx's answer, and a fortiori, the answer of the various communist parties, remains unclear. This vagueness can be explained in terms neither of reformism ("Let's wait for capitalism to end up profiting everyone") nor of voluntarism; instead, it results from the fact that something has not been understood concerning what is at stake in the singular economies of jouissance.

This analysis can be continued from another perspective, which can throw light on what seems to have been Marx's prime and definitive inspiration: his attention to the *relations* of production. This is the advantage of his analysis of commodity fetishism. Why, he asks, in capitalist relations of production, are the relations between commodities presented in a "mystical" form (Marx, 1867, p. 164)? In other words, why does the "definite social relation between men themselves assume here . . . the fantastic form of a relation between things" (ibid., p. 165)? This passage has been discussed many times and almost everyone has been struck by the term "fetishism", which, for Freud, is the paradigm of perversion; it marks the victory of the disavowal of maternal castration over its recognition. As is often the case, a truism excuses people from taking a path that seems to lead to places that are so obvious that they do not need to be explored.

Unlike them, I shall take this path. In his analysis, Marx highlights how relations between things have been substituted for relations between human beings, thus placing the difference between value and surplus-value in the background. Is it possible to go so far as to claim that this substitution would occur even in the absence of exploitation? Would it occur if workers were paid the equivalent of the value of what they produced? (This was one of the demands of Ferdinand Lassalle's programme, which Marx (1875) criticised.) In other words, *would commodity-fetishism disappear if exploitation disappeared*?

Although Marx's discussion of commodity-fetishism, in contrast to his treatment of surplus-value, has the advantage of pointing to our fascination with consumption, it also has its own weaknesses. In fetishism, commodities acquire a value that seems intrinsic to them, although their value is actually determined by the social relations between the human beings who produce them. The tension between the fantastic or mystical thing-value of the commodity could well be homologous to another tension: that between price and exchange-value. By approaching this tension through Lacan, we can bring out the weaknesses of the concept of commodity fetishism: in psychoanalytic terms, we can say that this is a tension between a commodity's "*agalmatic*" value and its exchange-value. Marx, of course, had a simple doctrine concerning exchange-value: in order for a commodity to have exchange-value, it must first have a use-value. Sugar that does not dissolve has neither form of value. Yet in this context, does the jouissance that is expected from a product count for nothing? This expectation would give an agalmatic value to this commodity, a value that would have no common measure with the cost of producing it. The product's brand (see N. Klein, 2000) could endow it with a price that is higher than that of a product produced at the same cost and with the same characteristics.[3] If *desire precedes the cause*, one product does not prevail over another because it includes surplus-jouissance as an intrinsic part of itself. What is primary, instead, is the desire of the potential buyer. Commodity-fetishism covers over this priority, for desire is said to arise from a cause that precedes it: the commodity's "intrinsic" value.[4] Only later is this desire put to the test of whether or not it is satisfied.

Fetishism does not directly imply an extortion of surplus-value, even if it may well mask this extortion. As a consequence, *the end of exploitation would not imply the end of commodity-fetishism. The endurance of the capitalist discourse* (*a* → $\$$, surplus-jouissance → lack-in-jouissance [*manque-à- jouir*] *is not only the result of the extortion of surplus-value by a private power.*

Lacan (1973a, p. 381) said that the symptom "only takes on its revolutionary" – or insurrectional – "effect when it is not being conducted by the so-called Marxist baton"; the symptom's status is decided, instead, by the various threads that I have been examining. In 1966, in "On a Subject Who Is Finally in Question", one of the intercalary texts in the *Écrits*, Lacan established Marx's precedence in relation to the symptom. I have already quoted from this text and shall do so again, this time placing the citation more fully in its context:

> It is difficult not to see that, even before the advent of psychoanalysis, a dimension that might be called that of the symptom was introduced, which was articulated on the basis of the fact that it represents the return of truth as such into the gap of a certain knowledge.
>
> *(1966c, p. 194)*

Immediately afterwards, however, Lacan distinguishes Marx's symptom from Freud's:

> Freud sets himself apart from the rest by clearly linking the status of the symptom to the status of his own operation, for the Freudian operation is the symptom's proper operation, in the two senses of the term. Unlike a sign – or smoke which is never found in the absence of fire, a fire that smoke indicates with the possible call to put it out – a symptom can only be interpreted in the signifying order. A signifier has meaning only through its relation to another signifier. The truth of symptoms resides in this articulation. Symptoms remained somewhat vague when they were understood as representing some irruption of truth. In fact, they *are* truth, being made of the same wood from which truth is made, if we posit materialistically that truth is what is instated on the basis of the signifying chain.
>
> *(ibid, pp. 194–195)*

This is a crucial statement. It is difficult not to read it as Lacan's objection to Marx immediately after his tribute to him. Marx and Freud are allied against Hegel; they refuse the latter's argument that the work of truth – of the particular – is absorbed into absolute knowledge. Freud, however, is also to be distinguished from Marx. For Marx, the symptom is the symptom of a truth: a strike is the symptom of the truth of capitalist exploitation. This exploitation is, in turn, the symptom of the truth of the "free" contract between the capitalist and the proletarian. For Freud, the symptom *is* truth. Because Marx missed this subtle difference, his conception "remained somewhat vague".

In presenting Freud's thesis on the symptom and his account of how the Rat Man's major obsessional symptom is dissolved, I have emphasised that the sense of the symptom includes a dimension that is related to transference. This may be a common observation: interpreting the symptom will have no analytic effect if it is imputed to the analyst as Other, without being appropriated by the subject. We must therefore decide firmly that the question of meaning or sense – and not simply of signification, which only concerns the statement [*énoncé*] – includes the question of how the relation to the Other helps determine the message. In interpretation, the Other and the subject must also not be commutative; it could even be said that *because* of interpretation, they can cease to be commutative. Interpretation must extract the subject from this reversibility, from what Lacan (1976–1977, 15 March 1977) calls a "double meaning" or "double direction [*double sens*]. For example, a man says, "You are my wife" and a woman replies, "I am your wife". The consequence of interpretation is to show, to both the man and the woman, that "my wife", in the first statement, and "your wife" in the second may denote the same woman, but nevertheless have nothing to do with one another. To say that the symptom is truth means that its formal envelope of signifiers always, in itself, conveys the message that this single denotation involves a non-equivalence. "My wife" and "your wife" do not coincide, even if they designate the same person.[5]

Two remarks can be made about this. First, in "On the Subject Who Is Finally in Question", Lacan shows how Marx and Freud differ in relation to the symptom. Yet in saying that the symptom is truth, Lacan (1966c, p. 194) adds that "it represents the return of truth as such into the gap of a certain knowledge". In this way, he emphasises, like Marx, the impossibility of absolute knowledge, but he also shows that this gap concerns the real rather than truth. It involves not an adequation between the thing and the idea, but the impossibility of this adequation. The "gap", as real, conditions and authorises the "return of a truth". As Lacan himself says, he is siding with Kant against Spinoza, and Marx against Hegel.

Second, meaning must not be confused with signification. Meaning is not the entirety of the successive significations taken by the symptom in the work of association; if it were, then the inflation of meaning could unfold ad infinitum. The symptom does indeed have a sense, but it is only accessible if we grasp the angle from which the Other, in giving the object, has established this sense. Grasping this angle is one of the conditions for putting an end to the commutativity of meaning. The subject recognises that his desire is the desire of the Other, while separating himself from the Other's jouissance (which is also his own jouissance, since "*I* is an *other*" [Rimbaud, 1871, p. 115]).[6] Sense involves direction and could thereby become equivalent to orientation.

To find the sense is to find the symptom's orientation, its clinamen,[7] with which I can then identify. Identifying with the sense of the symptom is the decisive moment, for this sense can never be made objective. We cannot say, "I know the meaning of this symptom"; if it becomes objective in this way, it becomes marked by religion. It would be religious to say, "I know [*je sais*] the sense"; this would be radically different from the atheism of the assertion, "I am and follow [*je suis*] the sense". It should be noted that to "be sense" is nothing less than an arbitrary decision; in order for "being sense" not to be arbitrary, it would have to figure the real.

Finally – and this remark knots the symptom to discourse – every symptom is particular. When it is "resolved" – a term that includes the semantic resonance of "resolving" to do something – it becomes singular.[8] For Lacan, however, there is one exception to this rule: the proletarian. In "*La troisième*", Lacan (1975b, p. 187) argues that the proletarian is the only social symptom. The proletarian has been stripped of everything, becoming a "man without qualities", who can be identified with the subject as a lack-in-jouissance. This worker is the universal subject of "The Internationale": "we are nothing; let's be everything [*soyons tout*]". However, there is a problem: this way of understanding the proletariat swings from having nothing to being nothing, and its status cannot be resolved by reaching a state of "whole being" [*l'être tout*] or of a being who is "everything" [*un être tout*]. The proletarian is a social symptom, but a symptom can only be resolved through its particularity.

This is stated explicitly in *R.S.I*:

> If we don't make man into whatever conveys an ideal symptom, if we define him in each case on the basis of his unconscious and the way that he gets off on it, the symptom remains in the same place where Marx put it, but it takes on another sense. Not a social symptom, but a particular symptom.
>
> *(Lacan, 1974–1975, 18 February 1974)*

This is Lacan's only definition of political action: the social symptom is only to be interpreted in terms of each person's particularity. This implies that the jouissance of having nothing and being nothing must not be left unquestioned. This questioning, however, can lead to a remark that verges on sacrilege: whole being or being everything could well make "The Internationale" the anthem of the capitalist ideal.

These considerations enable the social symptom – in a way that is slight but valuable – to establish a connection between political action and discourse, the social bond. The change in direction and meaning of the symptom – from the social to the particular[9] – does not make this connection obsolete. First, if we return to the passage from "*La troisième*" in which Lacan (Lacan, 1975b, p. 187) introduces the proletarian as a social symptom, he indicates explicitly that the individual, rather than the subject, is a proletarian. If the individual is the subject minus its unconscious, we can grasp more easily the significance of restoring to each of us our unconscious and our way of getting off on it. One avenue for political action would therefore be to restore to Hyde and Dark the unconscious that they have been deprived of by the doctors of chemistry and capitalists, who are themselves impelled by a passion for ignorance. It would also be tempting to present the proletarian as the lack-in-jouissance of the subject figuring in the upper left corner of the capitalist discourse, but there is a difficulty with this: the subject is not the individual. Such an equivalence could only be valid, and unfairly valid, in the capitalist discourse, if we remain within this discourse.

There is another perspective remaining here. If each individual, as Lacan (1975b, p. 187) says, "is really a proletarian", it is because s/he "has no discourse with which to make a social bond, in other words, a semblance". Does this mean that the proletarian would be outside discourse, or that the capitalist discourse is one in which there is no place for the semblance? First, we should remember that the semblance is the name given to the figure who cannot be named or name himself: the father (see Lacan, 1974a). The father can be named, but only through a semblance; no one has the power to be both the father of names and to have "father" as name.

The semblance thus enables the subject, by resorting to the signifier, neither to fall into the abyss of the absence of a name – a hole that cannot be brought back into the symbolic – nor to efface the real of this hole by delusion or hallucination. The capitalist discourse, like the others, is a discourse of the semblance. Although the proletarian does not appear as such in this discourse, s/he is present in it indirectly, as a consumer ($\$$) or as a worker (S_2). The capitalist discourse tends to fashion a virtual subject: one that, being cut from its unconscious, imagines that it has become unmoored from the real. In *The Society of the Spectacle*, Guy Debord (1967) located this aspect of capitalism definitively and almost prophetically.

Concrete manifestations of this discourse reduce the subject to a lack-in-jouissance. This subject's only future involves the forced choice of diminishing this lack through surplus-jouissance. Here the capitalist discourse displays its *diabolical* quality, for the economy is governed by the principle "of the extensive, and therefore insatiable production of the lack-in-jouissance" (Lacan, 1970, p. 435). Thus, those who are exploited are led to "compete on the basic principle of exploitation, in order to harbour their indisputable participation in the thirst of lack-in-jouissance" (ibid., p. 435). While the extensive production of the capitalist economy is offering more and more commodities to fill the lack-in-jouissance, this lack continues to grow, and with it the thirst that makes this lack manifest. This formulation stands in flagrant contradiction to the Pareto axiom, which posits that a drinker's thirst will be quenched less with the second glass than with the first. On the level of physical need, this is certain; on the level of the drive, this is erroneous. Thirst is addictive: the more I drink, the thirstier I become. Paradoxically, I drink in order to quench my thirst, but I cannot do so without the jouissance that *is* thirst. It is thus that, by producing these objects *a*, the capitalist discourse develops a "thirst *of* the lack-in-jouissance" (ibid., p. 435, my emphasis), and the preposition "of" can be understood in two senses. Thirst *is* lack-in-jouissance, and thirst is a thirst *for* the object that embodies this lack. Thus, this "thirst of lack-in-jouissance" operates on an inverted ladder of satisfaction, hollowing out a feeling that "this isn't enough, it's never enough", and thereby separating a subject from any satisfaction. This situation resembles a train that will never reach its destination because it is going in the wrong direction.

The subject is thus only a lack-in-jouissance in the capitalist discourse, and even there, it only approaches this condition asymptotically. If it were entirely this lack, then it would have to "lose its unconscious", in the way that Christians speak of "losing one's soul". Perhaps by abolishing itself as such, the subject would reappear as a symptom, the sign that something does not work in the capitalist discourse. Yet if we follow Lacan rigorously, the proletarian can only come into existence as a social symptom.

For this reason, there is no continuity between the subject, which is reduced to lack-in-being, and the proletarian as social symptom. A Marxist would say, "This is the proof that class consciousness is not automatic!" Yet the lesson goes beyond this: there is no relation between the historical figure of the proletarian, who becomes a social symptom, and the reality of the subject. The subject must give form to its own particular symptom; it must not seek vainly to become subjectivated as a proletarian. This is an absolute condition for preventing class warfare from becoming for Marxists what the *Parousia* is for Christians.

Lacan rightly pointed out the irony of this shoddy Eden, which is not without a certain piquancy, because of the anecdote about Marie-Antoinette's cynical remark that starving peasants should eat cake. There is no better way to announce the dawn of capitalism: 1) there is no bread, and thus no jouissance; 2) therefore we should eat cake, thereby getting more jouissance; 3) cake isn't all that exciting, etc. It should be noted that in the first step, "no bread" denotes both real privation – there is no money to buy bread, and even no wheat to make it – *and* a lack of interest in bread, since it is not as good as cake. Marx located the source of this problem not in the thirst of lack-in-jouissance, but in unlimited exploitation, for which he employed his famous trope of the chariot of the Juggernaut (see Marx, 1867, pp. 392, 799), under whose wheels worshipers threw themselves, thereby proving their faith in a manner that would have pleased Pascal. This image resonates with Lacan's (1937, p. 89) allusion to Moloch. These references involve incarnating the insatiability of both capitalism and the superego, through a reference to the "dark" side of God, who will always require more sacrifices. God drinks like a drunkard at the beginning of religion, and we find this again in the subject who does the same at the end of capitalism.

We know that Lacan (1973d, p. 275) analysed the question of sacrifice in relation to the "dark god" of the Nazi holocaust. This "final solution" tried to put a stop to the cycle that goes from thirst to lack-in-jouissance. The Nazi ideology of sanitisation was delusional, but also implacably logical. Nazis transformed the figure of the "Jew" into the embodiment of surplus-jouissance: the commodity that capitalism produces in order to create ever more thirst. The "Jew" does this by capturing the "Aryan" proletarian, who thereby becomes the "victim", in an economy of jouissance that excludes any satisfaction. Nazism was not the highest stage of capitalism; instead, it was an attempt to use death to go beyond capitalism. This explains the unthinkable mixture of far right and far left that sometimes appears.

Yet, what are the roots of the belief that sacrifice is required? As we have noted, the discourse of the master requires the master to sacrifice his jouissance, thus distinguishing himself from the slave. Yet the workers, by selling their labour-power to survive, also renounce "jouissance" in a very particular sense: the enjoyment or usufruct of the use-value of their labour-power. This connection suggests that it is necessary to renounce use-value and its enjoyment, thus making an access to jouissance possible, on the basis of the specific dialectic discovered by Freud and articulated by Lacan, a dialectic that established our linguistic being. Jouissance, which comes to be defined as what serves no good purpose, is excluded from the useful.[10] Is this renunciation the essence of sacrifice?

What makes this question even more worth examining is that, in a rather striking passage from *Capital's* unfinished chapter on social classes, Marx (1894, p. 1025) asserts that there is a homology between capitalists and proletarians, both of whom are owners.[11] The first own capital while the second own labour-power; they must both renounce the use of this "property" if they want it to be "capitalized on".[12] It is tempting to consider this renunciation as the first stage of the sacrifice whose aim will end up in a subjection to Moloch or Juggernaut. This would be an Orwellian vision, in which the tortured Winston Smith can only escape torment by loving his torturer. Neither Marx nor Lacan takes this position, but Lacan's disagreement with Marx centres on the latter's conception of surplus-value as something that can be counted. If surplus-value is the gap between the value of the goods necessary for training and maintaining labour-power, and the value produced by this power, Marx thinks of this gap in terms of an energetics of jouissance, implying that jouissance can be measured as an exchange-value, so that the subject's relation to jouissance could be regulated through the "right" distribution of surplus-value. His arguments seem to presuppose that the debt that the subject contracts as a being of language introduced into the "marketplace" of jouissance can, as a consequence, be paid off.

This argument can be disputed. Capitalism profits and proliferates from the "thirst of lack-in-jouissance"; if this lack is real, *it is not possible to exit from capitalism through a new distribution of surplus-value. This can only occur through a mutation in the subject's relation to jouissance.*[13] The basic principle of renouncing jouissance during a first moment can easily be translated into a requirement not to sacrifice everything on the altar of use-value. Somehow, we have expected that the exhaustion of use-value could magically satiate the superego. In a second moment, we must think through an alternative to sacrifice in order to escape the economy of jouissance that is specific to the capitalist discourse, an economy that still characterised the "real socialist" countries. In these countries, the recurrent debates over material and ideological motivations ran aground because they were marked by the Manichaeism that is internal to the capitalist discourse.

Indeed, as we know, Marx's reliance on energetics in economics – which may well contradict his political, historical and philosophical doctrines, and especially his contention that the relations of production are determinant – had an impact on his monetary theory. Marx's blind spot was to take price as the *duplicatum* of value, and Keynes, the friend of Wittgenstein, located this weakness and found a way to transform it into an antidote for capitalism itself. This is not to say that the *duplicatum* theory is not true "in the last instance",[14] but it forecloses the question of credit: the question that introduces the possibility of making money (M-M′) by means of a money that is only fictive. It thus appears that the social bond, and in direct terms, transference, are part of the conditions for this virtualisation, which has real consequences. The true disruption of the relation between money and value does not occur in the stock market; crashes always enable things to fall back onto their feet, or rather, onto the feet of the small investors. It occurred, instead, in the socialist experiment, in which the linkage between prices and value was completely undone. Perhaps this occurred, in part, in accordance with the principle that "to each [shall be given] according to his needs" (Marx, 1875, p. 347); more fundamentally, it was done out of a fatal mistrust of the symbolic.

Symptom and sinthome

In German, the term "*Kultur*" condenses the art of history and the history of art, while the French terms, "*civilisation*" and "*culture*" keep these elements distinct. Psychoanalysis can maintain that this combination of civilisation and culture is inevitable, because of an axiom that I shall state immediately. This axiom could be inscribed above the door from which all the woes of the world emerge, one by one: there can be no worthwhile satisfaction of the subject without the satisfaction of the other. This adage has nothing to do with oblativity, which only puts a coat of varnish over our fundamental malevolence towards the other, without realising the vanity of doing so; it cannot discover that the reverse of this malevolence is a benevolence regarding the self. Yet as long as this realisation has not occurred, this axiom only indicates an ideal direction. To make it more practicable, we must not get bogged down in a theory of the symptom that will lead certain crucial experiences – those that include but are not limited to psychoanalysis – into an impasse. These experiences prepare and authorise an identification with the symptom.[15]

In her work on phobia, Isabelle Morin (2009) distinguishes between a period that, in terms of structure, comes first, one in which the phallic function and secondary repression have not yet come into play. I would argue that what she says about phobia is also valid for the symptom; its primal emergence results because a body – which will turn out, despite certain vagaries, to be my own – is pre-empted by language. As I have shown, this mapping of language brings in Russell's paradox, which sets up a division between the master-signifier – which provides a quilting point in the use of language – and the second signifier, which makes a cut in the use of the body. In the present context, what is important is that jouissance comes into existence in the process in which things are nihilated [*se néantisent*]. They supposedly become "virtualised", for we cannot forget that the second signifier is not substituted for things; it only makes a cut in them and serves as an edge, thus constituting the drive. The problem is that the drive is acephalic: the master-signifier – the One that could order it into a set of signifiers – is not a part of the drive. Yet on the side of the master-signifier, the problem is just as serious, since the nihilation of things does not stop at the threshold of the body, which is now inhabited by language, and is thus also nihilated. In this conjuncture, the symptom is the body's response to language. It is an eternal response, which constitutes life itself: thou shalt not kill. *The subject wants the Other to be at its disposal. The subject does not want to be at the Other's disposal* (see Bruno & Sauret, 2006). This structural dissymmetry is neither acquired nor innate.[16]

In other words, the symptom, in its fundamental articulation, marks the lack of existence of the sexual relation. If such a relation were possible, it would imply both that the subject would want to get off on the Other and that s/he would consent to the Other's getting off on her/him. Instead, the symptom is a sort of uprising or insurrection, but only on the condition that it does not march either to the "Marxist baton" or to certain psychoanalytic ones.

In order to grasp the insurrectional quality of the symptom, I shall examine "constituted symptoms": these derive from the repression of the subject's will to get off on the Other. In them, we can see the place of anxiety, which signals a fear of being at this Other's disposal. Through the castration of the Other – and first, of the mother – the subject ensures that she is not at the Other's disposal. For example, a young woman in analysis regularly experienced tachycardia on her way to her analyst's office. This is incontestably a symptom and it would be reasonable to say it is the substitute for a relation that does not exist, just as a fetish is the substitute for the mother's missing penis. From this perspective, the symptom masks the nonexistence of the sexual relation. In the course of the analysis, however, it turned out that this tachycardia had already appeared when, as a little girl, she had accompanied her father on visits to dive bars; in order to buy her silence and reward her for her collusion with him, he gave her candy, which she then started to ask him for. Years later, during her treatment, this symptom returned when she was considering whether to ask her father for money to buy a house. We can thus see very clearly that, in the phase when the symptom of tachycardia first appeared, it was linked to demand and showed that the analysand's will-to-jouissance, a will directed at the Other (in this case, the father) was being repressed. From that moment on, such demands could only be made through this symptom. By the time that she reached adulthood, the demand had been repressed and had been replaced completely by the symptom. Her repression was only lifted through a demand to the analyst. This repression, of course, was part of the repression of the Oedipus complex, the libidinal bond with the father, which was then reactivated in the bond with the analyst.

Yet if we give Freud's final theory of anxiety its full weight, we should conclude that this anxiety results from the consequences of the subject's will-to-jouissance. Her determination to get off on the father would make him passive, thus threatening to render him unable to castrate the maternal Other. For this reason, the conception of the symptom as the equivalent of a jouissance that would replace the jouissance of the impossible sexual relation and would fraudulently authorise its existence is doubly incomplete. First, this conception does not see that the libidinal bond with the Other is not the sexual relation. Such a relation would require precisely the kind of commutativity that the symptom refuses. This refusal, however, has to be interpreted in order to be discovered. Second, this conception also does not see that the key to repression lies in anxiety: the anxiety that the real father – the father who has not submitted to the subject's will-to-jouissance and is therefore immunised against castration – be annihilated.

Another woman, near the end of her analysis, mentioned her father's answer when, as a little girl, she had asked him, "why did you marry Mommy?" He told her that her mother was the most beautiful of women and that he loved her. The mother herself had confided several times to her daughter that she experienced nothing during physical relations with her husband, a remark that the analysand took to mean, "Your father will never be able to make me come". She then mentioned a memory to her analyst. Once, while she was still a girl, she had found an unused sanitary pad in her parents' bed. When she asked her mother what this was, the mother answered, "It's for your father when he has a cold". Later, she presented herself in analysis with a persistent somatic symptom: vaginal secretions that occurred for no organic reason. In this session, she discovered the meaning of this symptom: "Through it, I wanted to make my mother come, since my father couldn't do so. At the same time, my vaginal secretions were also the equivalent of semen. In wanting this, I was identifying with my father".

Although the symptom is overdetermined, its meaning, which is what has been dissolved within the symptom's formal envelope by the enunciation, is singular. In this case, meaning is strictly related to the analysand's vaginal secretions. This sequence can, of course, have other possible meanings: it could involve showing the father's impotence, taking the mother's place, etc. and all of these could be pushed to the point at which we could say that the symptom masks the nonexistence of the sexual relation Yet if we stick to what this analysand says and avoid trying to play the role of ventriloquist, the symptom has a single meaning: she is seeking to rehabilitate the father so that he can maintain his place as agent of the mother's castration. In this way, he could ensure that the maternal Other would not get off on the subject. The symptom would thus signal the sexual nonrelation. Every symptom is fundamentally a call, which cannot primarily be articulated, to something in the father that cannot be castrated: its first task is to limit the will-to-jouissance that is imputed to the maternal Other, and second, it must limit the subject's own will-to-jouissance. The condition for the symptom is that there must be another plane, on which this x that cannot be castrated can nevertheless be named. As a consequence, this call can only be articulated through an equivocation, a statement that comes neither from the subject nor the Other, but from the real of the freedom that is contained within structure.[17]

This analysis does not move us away from the problem – which also offers us an opportunity – of how to move from the social symptom, in which the individual is a proletarian, to the particular symptom, which cannot take the form embodied by the statement, "I am a proletarian". The social symptom is the symptom of the capitalist discourse, which means that the only way to dissolve its formal envelope is to leave the capitalist discourse. This can be done, first, by subtracting the subject from the thirst of the lack-in-jouissance; this thirst transforms the subject into a proletarian, stripping it of everything, and indeed the relative impoverishment of the "middle" classes in the wealthy industrialised countries is not a fiction. Yet, *nec plus ultra*, capitalism hopes to ensure its durability not by formatting consciousnesses but *by cutting the bond between the subject and the unconscious*, between $\$$ and S_2. This cut can be read in the matheme through the absence of a connection between $\$$ and S_2 on the upper line.

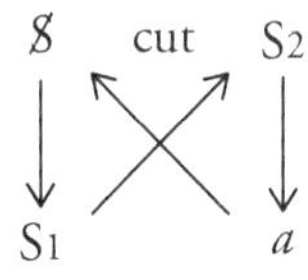

Once the association between the subject and the unconscious has been broken, the dialectic between the unconscious and the drive can no longer take place. Thus, the following sequence occurs: the unconscious is unplugged – the drive is unleashed – Stop – SOS *Kultur*. We would reach the epiphany of a new kind of racism, one that would be less marginal: above, we would be mindless; below, we would be primates. This perspective is especially threatening because it imitates, as if in a deforming mirror, the outcome of analysis. We can measure this danger through an ambiguous phrase: "being cured of thinking". Is this the separation from the unconscious, as brought about by an analysis, or is it instead something that might be stated as "I don't want to know anything about your little feelings" (a cynical maxim that has always been used to attack any thought that refuses to reduce itself to some kind of sales pitch)?[18]

In 1975–1976, in his seminar on James Joyce and related writings, Lacan (2005b) distinguished between a "symptom" and a "sinthome". Without going over this in detail again, I would like to emphasise that it enables us to envision a disconnection from the unconscious (in "Joyce the Symptom", Lacan (1982a, p. 141) refers to it as "having cancelled his subscription to the unconscious"), which would not be synonymous with unmooring oneself from the drives. This provides an answer to the old question raised by *The Four Fundamental Concepts of Psycho-Analysis*: at the end of an analysis, "How can a subject who has traversed the radical phantasy experience the drive" (Lacan, 1973d, p. 273), a drive that is no longer incarcerated in this fantasy? This question can even be asked in another, exaggerated way: because we have ceased to be perverse, how can we not imagine that we are outside the law? Lacan's answer in *The Sinthome* involves claiming that Joyce's art of writing involves both no longer subscribing to the unconscious – a condition that an analysis, pushed to its end, enables one to achieve – and "making-up for" (Lacan, 2005b, p. 71) the phallic function, which had failed in his case. This means first, that with this sinthome, the art and process of writing have a decisive weight; they are important because writing, unlike language, is not representative but figurative,[19] and the art of writing moves us from a particular to a singular symptom.

Second, this means that, contrary to the dominant readings of Lacan's work on Joyce, the definition of the sinthome as a "substitute that makes up for" [*suppléance*] the Name-of-the-Father does not mean that the sinthome is the general term, and that the Name-of-the-Father is merely a particular case of it.[20] It serves to make up for the Name-of-the-Father because it does this *in every case* – not only in psychosis, but also in neurosis and perversion. It makes up for the Name-of-the-Father's inability to open onto the right – feminine – side of the table of sexuation: the side where phallocentrism fails, and where poetry becomes possible.

A key question can be found here. An analysis is finished when something comes to replace the knotting of the symbolic, real and imaginary by the Name-of-the-Father, a knotting that has involved a recourse to the Other. Instead, there is a new knotting by the sinthome: the subject can be *authorised through his/her sinthome*. Under what conditions of civilisation could such an operation become practicable, as a priority, for the subject? This returns us to a question that has already been posed: the distinction between a generational being as a son or a daughter and the being of the symptom.

Notes

1 Freud (1916–1917, p. 261) describes the symptom as follows:

> A lady, nearly thirty years of age, . . . ran from her room into another neighbouring one, took up a particular position there beside a table that stood in the middle, rang the bell for her housemaid, sent her on some indifferent errand or let her go without one, and then ran back into her own room.

This enigmatic obsessional symptom became clear when the patient mentioned her husband's impotence during their wedding night. To hide his failure from the housemaid, he had poured red ink on the bed sheets, but not at the location where one would expect to find bloodstains. Now, in the room to which the patient summoned her housemaid, there was a tablecloth with a big red stain that the latter could not miss seeing, given the position the lady took.

2 [*Translator's note*: "Figuration" is to be distinguished from "representation" here. "Representation" refers not to the adequation of word and thing but instead to a situation in which one term marks the place of another (for example, a signifier represents a subject for another signifier). "Figuration", on the other hand, concerns the process by which elements of jouissance are shaped or encrypted (as in the writing of letters) by the unconscious. The French verb "*figurer*" can refer to the action of giving something a visual shape in drawings, paintings and sculptures; here it also includes the visual aspect of dreams. This distinction leads to a change in the translation of Freud's term "*Darstellbarkeit*", which can be defined as the "Requirement imposed on the dream-thoughts; they undergo selection and transformation such as to make them capable of being represented by images – particularly visual images" (Laplanche & Pontalis, 1974, p. 389). The *Standard Edition* translated "*Darstellbarkeit*" as "conditions of representability" (Freud, 1900, p. 339); here, it becomes "conditions of figurability".]

3 Even more decisively, the development of financial bubbles in contemporary capitalism could be seen as a demonstration that expected gains – which do not take the real (or productive) economy into account – are what drive financial markets, putting into play an enormous financial mass valued in *tera*-dollars. See François Morin (2006).

4 We recall the difficulty Marx had in addressing the question of the price of works of art. [*Translator's note*: for a discussion of this, see Ali Alizadeh (2017).]

5 Lacan owes a great deal to Frege's account of how one denotation [or *Bedeutung*] can correspond to several "modes of presentation" of an object, that is, to several *senses* [or *Sinne*], and this includes the point of view of the presenter; for example, one geometrical point can be defined in different ways [*Translator's note*: (see Frege, 1892, p. 152)].

6 This can also be read in reverse of the usual way, e.g. by identifying the "Other" with "I" rather than "I" with the "Other".

7 [*Translator's note*: on the concept of "clinamen", see Lacan (1973d, p. 63, 1975a, p. 58) and Mladen Dolar (2013).]

8 This singularity, by rendering null and void all forms of comparison, is surely the only way to get out of envy, which Melanie Klein held to be the obstacle that remains essentially insurmountable at the end of analysis. Only by renouncing his/her position as subject can the envious – unlike the jealous – subject replace the other who is believed to be fulfilled.

9 A definition of ideology can be deduced from this point: ideology is every mental operation that obscures the fact that social psychology is nothing but individual psychology.

10 A thinker like John Stuart Mill, who tried to rectify Bentham's utilitarianism in order to save its principal point, reveals the foundations of distributive justice, which can be

summarized as follows: everyone has a debt to the human community and justice consists in each person's repaying this debt (or at least reducing it to the lowest amount possible) by means of just action: an action that serves to confirm that the person is a member of this community. In this way, the virtue of a person is nothing other than his/her ability to act in this way. The guiding principle of this sort of justice is "punishment". Mill sees only one possible alternative to his conception, which he attributes to the utopian communism of Robert Owen: the idea that people are irresponsible. Mill is thus unable to see how responsibility can be dissociated from debt. [*Translator's note*: see Mill (1863, pp. 40, 81).]

11 [*Translator's note*: Marx (1894, p. 1025) writes: "The owners of mere labour-power, the owners of capital and the landowners, whose respective sources of income are wages, profit and ground-rent – in other words wage-labourers, capitalists and landowners – form the three great classes of modern society based on the capitalist mode of production".]

12 Similarly, the analysand also must give up some of the use-value of his/her property to pay for analytic sessions.

13 Readers familiar with the theoretical and ideological controversies of socialism might find this proposition reformist. That would be incorrect, because reformists believe – as much or even more than do revolutionaries – in solutions based on a more equitable distribution of surplus value; such an approach does not involve doing away with capitalism.

14 [*Translator's note*: see Althusser (1965, pp. 111, 113).]

15 Lacan introduced the term "sinthome", which makes use of the old French spelling of "symptom", quite late in his work, in his seminar on Joyce held in 1975–1976 (Lacan, 2005b). In an original way, he suggested that this is what mitigates the foreclosure of the Name-of-the-Father. Yet he then proceeds to present a more positive conception of the symptom, in which the symptom is no longer antinomic to its interpretation and in which, once this interpretation occurs, the symptom does not go away; instead, it is revealed as the salutary indicator of the impossibility of the sexual relation. Of course, this transformation changes the formal envelope of the symptom, which makes way for what can be called a style.

16 Only in masochism, which supposes that there is a *contract*, does the subject consent, *to some extent*, to being at the Other's disposal, for the sake of the jouissance of being the thing that is going to disappear, without the threshold ever once having been crossed.

17 The debate concerning the question of the greater or lesser degree of indeterminateness left by genetic factors is often confused with something very different: a freedom that has nothing to do with any kind of free will, and which comes from the presence of something that is logically undecidable in structure as such, or even from some "unfathomable" decision. This freedom of structure belongs only to the field of experience with which psychoanalysis is concerned, and which psychoanalysis demonstrates in a way that the hard sciences can only approach . . . asymptotically.

18 The consequences of this distinction between two conceptions of the symptom – one in which the symptom is the mark of the nonexistence of the sexual relation, and one in which its purpose is to hide this nonexistence – can be grasped in the way in which analysis is conducted. This emerged in a discussion of a paper on Calamity Jane presented by Isabelle Morin at the "*Midi-minuit des écrits de psychanalyse* [Psychoanalytic writings from noon to midnight]", a conference held by the *Association psychoanalyse Jacques Lacan* [Jacques Lacan psychoanalytic association] in Paris in 2005. Two opposing readings emerged. For Morin, Calamity Jane's decision to give her daughter up for adoption was the sign of a "love beyond the object". Discussants disagreed with this, suggesting that Jane's decision was more probably determined by a rejection of the castration that would have been imposed on her in the task of rearing the child. While it would be difficult to think of Calamity Jane as someone who had been able to remove herself from the peristalsis of jouissance, is it certain that she really rebelled against the castration of the maternal Other? By allowing her daughter to be adopted, she may well have been protecting her from the painful outcome that her mother had not spared her. It is

certainly possible that her decision expressed a belief that this course of action would allow her to protect her daughter from all or part of the trial of castration. However, it also, and especially, expressed her attempt to prevent her daughter from having to pay for Jane's own relation as a woman to jouissance, a relation that she knew to be nothing less than exemplary.

19 Writing is on the side of the real and its own play prevails over its function of transcribing language. Without writing, the materiality of the signifier is forgotten.

20 This is asserted quite clearly by Miller (2005, p. viii): "[Lacan's] calling into question of the limits of the Oedipus complex and of the paternal myth continued . . ., going as far as to reduce the Name-of-the-Father to the level of a symptom and utensil".

6

EXITING FROM CAPITALISM

Can we take leave of capitalism, and if so, how? For Marx, capitalism is a mode of production in which labour-power has been transformed into commodities. Surplus-value could only be theorised after the arrival of capitalism made it possible – at least ideally – to give a numerical value to the socially necessary labour-time used to produce a commodity. This value could then be compared to the value that is necessary for training and maintaining labour-power. Marx's political ideal was that private ownership of the means of production had to be abolished, so that surplus-value, which will always be appropriated, will give rise to a new logic, in which the rate of profit will not be at the service of a sort of parthenogenesis of money, but will serve each person's economic development and satisfaction, first "according to his ability" (socialism) and later, "according to his needs" (communism) (Marx, 1875, p. 347).

This vision is coherent and the concept of surplus-value, upon which it is based, is scientifically valid, as capitalists were the first to recognise. What, then, can explain the failure of two great and very different revolutions, the Russian and the Chinese, after they had aroused such immense hopes? Historians have begun their own expert work, which will probably continue for a long time. It would be pretentious and ill-timed to start drawing conclusions, as if they would enable us to leave the question behind us. It would also be simplistic to yield to the idea that capitalism is the natural mode of production, and that Russia and China were finally converted to it, after decades of indulging in an ideological mistake. This would be like claiming that the France of the First Empire and the Restoration was simply returning to the normality of feudalism, after having wandered in the desert of the revolution. It is both possible and desirable, however, to draw certain conclusions about these two major experiments on the basis of the preceding analyses of the splitting of the subject, the discourses and the symptom. My first – rather trivial – remark runs the risk of being judged to be of secondary importance. People will accuse me of being short-sighted and narrow. I would say, instead, that I am placing the ashes under a microscope: not only Stalin and Mao, but also Ceausescu, Pol Pot and many others were certainly psychotic. They were capable, with their left hand, of encouraging revolutionary enthusiasm and, with their right hand and with all the innocence of a paranoiac, of sending hundreds of thousands of people to their deaths. Neither Soviet nor Chinese communists were spared, and they were often the most persecuted. I have already quoted Lacan's claim that the psychotic seeks to contain the pulverulence of his delusion by taking the place of the master in discourse.

Thus, a question that is not trivial arises: why have societies that have attempted socialism and communism been unable to deal with psychosis, other than by allowing psychotics to establish dictatorships, in a way that, all things being unequal, led the entire experiment to be condemned? Perhaps the already well-worn notion of voluntary servitude could be put forward as an explanation, yet this is hardly sufficient. What should be examined, instead, is the overestimation of desire, which always gives a priority to the psychotic's fixed desire and its correlative valorisation of power. These remarks should not be seen as an attempt to segregate psychotics. Psychotic subjects have more than their share of the spirit that extends and enhances civilisation, but this spirit disappears as soon as they give up a questioning that has not been constrained by their generational being, and instead become frozen in a position of power that bars every other and does so both symbolically and in the real.

It may well be that "early" cultures did better than our own in offering psychotics a place that is powerful but remains marginal enough not to impinge upon politics as such. Religions – which are not, however, immune to mass exterminations – have perhaps also been able to channel the innocence of torturers outside politics. With the coming of capitalism, however, after a period of democratic conquests, these safety valves seem to have been closed, and as in the Roman Empire, the monomania of power has ended up rivalling the pursuit of money.

When the saints go marching in

For Lacan, it may well be that the "new man" or woman – who has received bad press – will be able to arise on the side of the mystics and the saints; capitalism cannot "fit" these figures any more than Cinderella's glass slippers could fit the wicked stepsisters' feet.[1]

Must capitalism be done away with or can we simply leave it? The answer is not obvious. In 1972, Lacan foresaw the blowout of capitalist discourse; shortly afterward, he wrote a striking phrase in *Television*: "The more saints, the more laughter; that's my principle, to wit, the way out of the capitalist discourse[2] – which will not constitute progress if it happens only for some" (Lacan, 1974b, p. 16). This statement is not finally, very original, and variations of it have been written throughout the centuries. The most eminent thinkers have always, whether rightly or wrongly, considered the saint and the poet as grains of sand in the coercive or segregative machine that pushes civilisations forward towards their impasses. Lacan's specific addition, however, is that this cannot be "only for some"; he excludes the possibility that an exit from capitalism will be progress if others are left inside it. Not surprisingly, this is a reference to the parable of the three prisoners from "Logical Time and the Assertion of Anticipated Certainty" (Lacan, 1945). Either they all leave together or they all remain prisoners. To say that the way out will not only be for some does not mean that everyone must be a saint in order to leave. There must, however, be enough saints to make the capitalist discourse obsolete, so that no one, anywhere, will be able to enter it. It would become a dead, uninhabited coral reef, a museum open on Sunday afternoon.

This reflection does not, in itself, tell us what a saint is. Belief or its lack can only be a trustworthy compass if we take seriously the theology that presided over the birth of the saint. The definition of a saint remains constant in Lacan's teaching: "the saint is the refuse of *jouissance*" (Lacan, 1974b, p. 16). "*Sicut palea*" (Lacan, 1968b, p. 8), to quote another passage in the same vein, where Lacan relies on Thomas Aquinas in order to sketch a picture of a psychoanalyst: these figures are not frozen in indifference or impassibility. Instead, they are open to their own impossibility. It is difficult to deny the family resemblance between the saint and the psychoanalyst. Think, for example, of a "minor" saint, such as Thérèse de Lisieux. Try also to take seriously the idea that "there is no better way of placing" a psychoanalyst "objectively than in relation to what was in the past called: being a saint" (Lacan, 1974b, p. 15). We can also note that Lacan (ibid., p. 15) chose the example of Baltasar Gracián for his "renouncing [of] personal brilliance". Once again, the saint is refuse. This implies that, for the saint, there is no jouissance in basking in the position of being a piece of trash; nothing, however, prevents the saint from catching up with this through ecstasy, if possible.

In this context, what is important is that saints act as a piece of trash, for their "business [is] *trashitas*" (ibid., p. 15), thus enabling any subject to take them as the cause of desire. Incarnating the object a, the saint sets up a discourse that goes against the capitalist discourse. The vector $a \rightarrow \$$ writes this "relation" on the upper line of the analytic discourse.

$$a \rightarrow \$$$

If the social bond follows this path, it cannot follow that of the capitalist discourse, in which the same vector, which is now diagonal, exaggerates the lack-in-jouissance by feeding the fantasy that the division of the subject can be suppressed by complementing it with a.

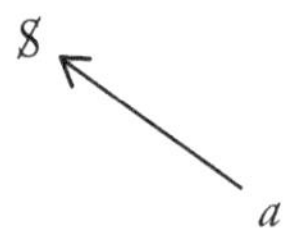

In the analytic discourse, on the contrary, this vector is marked as impossible, which means that the mutation of the subject in relation to jouissance is affected by the "abjectness" of this cause. Such a cause is both abject and produces abjectness. This mutation of the subject makes the capitalist discourse inoperative. Such a mutation should not, however, be idealised, for as Augustine recognised, the saint, in relation to God as jouissance, is always falling back into heresy. This is not a serious problem if we remember both that saints are not alone and can do nothing when they are alone.[3]

Let us suppose that our hope has been fulfilled: not a single person has not left the capitalist discourse and there are enough saints. We can link this with the symptom through the homophony between the French word "*symptôme*" and "*saint homme*", holy man. Let there be a *saint homme* for each according to his/her needs. If this reading of the future is correct, only the capitalist discourse will become obsolete, and the other discourses will remain. The discourse of the master is the one by which we enter language; we come into this discourse through an interior door, since everyone is already inside language. This leads to a rather incongruous question: when our holy people and our subjects of the unconscious come together, what sort of agreement would they have come to?

Nachtrag is not a deferred action.[4] At least initially, there has been no action at all, so nothing can be deferred. The action only comes into existence later, and acts by transforming the meaning of the initial moment. This is why "the meaning of the symptom depends upon the future of the real" (Lacan, 1975b, p. 186). One aspect of Lacan's treatment of time has not been sufficiently emphasised: because of language, our relation to time is never synchronic. Instead, it either takes the form of anticipation or occurs after the fact [*après-coup*]; thus, it introduces into science a dimension that departs from any postulates about the self-identity of time.

Let us try to grasp the symptom in terms of this dual temporality and take psychoanalysis itself to be a symptom: not a social symptom, but a symptom whose effect is as prosaic as possible on anyone who is undergoing or has undergone an analysis. With these two postulates, we can ask what the "dissolution" of the symptom means. The symptom comes into existence as an anticipation of the real: an anticipation of the impossible sexual relation, which would seek to reduce two to one, the not-all to the all, etc.[5] This symptom is then interpreted after the fact. Lacan thinks that interpreting the symptom does not involve stuffing it with meaning. Instead, we strip the real out of meaning, which can only imaginarise it. I began this section by quoting and agreeing with Freud's statement that the symptom has a sense. Have these considerations now rendered this formulation obsolete? If we define sense as what, on the basis of the symbolic and language, creates an image in the body in order to bring about the field of representation, then this formulation *has* become obsolete. In this context, meaning certainly misses what is real in the symptom. Yet there is another way to grasp meaning:[6] by distinguishing it from representation and connecting it, instead, to what enables the symbolic to be transmuted by the letter itself. This is not at all a representation by the signifier, and still less by the signified. It is generally a *figuration*, in the sense in which a figure is the thing itself. Without this figuration, painting, poetry or music would have no sense. This junction with the letter orients the subject along the curvature of the symptom: the real. This movement led Lacan to adopt the obsolete way of writing the French word *symptôme*: "*sinthome*".

If psychoanalysis is a symptom, then this has several implications. Psychoanalysis will succeed only at the price of abolishing the real. We must therefore hope that it will fail, because in doing so, it will remain a symptom of this real. The pervert's deal – in which the subject enters a passive mode as a bargaining chip in the demand that the Other also become passive – can only be proposed by the Other. Such a proposition has to be delegated to the Other because castration operates, first, at the level of the Other; this can assure the subject that there will be a limit to the passivity to which the Other would like to reduce him. Yet since the subject can only propose this perverse deal by putting her/himself in the place of the Other, s/he is exposed to castration. Structurally, this first odyssey can only have two results: 1) the subject can occupy the place of what cannot be castrated, which is necessary to certify that the Other can be castrated, *and* 2) the subject can move into the locus where castration ceases to operate, a locus that is no longer covered by the Other. Situating the priority of these two results is a true choice of *Kultur*: returning to the father[7] or going towards the feminine as unknown. This second result will preserve the first, although the latter's requirements will no longer be considered as absolute.

I can therefore desire that the real disappear; this would be a paradise and psychoanalysis would be a purgatory that would quickly be forgotten. In desire, is there something other than the desire for this disappearance? The real, however, does not disappear, and therefore gives us the occasion to desire, a desire that is brought to life by the ways of "making up for" [*suppléances*] that we have at our disposal; the dream is their natural prototype. Anxiety then becomes a risk, for it threatens us with the lack of lack. Can I live without the transitional object constituted by death? If life is full, can I live by forgetting death? In this context, it is invaluable to discover that only I am mortal and that the Other is not. The Other, beyond being the place of the "treasure trove of signifiers" (Lacan, 1960, p. 682), beyond being its living support, beyond Mount Olympus and its abstractions, is the white goddess, and it exists. It is the infinite element from which my finite body, as a living and speaking being, is made.[8]

Association *vs.* Institution

Near the end of volume III of *Capital*, Marx writes:

> Freedom, in the sphere [of the productive processes] can consist only in this, that socialized man, the associated producers, govern the human metabolism with nature in a rational way, bringing it under their collective control instead of being dominated by it as a blind power; accomplishing it with the least expenditure of energy and in conditions most worthy and appropriate for their human nature. But this always remains a realm of necessity. The true realm of freedom, the development of human powers as an end in itself, begins beyond it, though it can only flourish with this realm of necessity as its basis. The reduction of the working day is the basic prerequisite.
>
> *(Marx, 1894, p. 959)*

Marx's remarks are rather general and, in a certain way, almost ordinary. Yet they are interesting because they remind us implicitly that, in one sense, the capitalist mode of production is civilising: it is a condition by which the productive process can diminish the pressure of necessity. Once this task has been accomplished, however, it must disappear, to make way for a mode of production in which the "associated producers" could emancipate themselves from the "blind power" that had, until then, "govern[ed] the human metabolism with nature".

The problem is stated clearly but resolved less clearly: at what threshold does freedom begin? Surplus-labour, the source of surplus-value, will not disappear. What will change will be the mode of appropriating surplus-value, which will be collective rather than private. Does freedom begin with this change? Yes and no. At this level, freedom is still subordinated to the "empire of necessity". "The true realm of freedom" only begins when material production is accomplished in a way that is satisfying for everyone, and when it becomes possible to envision the primacy of free time over the time of obligatory labour. This condition remains unquestionable, but the perspective needs to be defined more fully, for the work that is called "free" remains without content. Furthermore, in another text in which Marx (1875, p. 347) envisions the communist "utopia", labour is defined as "a vital need". At least this way of putting the question keeps us from waiting for the poverty of minimal consumption to produce a solution, because even if dry bread and water could open the way to the kingdom of God, they run the more certain risk of programming people so that they cannot defend themselves against boredom, for they would tend to have no drives. Finally, in any event, this freedom, which is expressed by the formula, "From each according to his abilities, to each according to his needs" (ibid., p. 347) will, as the passage from *Capital* reminds us, remain based on the "realm of necessity".

This may be the moment to raise the question of the desire of the scientist and theorist. It is certain that Marx was able to resist boredom and was left indifferent by the trappings of power and wealth. As Lacan (1970, p. 434) says in "*Radiophonie*", surplus-value is "*Marxlust*, Marx's surplus-jouissance". This cannot be questioned seriously. If we seek to open up the paths for this research, how can we not see that the problem of surplus-value – once its discovery has given capitalism both its sceptre and its cross – is how to redistribute it? From this perspective, what is involved is not taking from some in order to give to others, but taking from everyone, so that the fact of possessing cannot be transformed into a thirst for possessions. The "theologians" of the economy of expense, especially Georges Bataille, saw this requirement, without being able to give it a suitable form. The goal is not to promote an economy of privation for everyone, which would be paired with an economy of waste for a God who has no needs. Instead, the diagonal vector of the capitalist discourse, $a \rightarrow \$$, needs to be broken, for it traps desire in an alternation between a "bulimia of consumption" and a destructive anorexia. Within the capitalist discourse, there can be no way out of this alternation. In a sense, the romantic poet became the bard of capitalism when he wrote that "One single being is wanting . . ." (Lamartine, 1820, p. 101, translation modified). From "I have a pair of

Adidas, therefore I am" to "A pair of Nikes is wanting . . .", it is clear that placing love in the consumerist prayer book has ennobled this book, but at the expense of love; the partner's departure, whether voluntary or not, becomes the cause of the poet's depression.

In the passage from volume III of *Capital* cited above, there is an invaluable expression: "associated producers". This is the green fruit that will ripen into the contradiction that I have drawn attention to, and which we must not forget if we do not want to remain stuck in the same place: what can be done about going beyond the labour that belongs to the realm of necessity if we do not make free, unconstrained labour the primary need of life? We know that Freud treated the desire to sleep as the first of all desires. Would the society that we dream of therefore be a society that is asleep? Rather than criticising the romantic poet, perhaps we should embrace him. When the poet writes "One single being is wanting . . .", he is indicating the way out of capitalism by making the other, the "associated" other, the figure who must be present as subject if our desire is not to be reduced to a desire to sleep. Perhaps the principle of "association" could thus be a way of refusing the diagonal arrow $a \rightarrow \$$ in the capitalist discourse.

Here are the minimal consequences of this principle.

1 $\$$ is no longer cut from S_2. The subject is no longer cut away from its unconscious.
2 Relying on the re-establishment of this junction, the subject accepts the impossibility of the vector, $a \rightarrow \$$. In other words, the foreclosure of castration ceases.
3 The subject can then cease to subscribe to the unconscious, to the extent that the latter will no longer be what produces him or her, as it does in the discourse of the master.

Whenever we say "association", we imply that people have decided to associate with one another. In the Lacanian psychoanalytic movement, the first and foremost association was the *École freudienne de Paris*, which Lacan himself founded in 1964. In this particular case, the foundation resulted from the desire of the analyst; Lacan's objective was to constitute a school that would be congruent with the purpose of psychoanalysis and would function on the basis of this purpose. In 1980, at the end of this school's history, Lacan himself dissolved it, for the explicit reason that it was functioning *against* psychoanalysis; the institution *had taken precedence over the association*.

It should also be noted that at the moment of this dissolution, Lacan presented himself as the one who, by withdrawing, would free the school's component elements. He was referring to the structure of the Borromean knot, in which the cutting of one circle frees the others. However, there was one difference in this particular case: unlike the Borromean knot, Lacan was the only circle that could free the others through the cut. This is far from being a negligible consideration, for it leads us to the idea that an associative structure can only be Borromean if each of the individuals who compose it is a founder of this association. "Founder", in this context, means the bearer of the only desire – the desire of the analyst – that is not a demand for identification. The next step would be to ask whether this association became an institution precisely because it had a single founder and *n* members. I shall leave to future historians of psychoanalysis the task of treating this question dispassionately. When erosion and fossilisation have done their work, the archaeologists will come. In legal terms, an association is necessarily and by definition an institution. Perhaps, furthermore, the association that had been dissolved left a sediment in the institutional configuration to which it had belonged.

The opposition between association and institution can be deduced from Lacan's final texts.[9] Yet, the prototype of this distinction can be found in the binary opposition between group psychology (*Massenpsychologie*) and collective logic. Very early, and at least as early as his famous article "Logical Time and the Assertion of Anticipated Certainty", Lacan (1945) distinguished his conception from the cynical and grumbling belief that psychoanalysis is something like a "sculpture of the self".[10] Lacan's entry into the psychoanalytic literature is often traced back to his fruitful and astute treatment of the mirror stage. The most important of his "youthful" ideas, however, is his conception of the act as an anticipation that is based entirely on two principles: an act is not the result of an abstract deduction and it implies taking the other as subject into account. Taking the subject into "account" has nothing to do with altruism, since it involves "counting" on this other. Lacan's early work, which still belonged more to psychiatry than to psychoanalysis, is already marked by a concern that never ended: the importance accorded to listening to *and* hearing the patient's message. This concern breaks completely with the idea, which, unfortunately, is still very much alive, even within Lacanian analysis, that the patient or – to put it bluntly – the analysand, can be reformed even when the practitioner does not hear her/his message. What immediately characterises this collective logic is that, in a very strange way, the fable of the prisoners treats the other's "doing" [*faire*] or "non-doing" [*non-faire*] as a saying [*dire*], even if saying is not always doing. In collective logic, no process of identification with the other turns this figure into an Other.

Louis Althusser pointed to a very important problem: an institution transforms the association between one and (another) one by hypostasing the One into an entity, which thereby becomes a norm that is independent of the associates. A sort of sleight-of-hand occurs, which obliges each of the associates to obey this One – even if the One has never given a command – while each of them believes that s/he is only obeying her/himself. It is easy to show how this trick is performed. All that is necessary is for some random person to become less the master than the "leader" (I won't mention the German word for this); he will then impose his own desire through a structural fraud, since the condition for following him is to believe that we do not have to follow him. Certainly, by setting himself up as One – while issuing frequent denials of what he is doing – he will confront the associates with what he considers to be their cowardly avoidance of any confrontation with the desire of the Other.[11] This desire must be cajoled and nourished, for if the Other did not exist, what would my desire be made of? This reasoning is impeccable, except that what belongs to me is the fulfilment – or not – of this desire, which turns my dreams into something simultaneously impersonal and intimate; once these dreams crystalise when I awake, I may be able to sign them in order to appropriate them.

The institution thus adds ideology to association. The practical question is whether this turn is inevitable. Even if we suppose that an association is explicitly governed by the principle that no one can enter it without (re)founding it, it is still necessary to avoid a principle that has no content. Since this content is the discursivity that characterises the analytic bond, the desire of each person in such an association can only be a desire without a demand: a desire that is regulated in terms of each person's satisfaction, a dephallicised desire. This, in any case, was Lacan's (1982b, p. 307) dream in the "*Note italienne*" where he suggested it would be possible to form an association that would be composed only of *AEs* [Analysts of the School].

The difficulty with this position is not so much its extreme requirements as its "set-theoretical" formalism, which thumbs its nose at hybridisation in its synchronic and, even more fundamentally, its diachronic dimension. An analysand who is not an analyst can belong to the group, even before the desire of the analyst comes to her/him, if it ever does. S/he can be a member of it because her/his presence is the condition for testing that very desire of the analyst. Consequently, the historical question concerning the privileged place of exception that Lacan occupied in his school returns in a new form: if a single member is not a founder – if he has not become a member by having demonstrated that the desire of the analyst has acted upon him, does this mean that the association is becoming sedimented into an institution? Does this inevitably signal the moment when a reversal will take place, and the institution will come to control the association? Should we then consider that the founding criterion was not correctly based on the desire of the analyst? This may be and is even without any doubt the case. The young generals of the French Revolution put a definitive end to the idea that establishing an oeuvre is a prerogative to be undertaken only at the end of one's career. In addition, this would involve recommissioning the idea of infallibility, making it conceivable and attainable for an association of analysts to display their desire out in the open, proudly, as if it were the badge of honour of a military decoration. The problem needs to be approached differently: no association can be pure – purged entirely of the institutional. For this reason, associations need to be sufficiently aware of the moment when they are about to pass the point of no return: the point beyond which conflicts of interest cannot be dealt with because – to use Melanie Klein's important distinction – they involve envy, which is insurmountable, and not only jealousy.

In this context, the solution becomes dissolution; this would be a way of removing associations from their institutionalisation, at a point at which the latter threatens to undo the associative foundation. Rather than waxing lyrical about institutionless associations, an objective that is as idealistic as the aspiration to be a subject without identifications, we must consent to associations in which the discourses of the hysteric, the university and the master will have a – subordinate – place.

This is certainly not a traumatic dream: a dream that is doomed to being repeated constantly. When we reread Marx's texts on workers' associations, which he considered not as a force for overthrowing the state but as a result of its withering away, or hear the statement attributed to Lenin to the effect that "Any cook should be able to run the country", we see how they thought that such institutions could operate smoothly. The reshuffling of positions becomes a permanent means of dissolution, and dissolution becomes an act that gives such reshuffling another chance. We know, however, that reshuffling can itself end up involving only a Stendhalian "happy few",[12] or turning around a fixed hub.

Finally, and perhaps especially, in order to avoid turning what is new into what is always the same, we need to take what Lacan called "swarming" [*essaimage*][13] seriously. This includes being aware of what has happened in the Lacanian movement since his death: the emergence of a constellation of associations whose only sun had been extinguished – "Other at last", as Lacan (1980c, p. 135) said before he became it.

An analysis, as both experience and experiment, is founded on the rule that an analysand must say everything or must speak in spite of everything. To make this contention more concrete through a rule, the sexual encounter between analyst and analysand is forbidden; the consequence of this rule is that if such an encounter takes place, the experiment of analysis comes to an end. The fault lies less in sexual activity itself than in the imposture of claiming that such activity is compatible with analysis and would even be a way of continuing it. From this single example, we can deduce the difference between morality and ethics: morality would have it that a healthcare professional should not take advantage of his position of authority by seducing the person under his care or allowing himself to be seduced by her/him; ethics argues that giving up the rule of abstinence means giving up the desire of the analyst.

In this field, psychotic subjects – whether or not they are analysands or analysts – may be the best able to question the modes of transference, not in psychoanalytic action but in political action. This action involves deactivating the capitalist discourse: making it obsolete because it no longer has any agents. Ideally, we could think that reformism – which always involves the primacy of ethics over politics – would be enough to bring about this transferral. Political action would consist in winning potential agents over to the maxim: act according to your ethics and don't worry about the results. This formulation is rather close to what would be involved in psychoanalytic action, but there is one problem with it. Since any maxim can only be imposed by suggestion, an agent's adoption of it would reproduce the primacy of political over psychoanalytic action, which is the opposite of what is being sought.[14]

I have just mentioned the psychotic subject precisely because for him/her, the Name-of-the-Father is foreclosed. This foreclosure prevents morality from operating, for the basis of morality is the possibility of identifying with the counterpart and saying, "I don't want to do to the other what I wouldn't want him/her to do to me". The Name-of-the-Father underlies the possibility of identifying with an other who has submitted to the law of castration; the law, in turn, decrees that every x is either a man or a woman, and that no son or daughter can be the brother, sister or father of his/her own father. If the psychotic subject lacks such morality, how can s/he be located? The psychotic subject may be able to submit to morality as a convention, without genuinely adhering to it. S/he can only locate her/himself through the symptom, and can do so in a way that can show the core of the symptom, stripped of any phallic embellishment. This core is the statement, "I want to get off on the Other without the Other's getting off on me". For the psychotic, the question is how to welcome becoming not-all, the margin in which castration does not operate completely, and in which s/he can touch the real. This not-all would allow the psychotic not to be forced into a push-to-woman [*pousse-à-la-femme*].[15]

For the psychotic, there can be a temptation here to realise the phallus – which one cannot have symbolically (if one is a man) or which one cannot entirely be symbolically (if one is a woman) – by becoming the living totem of a community, a country, a family. The paranoiac has a special talent for this and finds it attractive. The schizophrenic sticks to a collateral tyranny, from which he tries in vain to detach himself, for he can choose neither the Other nor himself as the tyrant. Finally, those who suffer from mania and melancholia have difficulty mourning for what they haven't lost. Otherwise, if ethics triumphs and the subject decides to identify with the symptom, to the point of being able to make up for the Name-of-the-Father, from which s/he did not have to suffer, but which s/he also did not know how to use, the solution s/he invents will express an authentic primacy of psychoanalytic action over both political pragmatism and idealism.

As we have seen, Lacan, when speaking of the consequences of the capitalist discourse, referred to the foreclosure of castration. This foreclosure does not differentiate between neurotics, perverts and psychotics, since it subjects all of them to a discourse that amputates them, as subjects, from their relation, whatever that may be, with castration. They are all deprived of access to an unconscious that could enable them to deactivate their fantasy or their delusion.[16]

Gelassenheit

This is the term that Lacan used when Catherine Millot (2001, pp. 12–14) reported her experience of the "emptiness" of death to him.[17] "*Gelassenheit*" can be translated as "releasement",[18] "serenity" or "letting be" (ibid., p. 12). It is tempting to set it in opposition to foreclosure – including this term's legal sense – which indicates that something has been rejected: thrown outside the field of the symbolic, after a phase in which allowing it in would have been possible.

Does "letting be" permit the advent, not in the symbolic but in lived experience, of some bits and pieces of the real which, because of a temporal shift, have not been able to make an imprint in the wax of the symbolic? In her book, Millot (ibid., pp. 31–39) mentions the poet Henri Michaux's experiments. Michaux made a deliberate attempt to reach this experience through drugs, and was not content to describe afterwards what happened to him. Instead, in the real time of the experiment, he made graphemes that circumvented language, enabling what could not be symbolised to be "written". Becoming a living seismograph, he hoped to enlarge knowledge, taking it beyond the borders of the linguistic and the symbolic.

Alain Didier-Weill (2003, p. 32) examines the same kind of problems in reference to Emmanuel Levinas' (1961) book, *Totality and Infinity*: "The newborn baby's absolute passivity is the position by which the human who is to come offers, in its finitude, a place where what is infinite in the Other can be inscribed". The problem here is to understand the status of "what is infinite in the Other", since in order for the subject to be constituted, a step must be taken that goes beyond this original passivity: an "act through which the subject responds" must constitute what Freud calls primal repression (ibid., p. 32). This act involves an abolishing of the *signifiance* that had been primally welcomed or received in an operation homologous to the invention of zero in mathematics (see Seife, 2000). We could suppose that the original receiving of *signifiance*, before it is cast out, in fact produces no signified-effect. Perhaps, instead, this effect would only occur at the moment of the expulsion, which itself provokes whatever was welcomed to begin signifying. In any case, I myself am inclined to think that the constitutive division comes about when the "half a subject" (see Lacan, 1991, pp. 62–66) objects to accepting an original passiveness that would fully deliver the subject, "as a whole", to the jouissance of the Other. If this is correct, then the subject would come into existence at the same moment as the symptom; these two advents would be two sides of one and the same event.[19]

This can shed light on two points. First, the foreclosure of castration that Lacan links to capitalist discourse means that – whenever contingency emerges – this discourse prevents unconscious knowledge from shaking the subject's assurance of being. It thus ends up foreclosing the space-time in which the law could cease to appear as the immutable commandment of God or nature. This is the space-time in which castration could cease to be abstract, and one could go beyond it. It is certain that there is always an irreducible place in the psyche where castration has not acted; Freud located this in his case history of the Wolf Man. When what is impermeable to analysis in this place has been located, then an end to the talking cure can be envisioned. Second, the foreclosure of castration has nothing to do with the foreclosure of the signifier of the Name-of-the-Father; this first foreclosure does not necessarily make the Wolf Man a psychotic. If we look for psychotics among the "neurotics" discussed by Freud, it would be better to focus on Woodrow Wilson (Freud & Bullitt, 1966), with his abstract and "unreasonable" love of power: his marriage, without any possibility of divorce, to power. This "marriage" enabled him to simulate a discursive position as master and was accompanied by a disavowal of this position, which was authentic precisely because it was true. In this travel-free odyssey, the worst is generally what becomes most certain.

To return to *Gelassenheit*, Catherine Millot seems to have perceived correctly that the father's position enabled the place of this experience to be brought out; at one moment, her father authorised her not to go to school, thereby allowing her to subtract herself partially from the Law. She writes that:

> On that day, my father had the paradoxical function of exempting me from the law that is common to all, of permitting me not to be wholly submitted to it. If it is true, as Lacan claims, that love is giving what one does not have,

> my father gave me the gift of his love, for he gave me what he did not have at his disposal: the power to exempt myself from castration. And if it did not fall within his scope to subtract me from it entirely, it is nevertheless certain that he gave me a little leeway with the ability not to take the norm for the law.[20]
>
> *(Millot, 2001, p. 142)*

This is a decisive remark, for it separates the submission to castration from the consent to something beyond the law, but which is not disorder pure and simple. This emphasises two requirements. First, there is no law without an interpretation: not an interpretation of what the law means, but a decision about what is and what is not law (see Agamben, 2003).[21] Second, beyond the Law, there is the space for an experience that does not fall within the jurisdiction of any law. At this level, the classical debate between *nomos* and *nomina* has no object, and this brings us back to the question of the "oceanic feeling", a term that indicates that it touches the infinite, and not only in a metaphorical way.

Through the context in which it occurs, we can see that this experience – which is little more than embryonic when we approach it only as a "feeling" – does not require the subject to be psychotic, and thus to have no relation with the naming [*nomination*] of the father. Instead, it would be better to distinguish mystical experiences from astrological and cosmological delusions, which have an inhibiting power that is as effective as ordinary forgetting. (Mysticism, in this context, needs to be differentiated from any religious connotations; it would include, for example, the experiences of the "experimenter", Henri Michaux.) To keep to related references, we know that the writers in the *Grand jeu* group, particularly René Daumal (see 1938), gave a pivotal place to this experience, while working to preserve its secular status. Likewise, the writers associated with *Acéphale* – Georges Bataille (1986) and a few rare people whom he had chosen – sought to force open the gateway to infinity by making Eros collide with Thanatos. If we take Teresa of Avila – who reached an ecstasy that was stronger than union – as the great paradigm of mystical experience, we can see that her very strong anchoring in the phallus enabled her to bear the painful aspects of this experience.

There are, however, great poets, such as Hölderlin and Celan – as well as Artaud – who cast themselves adrift from the phallus and found that this did not lead them to ecstasy. Instead, at certain moments, it immersed them in an unimaginable anxiety. Through writing, however, they succeeded in transmitting what someone like Teresa of Avila had difficulty in being able to say: the imperfection of God that founds life. We recall a line from Hölderlin (1801, p. 156/157) that was so enigmatic to his contemporaries: "*bis Gottes Fehl hilft*/Till God's being not there helps him."

On messianism

We can see a decisive issue coming to the fore: what is the rightful place of the transcendent, which was explicitly disregarded by Enlightenment thinkers because it was too closely related to religious obscurantism? Can the transcendent accommodate any form of social bond or is it always a monadic activity?[22] This is a difficult question, but – to start somewhere – I would say that a monadic stance in which all other subjects are cast aside seems to be the prerequisite for having a one-to-one relationship with God, with a "personal" God who, as experience shows, may reverberate through an ecclesiastical organisation that is more devoted to making sure that only one head rises above the others. It may even be that, although dialogue is an unusual occurrence, it can take place – however unpredictably – between an analysand and an analyst, and such exchanges always have a transcendent dimension. Beyond this, there may just be some finely-tuned misunderstanding.[23]

In his book *Specters of Marx*, Jacques Derrida (1993, p. 74) refers to the possibility of "a messianic without messianism". In a later response to Marxist critics of the book, Derrida elaborates on this idea as follows:

> I find it hard to decide whether messianicity without messianism (*qua* universal structure) precedes and conditions every determinate, historical figure of messianism . . . or whether the possibility of thinking this independence has only come about or revealed itself as such by way of the "Biblical" events which name the messiah and make him a determinate figure.
>
> *Derrida (2002, p. 255)*

What is being theorised in this controversy? Without seeking to choose between a messianicity with or without messianism, and without being too preoccupied with Léon Daudet, who ironically used the term "messianism" against Marx, it may well be necessary to examine the figure of the messiah. The Aramaic etymology of "messiah" refers to the "anointed one" and confirms that this figure has been given a divine mission. Yet if we remove the messiah's ecclesiastical logo and approach Jesus as an "important passand" rather than as a figure who was sent by God, then this can have implications for the bond with another subject that the analytic discourse itself promotes. This bond takes on a dimension that, unlike Freud's statements in his exchange with Romain Rolland, does not exclude the idea of the infinite.

What serves as the foundation of this bond? While Freud (Meng & Freud, 1963, p. 126) thought that psychoanalysis needed to be protected from priests, he also saw quite clearly – or at least said this in a letter to Oskar Pfister on 25 November 1928 – that psychoanalysts can be defined as "secular pastors of souls".[24] The pastoral metaphor would seem to be insignificant, if we forget that it could lead the analysand to change his/her identification with the herd. The bond between the analyst and the analysand is held together by transference; it only takes on its true significance when the analysand detaches him/herself from this couple. Hence, we can grasp how, in the analytic discourse, the vector between the two is qualified as "impossible". Things could go otherwise, however, in the experience of the pass. The pass is a mechanism that Lacan (1968b, 1978a) invented in 1967; it seeks to provide a way to authenticate the desire of the analyst. It comprises a "passand [*passant*]", the analysand who takes part in this, and two "passers [*passeurs*]", who each receive the passand's testimony about his/her analysis, independently of one another. They then transmit the testimony to a committee (the passand is not present for this). It can be argued that, in this experience, the bond between the passer and passand eludes, in principle, the alienating dimension of transference that occurs in analytic treatment. The passer is not a pastor.

We can now return to the question of what founds the bond with the other subject in analytic discourse. The passand testifies to a movement through and beyond the experience of *Hilflösigkeit*, a helplessness for which there is no solution (see Freud, 1926a, pp. 141–142). This is a moment in which I am out of "sync" with the other, and even a moment in which I am deprived of my ego, which is the product of an identification with the image of the other. At this juncture, the treatment proves the power that it has – or has not – had, for this helplessness is what provides a buttress for the subject. This buttress constitutes what is real in life, and death can only efface it in a false way, for *life has occurred*. Confronted with the passand, the passer is not the other who will palliate the absence of any solution to helplessness. Instead, the passer constitutes a sort of "secular address", which is necessary in order for the passand's testimony to go beyond the chains of solitude. Is the mystic's bond with God or with those who are still afraid of their *Hilflösigkeit*?

The work of the psychoanalyst Sudhir Kakar is relevant in this context. In Kakar, we find a questioning that indicates what is at stake when a non-religious transcendence is allowed to enter psychoanalysis. This transcendence involves neither a church nor an apparatus of initiation. Kakar locates himself outside any relation to the three monotheisms and their common ecclesiastical space (although the nature of the ecclesiastical model varies greatly from one monotheism to another). His reference to the *darshan* – looking at and introjecting the benevolent power of the guru through the gaze (see Kakar, 1982, p. 134) – may seem perplexing. The analogy between the guru's silence and the mother's silence (see Kakar, 1991, p. 66) may also appear puzzling, yet this is linked to the culture of India, where the mother's silence is associated with her presence; this situation is very different from what usually happens in the west, where her silence signals her absence. His praise of fantasy and its mythogeny, although written in terms that make it difficult to distinguish between poetic creation and Jungian anagogy, is even more suggestive. His interest in Bion, who dared to speak about the analysand's "divinity" (see Bion, 1965, p. 159) is also a good sign. It converges on the improper encounter, on the analytic couch, between the mystic, who "made the potatoes sing" and the poet who brought out the acid of the word "lemon" (see Clément & Kakar, 1993). What is unsatisfactory is his vagueness on the nature of the analytic bond: on what basis can one say that this bond is conditioned by a transference that is only valuable if it can be resolved, instead of being used for "worldly" ends?

In this respect, during the phase in which the analysand can envision an end to analysis, *Hilflösigkeit* will take forms that can be articulated; precisely because they can be articulated, they will be absolutely singular. The experience of the pass enables these forms to be collected, although we cannot know in advance what forms they will take; this increases the importance of what is at stake. This experience is still young, but it could lead to analyses in which the demon or daemon of transference will no longer be Satan. Instead, this figure will be the very action of sharing (the Indo-European word was *daiethai*) one's own time and the "time of the other".

The chariot and the sphere

In 1930, Ludwig Binswanger wrote an article that was translated into English under the title "Dream and Existence" (and published along with a lengthy introduction by Michel Foucault [1954]). We know about both Binswanger's friendship with Freud, which lasted from 1910 until the psychoanalyst's death (see Fichtner, 2003), and his gradual distancing of himself from psychoanalysis; his article testifies to this distancing. In its third part, he gives an interpretation of a dream, in which it immediately becomes apparent that the dreamer's associations (perhaps this was Binswanger's own dream) were not asked for; instead, it is interpreted according to a preformed ideological schema. As Binswanger notes:

> This is a most interesting dream in many ways. Notice the trichotomy of thesis (dreaming, tormented life in isolation), antithesis (death by total dissolution of individual life following total surrender to the overpowering objective principle of "otherness"), and synthesis (by "reclaiming objectivity in subjectivity"). The dream thus pictorially mirrors the psychoanalytic process as a progression from the individual's defiant persistence in his isolation, to the humble subjection to the (impersonal) "authority" of the doctor ("transference phase") to the "resolution of the transference".
>
> *(Binswanger, 1930, p. 100)*

I am deliberately not going to give the text of this dream, in order to accentuate the "chance" relation between it and its interpretation; it allows Binswanger to apply a grid that, following Jung's method, could be called "anagogical". Conceived in this way, the dream illustrates a process that, either partially or completely, is always the same. In this case, it could be said that it illustrates the ideal end of an analysis; the problem, however, is to know how this end can be reached other than by the analyst-interpreter's mental projection.

If we follow Freud, each dream should be considered as making present a particular movement from the jouissance of the drives to the unconscious, by satisfying the "considerations of figurability" [*Darstellbarkeit*][25] that enable the dream to become a form of writing that can be deciphered (Freud, 1900, pp. 339–349, translation modified). We can see the effect of this definition of the dream on Binswanger's conception.

The more interesting aspects of Binswanger's account lie in his attack on the theory of dreams found in Petronius, whom he describes as a "fine and free-spirited confident of Nero", but which also occurs in Lucretius, the great materialist poet (Binswanger, 1930, p. 96). This theory claims that dreams are not sent by the gods but that "Each man creates his own (*sed sibi quisque facit*)" (ibid., p. 96). Binswanger criticises Petronius' opinion, saying that he has "grasped only half the truth" and reproaches him for forgetting that although "man steers his carriage 'where he wishes'" – and thus he agrees with Petronius – "'beneath the wheels there turns, unnoticed, the globe upon which he moves'" (ibid., p. 96). He believes that this criticism places him closer to Freud than to Jung.

Concerning Freud, he is not absolutely wrong. For example, in his correspondence with Freud, Binswanger asks him whether the unconscious is the equivalent of Kant's noumenon. In other words, does the existence of the unconscious point to what is beyond phenomena? We also know that, to the great displeasure of Ernest Jones, Freud was always secretly disturbed by the occult. Following Lacan, we can say that this question suggests that there is a real that cannot be dissolved into phenomenal reality. Binswanger's argument is therefore not off track. Lacan's distinction between reality – which can be articulated entirely through language – and the real – which is incompatible with meaning, except through an act that can confer meaning upon it after the fact – goes in the same direction; this direction preserves psychoanalysis from being simply another antidote or just the best science of the soul.

The difficulty is that it is impossible to reach Binswanger's "globe" through his "chariot", and therefore he cannot avoid falling into the trap of spiritualism. To prove this, we need only read the key sentences of his article: "no one has ever succeeded and no one will ever succeed in deriving the human spirit from instincts (*Triebe*). These two concepts are, by their very nature, incommensurable, and it is their incommensurability that justifies the existence of both concepts, each within its own proper sphere" (ibid., p. 101). It may well be impossible to *deduce* the spirit from "instincts"; this statement is related to the problem, which Binswanger mentions, of the transference and how it is resolved. We can even agree that these are "incommensurable" concepts. Instead, however, of using these observations to measure the extraordinary and novel character of Freud's discovery, he concludes that only a spiritualisation of psychoanalysis can save it. To save it in this way, however, would be to eradicate both the drive – the limit-concept between the somatic and the psychic – and the signifier, which is material.

Binswanger's reasoning involves the same dehiscence – a coming apart or opening up – between an upper and a lower that, in the next section, we shall encounter in relation to Jesus. First, however, we should note what is at stake for the symptom here: if only the symptom *knows*, and therefore neither the subject nor the Other knows, then it is surely only at the level of the symptom as "medium" that we can grasp how impossibility inheres in the incompatible "relation" between the real and meaning.[26] On the basis of this, we can bring out a kind of knowledge that has no author, a knowledge that, unlike the ideal of science, cannot simply be formalist. "No author" does not mean "no signature". Finally, we should give Binswanger credit for having seen how the aporia of the relation between the human spirit and the drive touches on transference, which we know that Lacan related to what is transcendent in love.

The impossible supposition

In his erudite and perceptive book *Le pur amour: de Platon à Lacan*, Jacques Le Brun (2002) paid the finest possible homage to Lacan's interest in "pure love" by providing us with its history. He shows that its centre of gravity is located in the quarrel between Bossuet and Fénelon at the turn of the eighteenth century. At the heart of this confrontation, which ended in Fénelon's political disgrace, was the question of the "impossible supposition" (ibid., p. 44).[27] According to Le Brun (ibid., p. 53–54), this supposition originates in both a statement that Moses makes in Exodus[28] and these words of Paul to the Romans: "For I could wish that I myself were accursed and cut off from Christ for the sake of my brethren, my kinsmen by race" [Romans 9:3]. In other words, Paul envisions a situation in which, in order for his brothers to be saved, he would himself be separated from Jesus and deprived of salvation.

Le Brun discusses the different interpretations of this passage made by the saints and ecclesiastical authorities before Fénelon, in whose work we find formulations that presage the views that Bossuet would consider worthy of condemnation, and which were condemned by the Church when published in the *Maxims of the Mystics* (Fénelon, 1697b). Le Brun refers in particular to the following statement:

> We can also inspire in belaboured and truly humble souls an obedience and consent to the will of God, through what is, all the same, a very false supposition: rather than the eternal good that He promised to the righteous, He instead would keep them in eternal torment by His own whim, yet without depriving them of His grace and love.[29]
>
> *(Le Brun, 2002, p. 175)*

In this passage, three decisive elements mark out Fénelon's problematic:

1 A righteous soul can consent to eternal torment (as in Paul's statement), if this is God's will. With a slight change, this affirmation rectifies the canonical thesis that it is forbidden for a Christian not to want salvation.
2 However, God cannot want to condemn a just soul to eternal torment (the "false" or "impossible supposition"). Therefore, the righteous soul supposes wrongly that this is God's will.
3 Finally, even if a righteous soul can consent to eternal torment on the basis of a false supposition that this is God's will, this soul cannot be deprived of God's grace and love.

In the false supposition, we can see the shadow of Big Brother, a figure who tortures out of love, but this is not the essential point. If we follow Fénelon's distinction between condemnation to hell and the preservation of God's love for the righteous soul, and also the extreme criterion he uses in defining pure love as loving God *even while being* damned, a question remains: what if, when God condemns the soul to eternal torment, he *also* deprives it of his love? We thus see that the impossible supposition raises not one but two questions. The first can be formulated at once: is the supposition actually false? After all, nothing prevents God from being, for reasons beyond our understanding, the Supreme-Being-in-Evil, which Sade conceived of less than a century after Fénelon (Lacan, 1986, p. 215). The second, and even more burning, question is: could a righteous soul, in supposing wrongly that God wanted both to damn it and to deprive it of love, still consent to God's will?

Before examining the consequences of such questions for our own topics, two more remarks are necessary. First, in the *Maxims of the Mystics* (Fénelon, 1697b), there are several references to the impossible supposition. This seems to be the simplest version: "We should love Him [God] as much were He even – to suppose what is impossible – to see fit to take no notice of our love, or to wish to reward with eternal misery those who had loved Him" (1697b, p. 37). It is interesting to note that Fénelon considered this to be homologous to a remark by Saint Francis de Sales, which he goes on to cite: "'Purity of love consisteth in desiring nothing for self; in considering only the good pleasure of God, for the sake of which we should be ready to esteem eternal misery above the glory of heaven'" (ibid., p. 38). Francis de Sales was clearly not saying the same thing as Fénelon, because he does not include any sort of false supposition in his account; it is as if the "good pleasure of God" could in fact include damning a righteous soul to hell. In fact, Francis de Sales was not interested in whether God's will is good or bad; such a will simply *is*.

Second, if readers are once again wondering how this impossible supposition, however interesting it may be in its own right, could possibly be relevant to a book on the theme of Lacan and Marx, I would like to highlight the strange similarity – and even identity – between Fénelon's major signifiers and those of psychoanalysis: supposition, love, interest, soul, desire, will, resistance, equivocation, passiveness, division, jealousy, impossibility, loss, disapproval, etc.

⁂

Perhaps the best way to proceed would be to begin by taking three steps that will lead us to grasp the relevance of Fénelon's questions for psychoanalysis. The purpose of these steps is not to create the illusion of a teleology, but instead to recognise that the solutions and impasses that Fénelon articulated in terms of theology are also crucial for the Lacanian and Marxist fields. They are crucial because what is in question is nothing less than the status of jouissance: the jouissance of God and of the just or unjust soul.

1 This step involves articulating the relation between the impossible supposition and transference. What does the Other want? This central question, which Lacan examined in terms of psychoanalysis, is incontestably present.
2 This step, which is just as easy, introduces a side of God that concerns the will – whether imagined or real – of the Other. In this respect, it is worth noting that in Saint Francis de Sales' formulation, will is of the order of a real; God is not gauged in terms of a scale that weighs good and evil. Instead, God is identified with a will, and pure love is not supposed to judge the content of this will. In this context, passivity becomes a virtue of the righteous soul in its relation to God's will; in light of what Fénelon says about the effacing of the ego, one can wonder whether this passivity concerns the real side or the Other side of God.
3 Finally, the third step: if, impossibly, God wanted evil, which would reveal that the will of God is divorced from written law, how should Christians act?

Fénelon was also attacking quietists such as the Beghards, who believed that reaching pure love placed the righteous soul beyond the written law. This soul was no longer concerned by the written law and the Church's norms. In a sense, Fénelon's position was less courageous, since it held that the supposition of an evil God was impossible, attributing it to an error of the soul. He admitted that this error could have its source in God's jealousy and desire to hide his will; nevertheless, the responsibility for such an error is finally the soul's own. The aim of his relative cowardice is to preserve the value of the law, which is identical to God's will. In other words, if God did not love the righteous soul, then he would not be God, for he would be outside the law.

It is certainly a delicate matter to transfer these final considerations into psychoanalytic terms. They can, nevertheless, be located in a dialectic between the Thing (*das Ding*) and the father; in other words – and this is the guiding thread of my argument – this involves the confrontation between the symptom, on the one hand, and the Name-of-the-Father, on the Other.

Let us examine this point by point.

1 In response to the first question, "What does the Other want?", we should remember that Lacan's definition of transference detaches it from simple repetition. Beyond any duplication of infantile conduct towards the parents, transference includes the analyst's presence and its effect on the analysand. The fundamental condition for this presence is the introduction, in the analytic relation, of what Lacan did not call the "Other-supposed-to-know". Instead, he called it the subject-supposed-to-know. This does not mean that this subject is some sort of tracing of the contours of the analyst. Lacan insists that this subject plays the role of a third party in this relation; in the final phase of the treatment, the analysand is tempted to incarnate such a subject, before accepting, as a conclusion, that it be deposed [*destitution*].

How does this solution clarify and enable us to surmount the aporia of the "impossible supposition"? In analysis, this supposition can be detected in a fantasy that takes the form of a question: what if my analyst wants what is evil?[30] Such a fantasy is usually presented in whispers, and for the most part, does not affect the treatment; in cases of negative transference, it most often takes the form of an accusation that the analyst is stupid. The delusion that the analyst is fundamentally harmful arises almost exclusively in psychosis. Whether it takes the form of a fantasy or a delusion, no way out of this impossible supposition can be envisioned as long as the analysand remains trapped in the alternative that either the subject knows or the Other knows.

If it is the subject who knows, then we end up making it the equivalent of the Other, which had first been credited with knowledge, in a process that corresponds precisely to the theses of the quietists, the Beghards and other "false mystics". Fénelon had made a point of rejecting their ideas in order not to be taken by Bossuet and the Church for one of their defenders. Thus, in article XLIII of the *Maxims of the Mystics*, Fénelon (see 1697b, p. 103) explicitly disavows as false the notion that the "transformed soul" can "pass judgement on all the truths of Religion and not be judged by any person".[31]

If, however, the analyst is the subject who knows, we are close to Žižek's (1993b, p. 71) thesis, in *Tarrying with the Negative*, that "I am what I am only for the Other". From this point of view, Žižek's thesis is exemplary, for it allows the Other to determine the subject's being. In other words, absolute obedience to the Other's dictates would enable us to go beyond this aporia. Fénelon makes it possible for us to read this response implicitly in certain quotations from Saint Francis de Sales, who was not worried about supposing the "impossible". This immunity and indifference to the pathology of transference would signal an authentic adherence to pure love.

As we shall see later, the aporia of whether it is the subject or the Other who knows will remain as long as transference has not been resolved. If the soul obeys God passively and absolutely, what guarantees that God is not the devil? It is at this level that a solution is necessary in order to be certain that God's will is identical to the commandments of the law, as Paul stated them. The Church is founded on the axiom that they are identical, and therefore the soul can never separate them, however much it may have been transformed in its path towards salvation. This is how Fénelon reconciles ecclesiastical orthodoxy with the radicalisation involved in saintliness.

For psychoanalysis, such a "response" can be called religious because it delegates to the Other the responsibility for saying the subject's truth. In this context, it is interesting to note that in his book on Christianity and perversion, Žižek, without dealing with the psychoanalytic dimension of this question, implicitly criticises his own earlier conception. He does so when discussing the duping involved in displaying castration; through this duping – "I am what you say" – the subject simulates submission, thereby deceiving the Other. The position of Saint Francis de Sales is certainly not to be interpreted in this way, as I shall argue, but this feigning does indeed exist among the examples that Žižek mentions.

2 The second step is connected with the question of God's will. In relation to the question, "What does God want?", Fénelon's position is clear and always remains the same: God can want me to be damned, even if my soul is righteous. At the very least, he can jealously hide his will, so that the righteous soul will imagine that it has been damned. However, God cannot want the just soul to be deprived of his love, and therefore no soul can accept not loving God.

Fénelon's propositions concerning God's will are axioms, rather than theorems. As I have emphasised, Saint Francis de Sales does not ask whether God is just. God's will is neither just nor unjust but simply is, and this is the only way of positing a transcendence that cannot be qualified. As long as the debate does not reach this extreme position, there are only three choices. The first is Bossuet's, which is located in the master's political discourse, and holds that only the Church can make theological judgements. The second is the choice of the quietists, among others, who, while affirming absolute submission to God, make this submission into the source of their equality with God. This step exempts them from obedience to the Church, and for this reason, Madame Guyon was accused of quietism. Finally, Fénelon's position seeks to frame this transcendence. For a human being, it is impossible to understand and reach this transcendence, and Fénelon takes this impossibility into account. This problem led him to limit the freedom of God, who cannot want evil, and to preserve a certain freedom for human beings. The free and meritorious act remains indispensable, even in passive contemplation.

Fénelon's position may well claim to be more faithful to Christianity than the other options; it does not eliminate the fact that a human being is flesh as well as soul. This ingloriousness of humanity justifies and necessitates the mediation between the human and the divine. At the same time, his position has a limit, which may be the limit of Christianity, but which is transgressed by the saint: Fénelon can only posit God as Other. The real of God – God as unconscious – thus escapes him, even if this is at the heart of the problematic of the saint.

3 We now reach the third step, which concerns the dialectic of the symptom and the Name-of-the-Father. I have developed at length the thesis that only the symptom knows. The analysand can be caught in a dilemma: "Either I (the subject) know or s/he (the Other) knows". As long as the analysand remains in this position, there will be no satisfactory way out, except through a forcing that leaves intact the fantasy that had motivated the entry into analysis. For Lacan, equivocation was a paradigm of interpretation, whether the latter comes from the analyst or the analysand. All too often, however, such interpretation has been reduced to wordplay that has been cut off from the real. Interpretations only touch the real when the equivocation poses a question – who is speaking, the subject or the Other? – and imposes an answer – neither one nor the Other. What, then, is speaking, if not *das Ding*, the Thing, which, by the grace of the symptom, turns out to be the real messenger? Thus, the symptom escapes what seems to condemn the subject to a situation in which its being is spoken entirely by the Other, because the Other is the place where, primally, it speaks [*ça parle*] about this subject, in a kind of linguistic baptism.

The manifestation of the symptom says, "I don't want the Other to get off on me". This function is then paired with another position, "I want to get off on the Other", which results from my primary identification with the Other. "I don't want to be under its thumb and I don't want it to make me passive". In this situation, the only way not to become the slave of my own tyranny is the one that Freud discovered: the murder of the father, which transforms his will-to-jouissance into law. I shall not discuss the form of this discovery, except to recall that Lacan based it on a logical existence that is connected to the human being's linguistic status, without employing Freud's questionable anthropological myth. The Name-of-the-Father serves as a guardrail against a general tyranny, but by conferring the status of exception upon the father who bears it, it includes a consequence that becomes religious if it is accorded primacy or exclusivity: the expression "in the name of the father" refers to an Other who is supposed to be infallible.

The Name-of-the-Father neither prevents the symptom nor dissolves it; at best (or at worst), it hides the symptom. However, when the Name is foreclosed, the symptom is given latitude to act without the law. In the first of these two cases, there is a primacy of the Name-of-the-Father over the symptom. The second case concerns psychosis, where the problem for the subject is to procure a sort of prosthetic law, which would enable this subject to carry out the sometimes very difficult task of escaping from his/her own tyranny.

In this context, what kind of solution is offered by analytic treatment? To answer this question, let us return to Saint Francis de Sales and to what enables him to explain the impossible: that a saint would not be preoccupied with being damned, and even – scandal of scandals – with being deprived of God's love. Yet this can be inverted. Fénelon asks a question that his membership in the Church imposes upon him: how can a saint possibly want to be anathematised? While responding to this question, he rejects the possibility that God can deprive the just soul of his love. We need to ask the opposite question: perhaps saintliness involves the ordeal of encountering a God who is flawed or inadequate. The law does not thereby become a dead letter, since, as we have seen, it fulfils a secular task: it prevents the subject from succumbing to his/her own tyranny. Yet if the saint does not get through this ordeal, God remains the Other who knows, even if nothing knows, except the symptom.

In one of his final seminars, *The Sinthome*, Lacan (2005b) developed the transformation of the symptom into a sinthome. This movement, contrary to Freud's thesis, does not occur through sublimation; as Lacan (1971, p. 327) put it, Joyce "[went] straight in it to the best one may expect from psychoanalysis at its end". He detached the symptom from its pathological interior, keeping only its envelope (see Lacan, 1966d, p. 53): instead of being invaded by manic ideas, he wrote *Finnegans Wake* (1957), which is marked by a circular structure. Nothing is less certain than that he ever believed in the father. In this sense, he had an advantage over neurotics, whose movement from the symptom to the sinthome implies going beyond the defect of God. Neurotics must separate the Name-of-the-Father – which remains necessary if there is to be a law and a One – from the ransom required for this by religion. If neurotics succeed in doing so, their achievement can be written in the following way:

$$\frac{\text{sinthome}}{\text{Name-of-the-Father}}$$

Lacan thought and said that Joyce himself was able to overcome the lack of the Name-of-the-Father. Yet it remains to be seen whether this always happens in psychosis.

At the beginning of the nineteenth century, with the French Revolution vanquished and the Napoleonic adventure at an end, the Catholic bishop Louis-François de Bausset wrote a four-volume biography of Fénelon, the *Histoire de Fénelon*, published by the royal printer. Although de Bausset's position within the Church and his concern with avoiding ecclesiastical incorrectness led to a rigid and constrained presentation of the material, he forcefully, and on the basis of first-hand documents, presented the merciless combat between Bossuet and Fénelon. This was a difficult task. He clearly supported and wanted to rehabilitate Fénelon, but he also did not want to attack Bossuet, who remained one of the Church's great authorities. He therefore took a line that involved a maximal accentuation of the gap between Fénelon's doctrine and the quietism of which he had been accused. Condemning quietism and attacking its founder, Miguel de Molinos, he attributes an "abominable consequence" to de Molinos' doctrine: "a soul that had reached a state of perfect contemplation ceased to be guilty in its relation with God, and could abandon itself to the most criminal of actions" (Bausset, 1817, p. 203). Whether this portrait of de Molinos is true or false, we can see in it the contemporary face of the perverse guru, who uses God – or even psychoanalysis – to satisfy his drives. What escaped Cardinal de Bausset and remained unexamined in the theological debate is precisely the key proposed by psychoanalysis: that which is higher (the spirit) and that which is lower (the body of the drives) do not belong to two parallel worlds, which could be stitched together by religion. We can also see how Binswanger, by treating the human spirit and the "instincts" [*Triebe*] as incommensurable realities, signalled his abandonment of Freudian knowledge.

Notes

1 The master of Jansenism, Pierre Nicole (1671, p. 385), conceived of a "republic of saints", but I am not sure that this was ever anything more than a fictional utopia.

2 The form of the question itself is decisive and unprecedented. It is not a question of getting into "this" or "that", but of *getting out*. Here, once again, is the parable of the three prisoners! In this way, that story does not refer to a teleology, but instead to the future anterior from which the subject has to detach itself. From this perspective, it would be precipitate and naïve to think that the failure – a word that we cannot avoid using if we think of what was hoped for – of the two great Marxist revolutions of the last century has ended in a pure and simple rallying around the "natural" system, capitalism. Although they may be difficult to read, several clues lead us to think that we are witnessing the emergence of societies that are not clones of the illustrious civilisation of the "West"; their gestation may well not involve an absolute obliteration of China and the Soviet Union's revolutionary experience.

3 Should analysts be saints? Certainly not, when they are not at work, but even in the context of analytic practice, it would still be asking too much. The only requirement is that the analyst's pass – the passage from being an analysand to an analyst – *can* be authenticated (whether or not it actually has been). The end of analysis is a different matter. In any case, neither the pass nor the ending is a matter of grace, in the Jansenist sense, as some would have us believe; such people are like sirens who would enjoy seeing Odysseus detach himself prematurely from the mast of his transference.

4 [*Translator's note*: In *La troisième*, Lacan (1975b, pp. 185–186) describes how, when he worked in psychiatric hospitals at the beginning of his career – long before he had come up with his ideas about the imaginary, symbolic and real – he was already describing the symptom as a *Nachtrag* or "addendum". "*Nachtrag*" should not be confused with the Freudian term "*Nachträglichkeit*" or "deferred action".] Marie-Jean Sauret brought this to my attention.

5 As Lacan (1975b, p. 200) said, "The symptom is an irruption of the anomaly that is phallic jouissance, inasmuch as it lays out and opens up the fundamental lack that I consider to be the sexual nonrelation".

6 This distinction can already be found in *La troisième*, Lacan (1975b, p. 186): "The sense of the symptom is not what one feeds it to make it propagate or die off; the sense of the symptom is the real".

7 There has been quite a bit of nostalgia for the Name-of-the-Father in psychoanalysis of late; this is found to different degrees and in different forms in the work of a whole range of analysts (see Legendre, 1989; Melman, 2002). Michel Tort (2005) tries to lay this to rest, but unfortunately the severity of his judgements against Lacanian theory is more ideological than psychoanalytic.
8 Alan Ginsberg once asked "What is death?" and William Burroughs replied: "A gimmick. It's the time-birth-death gimmick" (Hibbard, 1961, p. 1).
9 Lacan made an impressive number of efforts to create a nonrelation between association and institution, thus breaking with the practices of old established organisations and societies: cartels [a form of Lacanian study group], the *Scilicet* journal [which published unsigned articles], the distance set up between *gradus* [or "rank", as in the designations such as "*AE*" or "Analyst of the School", etc.] and hierarchy [or the status and institutional power of rank] (see Lacan, 1968b, p. 1), and even the dissolution of the school itself. The most decisive of these efforts was certainly the pass, which authorises the analysand-subject to become a *passant* [that is, a "passand" (a neologism based on the combination of "pass" and "analy*sand*")].
10 [*Translator's note*: See Onfray (1993).]
11 Fortunately, the desire of the Other is not something that one can just avoid knocking up against.
12 [*Translator's note*: English in the original.]
13 See *Essaim* [*Swarm*], a psychoanalytic journal edited by Érik Porge.
14 In connection with this, it would be useful to explore the effectiveness, and relative success or failure of significant political movements, such as the one led by Mahatma Gandhi, in which ethics were more of a motive force than was the search for power.
15 [*Translator's note*: see Lacan (1973b, p. 466).]
16 A number of psychoanalysts have disagreed with Freud's (1918) diagnosis of the Wolf Man, taking him to be psychotic. Perhaps they are right. In any case, their position ends any discussion of the essential question that Freud asked: is it possible, even in neurosis, that there are points of foreclosure that concern castration, rather than the Name-of-the-Father? If so, does this provide a way to account for certain psychosomatic phenomena in neurosis? It is clear that such phenomena do not have the same central role as in psychosis, but they refer back – in their very marginality, which is sometimes quite insistent – to something that cannot be symbolized. Further, what is the theoretical reason that castration cannot be foreclosed locally, supposing that: 1) castration is not-all [*pas-toute*], and 2) it is to be distinguished from the division of the subject? Finally, could it not be said that the condition of the possibility of what is known as "depersonalisation anxiety" which, in neurosis, can indicate the beginning of the end of an analysis (even while continuing to be experienced in other contexts) is the crossing over of a boundary beyond which castration reveals its inability [*impuissance*] to guarantee ego-based identification? For more on this, see the discussion of "*Gelassenheit*" in Millot (2001).
17 [*Translator's note*: For an account of Catherine Millot's experience, see the translator's introduction.]
18 [*Translator's note*: *Gelassenheit* is a term used by Heidegger which is usually translated into English as "releasement". See Davis (2010, p. xi).]
19 On the concept of "event", see Badiou (1988). An "event" involves an original encounter with the real of time. This originality does not, however, occur without the division whose mark is the symptom. This is why I do not think that jouissance is, first of all, primary, or that what is called "feminine jouissance" would constitute the return of this primary jouissance, after the "accident" that would be sexuation located on the masculine side.
20 This passage was brought to my attention by Pascale Macary.
21 See also the discussion of Benjamin and Schmitt in chapter 4 of this book.
22 In the twenty-first century, the question of the transcendent has been taken up again in what promises to be a new way, for the transcendent is no longer completely fused with

the religious. Thus, in *Dis-Enclosure: The Deconstruction of Christianity*, Jean-Luc Nancy (2005, p. 177) sets the tone with his expression "transcendence *of* immanence". In the domain of psychoanalysis, the transcendent is also open for discussion, for example in *Les désarrois nouveaux du sujet* edited by Jean-Pierre Lebrun (2001). Starting with the observation that hierarchical society has been issued a "death certificate" (something that does not seem self-evident to me), he explores how there is no longer a fixed, exogenous point from which norms can be established. Along with this, he examines, quite rightly, the paradox whereby any fixed, endogenous point, from the moment it becomes the basis of a norm, is externalised. A full presentation of my disagreements with the solution Lebrun proposes is beyond the scope of this footnote. However, I would like to note that the chance of the transcendent is manifest in the unfillable gap between the *totality* [*tout*] organised by the Names-of-the-Father and the *non-totalisable* symptom. This transcendence is transference to the extent that the latter does not, on the basis of the nonexistence of the sexual relation, draw the conclusion that love is inane.

23 This misunderstanding is probably the rule of love, but what Stendhal (1822, p. 6) called "crystallisation" refers to the moment of encounter in which there is an epiphany of the real between two people who are to become lovers.

24 [*Translator's note*: In the English version of this letter (Meng & Freud, 1963, p. 126), Freud's term "*weltlichen Seelsorgern*" (see Noth, 2014, p. 263), rendered here as "secular pastors", is translated as "*lay* curers".]

25 [*Translator's note*: on figuration and *Darstellbarkeit*, see p. 167, note 2 above.]

26 The term "medium" is borrowed from Kierkegaard's (1843) discussion of art.

27 [*Translator's note*: On the "impossible supposition" of the mystics, also see Gorday (2012, pp. 14–15):

> then came the notoriously famous "impossible supposition": if it were God's predestinating will that we be in hell, however saintly we may be, we should prefer the delight of conforming to that will rather than the contrary position of being in paradise without conformity to God's will. The loving soul "would prefer hell with God's will to paradise without God's will." If God wants hell for me, I will out of love for him take delight in that eventuality – which is to say that out of love for God I will give up even the hope of my salvation! What makes the supposition "impossible" (in theory) is the orthodox view that God could never have consigned to hell a soul whose love for God was so perfect. Or differently stated in the orthodox view: if I truly love God, the knowledge that God intends me for paradise will be present as well. But the bare statement of the impossible supposition is a way of reinforcing the idea that love of God must be radical. It must be a love of *God*, not of my own salvation, if it is truly God that I love.]

28 [*Translator's note*: "So Moses returned to the Lord and said, 'Alas, this people have sinned a great sin; they have made for themselves gods of gold. But now, if thou wilt forgive their sin – and if not, blot me, I pray thee, out of thy book which thou hast written'" (Exodus 32:31–32).]

29 [*Translator's note*: This is from the thirty-third article of Issy (Fénelon, 1695, p. 19).]

30 As mentioned earlier, the "Rat Man" thought that one of Freud's brothers was a murderer.

31 [*Translator's note*: The French text cited here, from the "*Faux* [False]" subsection of article XLIII (Fénelon, 1697a, p. 39), seems not to appear in any English translation.]

FOUNDATIONS

> For it is not a vain matter that astonishment may greet the fact that the name of Freud alone, by virtue of the hope of truth it bears with it, is of an order to confront the name of Marx, the still undissipated suspicion, even though it is plain that its abyss is unfillable, that in the path opened up by Freud might be perceptible the reason why Marxism fails to account for an increasingly immoderate and insane power insofar as politics is concerned, unless what is in play is a reverse effect of its contradictions.
>
> —Jacques Lacan, "Founding Act"[1]

I

The long epigraph that appears under the title of this final part will exempt me from having to restate the aim of this book, which is now nearing its end: to remove the non-encounter between Freud and Marx from the ideological dross that is inseparable from a sense of frustration. Such frustration is born from the sense that the gap between them is unbridgeable. This has covered over attempts to answer a question: in what way is this gap, which is impossible to deny, becoming the sign of something that is real? Taking the real into account can throw light on how politics has been ravaged by a debasing inflation of power. In his hastily written *The Question of Lay Analysis*, a text that opposes both the medicalisation of psychoanalysis and the threat that psychoanalysis, as science, would be destroyed by an emphasis on therapy, Freud does not hesitate to place psychoanalysis beside Christian Science. Although the latter may be a sect, both it and psychoanalysis are ways by which "each man" can seek "to be saved after his own fashion" (Freud, 1926b, p. 236) and they should both be left free to pursue their respective quests. The only difference – a decisive one – between them is that psychoanalysis is not religious and wagers on science. This wager means precisely – and almost paradoxically – that it can free itself from techniques that have been conditioned by science: techniques that can easily be used by various powers, "bio-" and "psycho-" among others.

I have already opened up this can of worms by asking whether psychoanalysis could be a science in which the subject is not sutured. To take a step forward, rather than backwards, with this question, we can note that, as a form of theory or body of doctrine, psychoanalysis is much more vulnerable than the hard sciences to arriving at mutually-exclusive positions (espousing both the black and the white at the same time). It does not make use of strict experimental procedures, which, at least in principle, are supposed to put a stop to the kinds of theoretical "flights of fancy" that contravene well-established axiomatic foundations. Yet the science of physics finds itself with relativity on one side and quantum theory on the other, even if this explicative duality is not considered as a final position. It is not impossible that Lacan's titanic efforts to establish the foundations of Freud's discovery will not ultimately arrive at a kind of doctrinal consensus analogous to that in physics: one that unifies the community – although without removing all disagreement and tensions within it – by having all physicists agree on a very small common denominator.

However, whatever happens in that respect (because it is also possible that psychoanalysis will succumb to death by pulverulence), there will still be a fundamental "abyss" between the theory and the experience (rather than the "technique") that it makes possible. Only this experience – in the current state of things, analytic treatment and the pass – is able *not to suture the subject*. On the other hand, as soon as theory is transmitted, it supposes an Other that would guarantee it, thus undoing the "Freudian uprising" of the symptom. To take the minimal example, we can show that a round of string, once cut, is no longer closed; nothing, however, will prevent a subject like Wittgenstein from suggesting, as he did about Russell's paradox, that we should just pass it over in silence.

For psychoanalysis, it may well be practical to distinguish between theory and experience. Nevertheless, this distinction should give way before another opposition, one that will take us further: structure and experience. Not everything can be learned from either of these terms: this is the key to using them well. We are, however, allowed to say – and the reference to Wittgenstein here only *seems* to be the opposite of our first reference – that just as the image and reality must have a common logical form if the image is to be able to "depict" reality,[2] so structure must also have the same logical form as experience. I would like to make it clear that the term "common" does not imply truth; it can only imply the possibility that a truth will emerge. (This statement breaks with any kind of psychoanalytic nominalism.) To get a better sense of that which remains unheard of – or better, that which cannot be articulated – without analytic experience, it seems both appropriate and necessary to provide several concrete samples of this "mercurial substance", even at the risk of becoming a bit rhapsodic.

- A child of two-and-a-half begins to be toilet-trained. At this moment, the word "poo" emerges as a metaphor for the child's use of language, becoming the source of an incontestable sense of jubilation: the world becomes "poo".

- A woman dreams that she goes into a store to buy a jumper, which then turns out to be too small. Then, in the course of the day following this dream, she buys a jumper that fits her.
- Another woman dreams that she is "assaulted" verbally by her sister and allows herself to be mistreated. Then during the next day, when she has a problem with a colleague, she finds the resources to prevent the same thing from happening.

  In two of the preceding sequences, jouissance the name that Freud gave to the movement towards self-annihilation – comes to be *figured* in the dream, thereby moving into the unconscious; it passes into a knowledge that remains unknown but is by definition articulated. Therefore, it no longer has to be acted upon while we are awake. Because the dream has fulfilled desire, the field is left free for something else.
- A female analysand dreams that she receives some empty boxes from her father. The dream provokes anxiety in her. When she relates this dream, however, she interprets these boxes in a positive way: they make it possible for her to place whatever she desires in them. The legacy of empty boxes is therefore the good aspect of what her father has done for her. She decides to put letters in these boxes.
- Another female analysand wonders whether she still wants her father to die. In her analysis, she had learned that, as a girl, she had desired this unconsciously. Does knowing now what had once been desired imply that this wish has now been dissolved? Can we hypothesise that she no longer desires her father's death?
- Yet another female analysand wrote to me that if her mother's neurosis had really decreed her own fate, then her mother's husband and her own father would be equivalent. Yet this was not true for her: "my mother's husband" is not the equivalent of "my father", even if they are, in reality, the same person.
- A schizophrenic patient went to visit his parents without being able to put down his suitcase, because as he said, there was no empty space.

This list could be extended ad infinitum. These reported statements are factual, and I hope that it can be seen immediately that they sketch out a strange scene; the term "desire", which Freud and Lacan have bequeathed to us as a central concept,[3] flickers and fluctuates in ways that are difficult to pin down.

It is here that Wittgenstein's "dis-philosophy [*dé-philosophie*]" will turn out, for a third time, to be extraordinarily valuable, even if I do not agree with what he says in this context. According to the *Tractatus* (Wittgenstein, 1921, p. 76, 6.124), "logic is not a field in which we express what we wish with the help of signs, but rather one in which the nature of the absolutely necessary signs speaks for itself". It would certainly be possible to attenuate the a-subjectifying implications of this proposition – which can be read as both pro- and anti-Freudian – by emphasising that it is restricted to the field of logic. In any case, as Wittgenstein admits in his *Philosophical Investigations*, it is a requirement.

This way of diluting the subject into an anonymous thinking machine (even if it is not transformed into a substantive) is open, however, to an objection: the bodily organism, by being the place where the symbolic is incorporated, becomes the means by which the symptom, which exceeds the symbolic, transforms itself into an event. The symptom is a "body event" (Lacan, 1979, p. 569). I have tried to show two ways in which the symptom exceeds the symbolic: 1) it makes the gap between the drive and the unconscious manifest; 2) it brings out the dissymmetry between activity (I want to get off on the Other) and passivity (I do not want the Other to get off on me). Although Lacan came upon this doubling of the symptom and the symbolic relatively late in his work, it is a discovery that retroactively recasts the foundations of the entirety of psychoanalysis. Further, it is something that can be recognised on a completely different level, in terms of the relation between language and writing.

In terms of its semantic dimension, language can claim to be incorporeal (what theologians would call "glorious"). Lacan thus begins by showing the ways in which language is not incorporeal, because it is phonetic and acoustic. However, this leads to a second phase of showing how the representative-descriptive function of the signifier must be distinguished from its figurative function (as discussed by Freud in reference to the dreams).[4] This "figurability" refers less to speech than to writing. For example, because proper names are translinguistic, they are both included in and excluded from the symbolic. That is how the proper name allows the symptom to *ek-sist* in relation to the symbolic, although with the trade-off that, because it is equivalent to the exception that founds the rule of the symbolic, the proper name can, spontaneously, be deified. This is the opposite of what could be called the symptom's insurrectional quality, which excludes any kind of Other that would guarantee itself.

If there is a kernel of desire, a soul – in the topological sense – in the symptom, and this would include the symptom's defensive aspect – the defence of desire against the death drive, against the jouissance of being annihilated – then there are three major consequences for psychoanalytic experience.

First, it is necessary to undo the confusion between the symptom and its jouissance. This confusion is not rare and leads analytic discourse to swerve into the discourse of the master, which can be observed among both "post-Freudian" and "Lacanian" analysts. In the name of the opposition between jouissance and desire, analysts hunt down jouissance and end up putting the symptom to death, instead of leading the analysand to devalorise the jouissance of the symptom, so that this symptom can be transformed into a sinthome.

Second, we encounter, once again, the question of the transcendent. In *Television*, Lacan (1974b, pp. 28–29) used the term "transcendental" to characterise what is "novel" in analytic discourse, explicitly in the sense that the term is used in number theory: to describe any number belonging to a nondenumerable set (the prototypical transcendental number being π). The "novel" aspect concerns transference: "through the transference the subject is attributed to the knowledge that gives him his consistency as subject of the unconscious, and it is that [knowledge] which is transferred onto the analyst" (ibid., p. 29). How can transference be called "transcendental"? It is transcendental in the sense that the subject to which knowledge is supposed, by the very operation of transference, can never be affixed to the subject to which this knowledge has been transferred. This unconscious knowledge transcends every subject, whether the latter is the analysand, the analyst or God. In this respect, the vocation of the poet may well consist in becoming the voice of the saying [*dire*] of the transcendent, which cannot be reduced to any specific subjectivity. In other words, perhaps this transcendence makes itself most fully present in the desire that, paradoxically, belongs to no subject, and to which the mystics testify so well.

The third consequence is the last but not the least. Since the symptom is "a body event" (Lacan, 1979, p. 569) – a form that can be articulated by saying something – affect, in all of its modes, going "from anxiety to ecstasy" (see the title of Janet's (1928) book), could be defined as a corporeal state, as determined by its relation to the symptom. Thus, a young woman who had experienced an incestuous relation with her father had, since then, lost her "zest" for life. She recovered it when the real fact of incest was detached from the jouissance of meaning, which was still enigmatic, and which had been conferred upon this real in order to ward off the unbearable trauma.

II

These preliminary formulations are not superfluous, for they will make it possible to review retroactively the results that I have reached.

The Capitalist Discourse can be defined in terms of three parameters.

1 It entrusts the relation between the subject ($\$$) and unconscious knowledge (S_2) to a hidden master (S_1), thereby transforming the splitting of the subject into a sundering; this will always prevent the subject from realising that this unconscious cannot be mastered.
2 It institutes a mode of jouissance in which the "thirst of lack-in-jouissance" becomes the principle of an economy in which consumption serves as the motor for more consumption. Such a system transfers the *agalma* from the human being to capital.
3 It forecloses castration, that is, the matters of love. The "starting point" of capitalism, as Lacan (1974b, p. 30) says, was "getting rid of sex".

Such statements need to be clarified one last time. The origin of the expression "foreclosure of castration" can be found in Freud's (1918) account of the Wolf Man's infantile neurosis. Freud considers this to be a case of neurosis, which has never failed to bewilder Lacanian psychoanalysts, who are puzzled to find foreclosure connected to neurosis. Instead of considering this as an error in diagnosis, I have argued that it should be recognised as one of Freud's major discoveries. Whatever the particular psychic structure may be, every structure contains a blind spot in which castration does not operate; this spot can vary according to the subject. Capitalism is the discourse that gives precedence to this blind spot, by making it command discursivity; unlike it, the other discourses are organised in order to counter this blind spot. The capitalist discourse does this by "getting rid" precisely of the aspects of "sex" that can activate the castration complex. "Sex", in this context, refers to what can make the sexual relation fail, a failure that can perhaps lead to a true encounter.

I have sought to throw light on the matheme of the capitalist discourse through my readings of the *Strange Case of Dr Jekyll and Mr Hyde* and *Saint Joan of the Stockyards*. Stevenson's short novel depicts the sundering of the subject from his unconscious. Dr Jekyll is the bearer of unconscious knowledge while Hyde is the subject. This sundering is so radical that the moral of the text becomes, as the puritanical morality of Fanny Osbourne would have it, the death of the subject; Hyde kills himself by, and in, his unconscious. This strange ending reminds us that the eradication of evil (represented incontestably by Hyde) must turn out badly if "I", as subject, wants to know nothing about evil, even if this "I" is the bacillus that carries this evil. Instead, the "I" wears itself out through a racist mechanism: it imputes evil to the other. It would not be difficult, at our current historical moment, to locate precisely this segregationist simplification in the "clash of civilisations". This clash does more than stigmatise the Hyde of terrorism. It goes to the point of reviling and treating as treasonable a tendency of Jekyll's that actually demonstrates his courage: the courage to learn and to be tested by evil, a courage that is limited by his refusal to let Hyde be the true subject.

This same sundering occurs in Bertolt Brecht's play, with the difference that Joan Dark, despite her name, is pure good. This difference does not really affect the plot. It does, however, modify the way that the story is organised, since Brecht accepts Joan Dark as the true subject, who has been deprived of her unconscious knowledge, which is located in Pierpont Mauler. At the end of the play, Brecht exalts splitting over sundering, but takes the side of neither Mauler nor Dark, in a way that no doubt seemed heretical to more conventional "Marxists". Here, once again, the subject is the one who pays with her life, thereby paying the debt that she could not or did not know how to acquit in relation to the capitalist discourse. Mauler himself gets by, unlike Dr Jekyll, who dies as Hyde and thus finds himself posthumously in the place of the subject. At most, Mauler may suffer from the authentic pain caused by the loss of a woman whom he had begun to love. Yet this is where we can locate the author's tour de force: when we try to make an ethical judgement on Mauler, Brecht prevents us from deciding whether he is a talented and cynical fraud or has, despite everything, experienced spiritual changes. Are his actions determined by the exchange rate or by his sensitivity? Nothing can resolve this uncertainty. The only thing that we can be sure of is that in the capitalist discourse, Mauler is torn between S_1 and S_2, pulling the strings of his own puppet; he could only get out of this position by allowing matters of love to take precedence over everything else. This he does not do.

Let us return, finally, to the four thinkers who are all emblematic of a certain relation to Lacan, from the 1970s until today. Yet what can "certain" mean in this context? Can the same position really be imputed to all of them? Yes and no. I can answer yes because Althusser, Deleuze and Guattari and Žižek are all animated by the question of transference: will the subject who is entering transference be allowed to envision a way out of it? This question is the smallest common denominator among the four thinkers, and they give divergent responses to it. For Althusser, a subject can only exit from it by being a "bad subject". For Deleuze and Guattari, the schizophrenisation of transference makes a way out possible. For Žižek, who is either the most optimistic or the most pessimistic, there is no solution, except by deactivating the Other: reducing oneself to being what the Other says.

These three ruses are not the ones that are chosen by psychoanalysis, even if, in a sense, they are ways of criticising certain psychoanalyses. Any subject can separate itself from the Other who has brought it into existence; we can do this, first, by allowing ourselves to be guided by an assent to the symptom – which is the only real relief against helplessness. Second, this can be done by recognising our division between castration and womanhood, or what is beyond the phallus.

If distinctions between psychosis, neurosis and perversion are relevant, it is because each of these can become the basis of a particular mode of division. In psychosis, in order for castration to be brought back into play through division, this implies that the psychotic subject can count on something that could name him/her, in the place of and instead of the nonexistent Names-of-the-Father. If this does not occur, an unsymbolised castration will manifest itself in various elementary phenomena, from hallucinations to delusions. There is, however, another possibility, the least desirable of all: a psychotic subject will locate his delusion within a political architectonic. This subject will close off all castration-effects, employing a police state to fix things in their proper places.

For the neurotic, the mother's castration has taken place through the paternal metaphor; what must be avoided is a situation in which the means of this castration is taken to be a guarantee of women's privation. In the latter case, the Names-of-the-Father would become an excuse for submitting to God the Father, a figure that the psychotic subject could incarnate without any compunction.

In perversion, the recognition of the mother's castration is neutralised through disavowal; the consequence of this is to authorise a transference only to the same sex, a transference for which Lacan (1975c, pp. 84–85) wittily used the term "hommosexual". There is no question of risking one's love for an object that would not respond in specular terms; such an object would remind the pervert of castration, and he knows how to freeze what is at stake in that.

In these cases, the phallic function, on the basis of whether or not it operates, demarcates psychosis from neurosis and perversion. A long time ago, during the brief romance between Marx and Freud after May 1968, it was suggested that there is a homology between the phallic function and the function of money as general equivalent.[5] This was a structural short-circuit, but it contained an element of truth. Language organises the symbolic order, without being reduced to it – this is the limit of structuralism – and in this order, both the symbolic phallus and money are operators and emblems of the One and of its functioning in what is denumerable. History, through a witticism rather than a farce, set two theories of money in opposition, although they are actually two sides of the same coin. The first is financial capitalism, in which money is believed to be capable of producing more money (M → M′). The second is Stalinism, in which the linkage between price and value was entirely undone. Because of this, for a number of people of "good will", financialisation, which had been condemned for its speculative excesses, could "liberally" be taken as the best antidote for a disorder produced by sundering price from value; we know from experience that this disorder generated a ruthless order. It may well be that this good will – which, from one perspective, can be appreciated – reaches its limit and secretes a danger in missing that which, in history, has ended up producing this reversal: where M → M′ works for some and M-C-M′ works for others, there will be a temptation – which can never be eliminated – to replace some by others, or vice versa. This good will ended up in maintaining two separate versions of the status quo: the first enabled Stalinism to endure in conditions that made it perilous and difficult to choose another option. Another made the capitalist discourse endure by refusing to see that, even if the powerful deserve to be criticised, *the worst example comes from below*: in a servitude that has involuntarily become voluntary.

In this context, questions about the decisive status of the symptom became necessary, in order to place a radical distance between two conceptions, one of which will lock us into the capitalist discourse, while the other can dismantle it. Either the symptom emerges in order to mask human sexuality's lack of harmony and the objective is to get rid of it *or* the symptom is the inaugural marker that the subject is not a product that was "made in the Other". The purpose of psychoanalysis would then be for the subject to undergo a transformation that will lead to an identification with this symptom. According to this conception, the symptom, which has become a sinthome, knots the symbolic to the aspect of the real that remains outside the symbolic. This would happen if we follow and generalise the solution that Lacan proposed in relation to Joyce.

How then can we exit from capitalism, or rather make it exit from us? Marx, if we reduce him to the vulgate, which can indeed be found in his work, answers that the private means of production must be abolished. Historical experience has proven that this solution was insufficient and Marx himself glimpsed its limits, for example, in his discussion of fetishism. Lacan's critique of the concept of surplus-value, however, opens up a new perspective. He does not challenge the relevance of this extraordinary discovery; instead, he points out that it misses the force that makes capitalism effective: the relation to jouissance. This is both enormous and razor-thin.

At the end of this book, I examined several of Lacan's hints concerning the appropriate form of association for psychoanalytic societies; in doing so, I sought to rehabilitate a transcendent dimension that would no longer be tied to religion. This involves the kind of satisfaction that is acquired at the end of an analysis; this satisfaction is incompatible with the mode of jouissance inherent in the capitalist discourse. I have tried to mark out some of the components that could give us a direction to follow, components that are hardly more discernible than the traces of the wind in the reeds. This may be a message in a bottle, but the sea is smaller than it seems.[6]

Notes

1 Lacan, J. (1964a). Founding act. In J. Copjec (Ed.), D. Hollier, R. Krauss, & A. Michelson (Trans.), *Television/A Challenge to the Psychoanalytic Establishment* (pp. 97–106). New York, NY: Norton, 1990. p. 104

2 [*Translator's note*: See Wittgenstein (1921, p. 11): "What any picture, of whatever form, must have in common with reality, in order to be able to depict it – correctly or incorrectly – in any way at all, is logical form, i.e. the form of reality".]

3 Freud uses the terms "*Wunsch*" and "*Begierde*", although the latter appears much less frequently in his writing.

4 [*Translator's note*: on "figuration" and "figurability", see p. 167, note 2 above.]

5 [*Translator's note*: see Goux (1973, pp. 16–34, 55).]

6 As a final touch, a citation from *L'étourdit* (Lacan, 1973b, p. 454): "Because Freud did not use the discourse of the analyst to forge the bond that would have enabled psychoanalytic societies to sustain themselves, he located them within other discourses, which necessarily, block [*barrent*] his saying [*dire*]".

APPENDIX 1: LACAN'S PORTRAIT OF MARX[1]

In *D'un Autre à l'autre*, Lacan (2006a, p. 64) tells us that, when he was twenty, he read Marx while taking the metro. This was in the 1920s. Judith Miller has confirmed to me that Lacan read the old edition translated by Jacques Molitor and published by Costes (Marx, 1924–1939). You will not be surprised that he read Marx's great work in its entirety, rather than contenting himself with anthologised selections. It would therefore be incorrect to think that his interest in Marx dates only from two seminars, *D'un Autre à l'autre* and *The Other Side of Psychoanalysis* or to think that he was motivated only by the enthusiasm for Marx's work that marked the period between 1968 and 1970.

Who – or even what – was Marx for Lacan? This is the question to which I hope to give a first response, and it legitimates the use of the word "portrait" in my title. As you know, in "*Radiophonie*", Lacan (1970, p. 434) dared to say that "*Mehrwert* [surplus-value] is *Marxlust*, Marx's surplus-jouissance". I shall seek to present a portrait that is illuminated by surplus-jouissance. This may be what is necessary in any true portrait.

The references that interest us are those that concern Marx and the origin of the symptom; for the most part, they occur over the course of ten years of Lacan's teaching, between 1966 and 1975. The first is found in one of the interpolated texts in the *Écrits*, "On the Subject Who Is Finally in Question", which immediately presents us with the problem of *bringing out* both the homage that Lacan pays to Marx and his reservations about the status of the symptom in his work. Lacan writes:

> It is difficult not to see that, even before the advent of psychoanalysis, a dimension that might be called that of the symptom was introduced, which was articulated on the basis of the fact that it represents the return of truth as such into the gap of a certain knowledge. . . . One can say that this dimension is highly differentiated in Marx's critique, even if it is not made explicit

> there. And one can say that a part of the reversal of Hegel that he carries out is constituted by the return (which is a materialist return, precisely insofar as it gives it figure and body) of the question of truth.
>
> *(Lacan, 1966c, p. 194)*

His reservation can be found in his reference, in relation to this first step, to what he calls the "jump" constituted by the "Freudian operation" (ibid., p. 194). With this operation,

> Freud sets himself apart from the rest by clearly linking the status of the symptom to the status of his own operation, for the Freudian operation is the symptom's proper operation, in the two senses of the term. Unlike a sign – or smoke which is never found in the absence of fire, a fire that smoke indicates with the possible call to put it out – a symptom can only be interpreted in the signifying order. A signifier has meaning only through its relation to another signifier. The truth of symptoms resides in this articulation. Symptoms remained somewhat vague when they were understood as representing some irruption of truth. In fact, they *are* truth, being made of the same wood from which truth is made, if we posit materialistically that truth is what is instated on the basis of the signifying chain".
>
> *(ibid., pp. 194–195)*

In both cases, the symptom is the "return of truth". This provides the foundation, at least in this area, for Marx's compatibility with Freud; it is built upon an alliance against Hegel, who reduced the work of truth – the work of the particular – to a cunning of reason; this reduction was necessary in order to found absolute knowledge, a form of knowledge that has no gaps. Yet Freud's jump must not be made to disappear, and the effect of his difference from Marx's position can be stated simply: whereas for Marx, the symptom is the symptom of a truth, for Freud it is truth itself. I will therefore take the risk of placing the words, "With Marx" at the beginning of Lacan's sentence: "[With Marx] symptoms remained somewhat vague when they were understood as representing some irruption of truth".

Without this conclusion, there is no way of making sense of the gap, which Lacan emphasised in a second moment of this elaboration – in *RSI*, "*La troisième*" and his lectures in the United States in 1976 – between Marx's social symptom and Freud's particular symptom.

We can get a sense of this gap at the level of interpretation, for as Lacan (2011b, p. 45) says, in a sweeping statement: "A symptom is not cured in the same way in Marxist dialectic and in psychoanalysis". In psychoanalysis, indeed, the movement of interpretation unfolds by beginning with the particularity of truth and expanding into the demonstration of a real: that of the primal loss of being implied by the constitutive division of the subject. This is why, when interpretation seeks to reduce the symptom through knowledge alone, it fails: it feeds the symptom instead of resolving it. Marx's limit was to have incarnated this loss in the proletarian: the figure who has been "stripped of everything and the messiah of the future" (Lacan, 1974–1975, 18 February 1975). After having brought the real out into the open, he covers over the real aspect of the loss of being that is made present by the symptom. Perhaps the source of this limitation lay in his inability to detect where this loss of being insists in the return of the repressed. Yet this formulation is only a way of harping on the truism that Marx is not Freud. It would be more relevant to grasp that this limitation is a consequence of what Marx does a priori with the proletarian: he identifies this figure with the norm of humanity, the custodian of a meaning of the real. In this context, it would not be out of place to wonder what becomes of those who were once revolutionaries when this identification becomes oppressive.

Psychoanalysis does not treat the proletarian as the essence of humanity, into which the meaning of the real would crystallise; therefore, for psychoanalysis, the symptom remains where Marx located it – the place of truth – but takes on another meaning. For Lacan, it is not a social symptom, but a particular symptom. I would like to emphasise Lacan's prudence in assessing this gap. He is concerned less with refuting the existence of the social symptom than with constructing an axiom. This is an affirmative change, which in my opinion gives it its rightful significance: whoever makes the human being into the vehicle of an ideal future, while giving the symptom the place of truth, transforms the content of this ideal into a social symptom. This formulation knots Marx's doctrine to the effect of his desire.

This is not certain, but perhaps the distance between the discontents of civilisation and what Freud and then Lacan call the "Gospel According to Marx" should be located here. Perhaps in this context, we must also wonder what place the concepts of the superego and repetition would have in historical materialism. Whatever this place may be, I hope that, by examining the status that Lacan gives to the symptom that Marx invented, I have opened up the space in which I can introduce the kernel of Lacan's critique of Marx. This critique, which is explicit, bears not on his conception of surplus-value, which Lacan considers to be irreproachable – including the denunciation of capitalism that it leads to – but on what Marx does with it. Let us say that this involves two separate "fields": the Marxist field and the Lacanian field.

The problem can be framed simply and correctly by noting that Lacan accomplishes this task in *The Other Side of Psychoanalysis*, the seminar in which he set up the four discourses. There, the Danaides and their sieve become a metaphor for jouissance (Lacan, 1991, p. 72), which is primally lost in the attempt to repeat it; for this reason, the basic function of discourse is to signify this loss, to give a meaning to this structural entropy. It does so by forbidding the jouissance that, if it were not forbidden, would leave the subject entirely in the grip of the fallacy that this much-vaunted vessel – phallic jouissance – can be filled. This is the meaning, from beginning to end, of the Oedipus complex.

The homology between surplus-value and surplus-jouissance – the object *a* – intervenes here. Surplus-jouissance is brought about when discourse, by constituting the object *a* as non-subject [*hors-sujet*] of jouissance, confers upon this object the power to make up – by desire – for the jouissance that has been lost. Surplus-value is brought about when the transformation of labour-power into commodities produces an object that is composed of the loss of the surplus-labour. This labour, as Marx discovers, is not paid to the worker, thereby conferring an additional value upon this object.

This is the point at which Lacan disagrees with Marx. He reproaches Marx for striving to enter surplus-value into the account books: to reason in terms of an energetics of jouissance, as if the subject's relation to jouissance could be regulated by a new distribution of surplus-value. In more precise terms, it is as if the debt that the subject attributes to the loss of jouissance could be acquitted simply by destroying the "juggernaut of capital" (Marx, 1867, p. 799). For those who have not read *Capital*, this Juggernaut was the chariot of the statue of Vishnu, which trampled the faithful during the annual procession to the Jagannath temple. This implies that the cause of desire could be dissolved in a new distribution of its object. In what I am seeking to transmit to you concerning Lacan's portrait of Marx, I am not sketching a picture that has been contaminated by the post-Freudians. Instead, I am seeking to delineate the basis of our own situation: we are trying, through the procedure of the pass, to know a little more about the movement from the impasse of desire to a support that is found in being. This support, by being outside the subject, leaves us confused about our apparatus of identifications.

Now we can go directly into the final question, which involves Marx's position as the inspirer of revolution. Lacan's diagnosis can be grasped through a few illuminating sentences:

> It is odd to observe that a doctrine such as Marx's whose articulation onto the function of struggle, the class struggle, which he instituted has not prevented it from giving birth to what for the moment is, indeed, the same problem that confronts us all, namely the persistence of a master's discourse.
>
> To be sure, the present one does not have the structure of the old, in the sense in which the old is installed in the place indicated under this big M. The present one is installed in the place on the left, the one capped by the U. . . . What occupies the place there, which we will provisionally call dominant [on the upper left], is the S_2, which is specified as being, not knowledge of everything (*savoir de tout*) – we've not got to that point yet, but knowledge taken as a whole (*tout-savoir*). Understand this as what is affirmed as being nothing other than knowledge, which in ordinary language is called the bureaucracy. It cannot be said that there are no problems created there.
>
> *(Lacan, 1991, p. 31, translation modified)*

This stupifyingly lucid text, which dates from 17 December 1969, seems to confirm what I have been saying about Lacan's relation to Marx. The opposition between knowledge taken as a whole and knowledge of everything is extremely valuable. The first of these terms, which occupies the dominant position in the discourse of the university, does not mean that one claims to know everything. It is a guarantee that provides vulgar materialist Marxists with a sense of comfort: if we don't claim to know everything, then we are materialists. This is obviously insufficient. If knowledge is conceived of as a whole, it means that no place has been left for truth; to approach knowledge in this way is to contradict and even to annul the step that Marx took in inventing the symptom. If we relate this expulsion of truth to what we know about the consequence of expelling truth from analytic experience, we can explain why this form of knowledge, placed in the dominant position, is incompatible with the development of transference. This can also enable us to assess what can be called a false transference: a transference that will only end up being destroyed by hatred. Transference, the motive force of treatment, is only addressed to knowledge if there is a margin in this knowledge – a margin in relation to its "wholeness" – in which truth can act as cause.

A final question then arises: does the absence of a place of truth result from substituting the proletarian for the real of the loss of being? The proletarian both marks the appearance of this loss and closes it up. This is a crucial question. To answer yes would mean – and this is not to be ruled out – that just as the Hegelian dialectic becomes frozen in the misunderstood gap of knowledge, so also Marx's dialectic becomes paralysed in a tyranny of knowledge. In the course of the movement of history, this paralysis makes it impossible for it to reach the place of truth, "as we were perhaps hoping" (ibid., p. 32). From then on, more than ever, the sign of truth ends up being in the keeping of those who, in the discourse of the university, have taken over from the ancient slave in the place of the other: the "human material" (ibid., p. 32). The times are indeed a-changing. In the folds of the flag of the October revolution, what we now see is not the "golden dream" but an empty circle, from which the revolutionary emblem in the red flag has been cut out. This is a fact. Some will rejoice, and others will be upset by this; others will both rejoice and be upset. This may well give us a proper sense of the symptomatic character of this cutting out, which is both particular and collective, and we may even see in the contour of this void the living truth of Lacan's portrait of Marx: confronted with the discourse of the master, whoever he may be, some lack of satisfaction may persist.

Note

1 This article was presented at the Rencontre Jacques Lacan conference in Paris in 1991 and first published in Cahiers psychanalytiques ACF-Est, no. 3, December 1994.

APPENDIX 2: THE INSATIABLE[1]

> The object of psychoanalysis is not man; it is what he lacks – not an absolute lack, but the lack of an object. . . . It is not to scarce bread but to cake that a Queen sent her people in time of famine.
>
> —Jacques Lacan, "Responses to Students of Philosophy"[2]

I am not really qualified to talk about political economy, for I have only really read – and a long time ago – the work of Marx, especially the first volume of *Capital*. I was also surprised at first to find my presentation placed under the section "Speculation" – which could be understood as financial speculation. Since then, I have changed my mind. In looking over Jean-Joseph Goux's (2000) book, *Frivolité de la valeur*, I realised that financial speculation is very much one of the essential preoccupations of "neoclassical" economics. This is an interesting, although unconvincing, way of introducing a consideration of desire into economics. Through this book, I also discovered Vilfredo Pareto's exquisite expression, the "ophelimity" – the desirability – of a glass of water. Pareto begins with the incontestable observation that we take less pleasure in the third glass of water than in the first and deduces a law from this: the value of water decreases in proportion to its consumption. Yet the guide provided by the pleasure principle is misleading, and the entire clinic of desire goes against this pseudo-law. We have only to mention bulimia and anorexia to understand that the "value of the last unit consumed" can be higher than that of the first, or that the first can have no value, at least if value is measured, as Pareto does, in terms of a scale of consumption. In fact, the flaw in this neoclassical reasoning can be found not in the counter-example of the drunk who cannot stop drinking, but in his/her underlying axiom: I consume, therefore I desire. We can, however, understand intuitively, even without being Freudians, that "I consume, therefore I do not desire" is also an acceptable axiom.

I am going to try to take up such commonplace observations through a critique of Marx's conception of surplus-value, a critique that I shall develop on the basis of Lacan's remarks in his seventeenth seminar, *The Other Side of Psychoanalysis* (1969–1970) and his text, "*Radiophonie*", which he wrote in the first half of 1970, as well as of several other statements that he made two or three years later. My critique does not call the economic relevance of Marx's discovery into question; instead, it seeks to reveal the hidden side of this discovery, a side that founds capitalism, and to bring out the reasons for a misunderstanding that exists within the system in which we still live.

I shall first examine briefly what I am criticising, beginning with what Marx referred to as a "decisive point":

> The *value* of the labouring power is determined by the quantity of labour necessary to maintain or reproduce it, but the *use* of that labouring power is only limited by the active energies and physical strength of the labourer. . . . Take the example of our spinner. We have seen that, to daily reproduce his labouring power, he must daily reproduce a value of three shillings, which he will do by working six hours daily. But this does not disable him from working 10 or 12 or more hours a day. But by paying the daily or weekly *value* of the spinner's labouring power, the capitalist has acquired the right of using that labouring power during the *whole day or week*".
>
> *(Marx, 1865, pp. 130–131)*

This passage provides a clear exposition of the sale and purchase of labour-power, as well as the transformation of labour-power into commodities. It is relevant here because it can serve as a support for dealing with a problem that is more difficult than that of the expression of labour-power in terms of the yarn produced: the establishment of what Lacan calls jouissance. This is a prerequisite for understanding what he will then call "surplus-jouissance" or *Mehrlust*, a term modelled on Marx's term *Mehrwert*, surplus-value.

In order to talk about jouissance, it is necessary to find the right distance: to speak of it simply, without thereby leaving out any part of what is at stake in it. There are two requirements, which can sometimes pull us in opposite directions.

First, there is the origin of the term "jouissance" in Freud's work. In *Beyond the Pleasure Principle*, Freud (1920) discusses psychic processes that have been revealed through our experience, and which are not a part of the pleasure principle, or of its complement, the reality principle: the traumatic dream, the neurosis of failure, masochism and the compulsion to repeat. Through the death drive (Thanatos), he is able to order these facts and make them intelligible by linking them explicitly to a jouissance of annihilation. From the beginning of his teaching in the 1950s, Lacan relates this jouissance of annihilation to the principle of language. The thing produces the word, which consumes it. Act I.

If jouissance emerges with the signifier, the *lektón* of language (in linguistics, Lacan was a Stoic before he was a Saussurian), then this jouissance is immediately lost; the meaning-effect – whatever it may be – that is produced by the signifier does not concern the signifier's being. Lacan refers to contemporary logic, which recognises the impossibility of self-reference. I shall add, however, that what objects to this is not intrinsically language, but rather speech – which anticipates language. The word is less the murder of the thing than the de-reification of the speaker. Act II.

In *The Other Side of Psychoanalysis*, Lacan refers not to Pareto's glass of water but to the sieve of the Danaides, which enables him to describe a specific aspect of jouissance: it is like the water that leaks out while the sieve is being filled (Lacan, 1991, p. 72). Images must be distrusted, and this one is no exception, but, in any case, we can see that the sieve can never be filled, and this is a major characteristic of jouissance. As Lacan notes (ibid., p. 72), "once you have started, you never know where it will end. It begins with a tickle and ends with a blaze of petrol. That's always what *jouissance* is". It would be interesting to restore the series of figures, which includes Marx, Freud and Lacan, who created this category of the "insatiable"; "modern" – or "postmodern" – critics of the great "obsolete" ideologies would, in part, have us forget this category. The figure of Moloch is emblematic of the superego, just as the wagon of Juggernaut (under whose wheels worshippers of Vishnu were crushed) is emblematic of capital. It is therefore all the more surprising that Marx ultimately went in another direction.

Thus, jouissance is lost, and is not even preserved in masochism, despite the masochist's deference to Thanatos. What Freud calls repetition is the process in which the signifier, in its fundamental form as "unary trait" – 0–0–0 – becomes both a means of jouissance and the vector of its loss. Repetition functions as a homeopathic defence against the volatility of jouissance by repeating a loss. This can be observed in everyday life when, in order to remobilise desire, I repeatedly lose objects. I am using very few words to summarise monumental theoretical constructions: at the place of the loss introduced by repetition, the lost object, object *a*, arises. We can therefore speak of the object *a* as two-sided: on one side, there is entropy, while on the other, surplus-jouissance [*plus-de-jouir*] can be recovered. The double character of the French word "*plus*", which can mean both "more" and "no more", has often been noted. In renaming the object *a* "surplus-jouissance", Lacan was proposing a general theory of what Freudians call a part-object and Winnicott calls a transitional object. Lacan himself, in his own earlier teaching, had called it the object-cause of desire.

*
**

Act III. We can now approach Lacan's criticism of Marx. Lacan argues that "If, by means of this relentlessness to castrate himself that he had, he hadn't computed this surplus *jouissance*, if he hadn't converted it into surplus value, in other words if he hadn't founded capitalism, Marx would have realized that surplus value is surplus jouissance" (ibid., pp. 107–108). This is Lacan's major reproach: Marx treated surplus-jouissance as something that could be entered into an account book. It is strange and remarkable that this was the same reproach to Pascal, who wanted to enter the losses and gains of his wager into an account book in order to demonstrate that there was no risk in his wager. As Lacan notes in passing in *The Other Side of Psychoanalysis*, it is "worth the effort of playing double or quits with surplus-jouissance ... only ... if the A is not barred". (ibid., p. 100, translation modified.) In both Marx and Pascal, the result is that what is incalculable in loss, which is its determinant and irreducible character, is masked, along with its reverse side, insatiability.

All of this has a consequence that concerns capitalism: what Marx conceives of as the appropriation of surplus-value is only, for Lacan, the recovery, in the form of surplus-value, of the jouissance that the capitalist had to renounce in order to start the process (Max Weber's (1905) book, *The Protestant Ethic and the Spirit of Capitalism* provides valuable support for this argument). In reality, this appropriation should be located somewhere other than where Marx had situated it: in the reduction, which Marx endorses, of labour-power to a commodity. Exploitation, therefore, will end not through a new distribution of surplus-value, but rather by going beyond this reduction. Marx was certainly not naive enough to believe that all surplus-value could be spent in non-productive consumption (see Marx's (1875, pp. 343–354) criticism of Lassalle). End of Act III.

*
**

Act IV. Lacan wrote "*Radiophonie*" while he was concluding *The Other Side of Psychoanalysis*. Similar remarks appear in this text but in a new form, which would soon lead him to introduce a fifth, capitalist discourse, one that, as we shall see, departs from the structure of the other discourses. For Lacan (1970, p. 434), one point has been established: surplus-jouissance is necessary because jouissance is a "hole that has to be filled".

Through surplus-value, Marx filled this hole, at least to the extent that a hole can be filled. (I would like to indicate in passing that the function of fantasy is to provide a removable stopper, which does not abolish the hole.) This is why Lacan (ibid., p. 434) states that "*Mehrwert* [surplus-value] is *Marxlust*, Marx's surplus-jouissance".

Surplus-value is the cause of desire that capitalism takes as its principle – the principle of extensive production. Capitalist production, the M-C-M′ cycle, implies that consumption is always growing. Yet if this consumption could procure a jouissance that would bring the call for jouissance to a halt, this would slow down production and the cycle would come to a sudden stop. This has not taken place because this economy, through a reversal that Marx did not foresee, produces a lack-in-jouissance. The more I consume, the greater is the gap between the jouissance that I get and the jouissance that I expect to obtain. This is precisely the opposite of Pareto's theorem. Thus, to quote Lacan one last time, the struggle over how to distribute surplus-value "only leads those who are exploited to compete on the basic principle of exploitation, in order to harbour their indisputable participation in the thirst of lack-in-jouissance" (ibid., p. 435).[3] Perhaps this could provide a basis for explaining why, although price can only derive from value, it does not reflect value. Perhaps this could also enable us to enter into the enchanted – or bewitched – empire of financial capital, where credit gives birth to money. In the capitalist economy, the object *a*, surplus-jouissance, tastes like exotic spices that are sweet to the tongue but burn the stomach. This brings us to a question: how is this reversal possible? Thus, Act V begins.

***

I anticipated this a bit when I referred to the fifth discourse. I am not sure that Lacan's matheme for the capitalist discourse resolves the question that I have just asked. Yet at the very least, it brings out the right components – which, frankly, are rather surprising. In 1972, in his series of lectures *The Psychoanalyst's Knowledge*, Lacan puts forward the thesis that the capitalist discourse forecloses castration, which thus exempts us from the structure of discourse. In the capitalist discourse, the barrier of jouissance is abolished. In other words, something is missing: the apparatuses controlled by this barrier, which enable the hole to be filled in – even if the hole continues to exist – are missing. From now on, the recovery of surplus-jouissance puts an end even to the short break that we have been allowed in relation to the imperative to experience jouissance and our submission to its insatiable god. This change only increases lack-in-jouissance, and, thereby, the thirst of this lack. Enrichment turns out to be deprivation [*dépouillement*]. Integration, the tendency of the life drive to create ever greater unities (Freud's *Vereinigung*), turns out to be a force for segregation. In this context, the "new man" of the capitalist order is someone who possesses holy cunning; there is no more convincing portrayal of the new human than Brecht's capitalist, Pierpont Mauler in *Saint Joan of the Stockyards*. He turns out to be a saint because, in the name of a sudden aspiration towards asceticism, he sells his stocks before they go down; he is cunning because, in order to provide labour to his workers, he buys them back again before they go back up.

Notes

1 First published in 2004 as L'insatiable. In M. Drach (Ed.), *L'argent: croyance, mesure, spéculation* (pp. 141–145). Paris: La Découverte.

2 Lacan, J. (1966f). Response to students of philosophy concerning the object of psychoanalysis. In J. Copjec (Ed.), D. Hollier, R. Krauss, A. Michelson, & J. Mehlman (Trans.), *Television: A Challenge to the Psychoanalytic Establishment* (pp. 107–114). New York: Norton, 1990. p. 113.

3 On the basis of Marcel Mauss' ethnographic work on the potlatch, Georges Bataille (1933) had an insight into how an economy based on expenditure, while being the antithesis of an economy based on acquisition, would reveal the hidden nature of the capitalist economy: spend in order to increase the lack-in-jouissance. In addition, this was precisely the mode of operation that Bataille wanted to subvert by transforming it into a passion for pure loss, which he made into an ideal. Note that, in this article, Bataille also came up with an excellent definition of poetry: "creation by means of loss" (ibid., p. 171).

REFERENCES

Adorno, T. W. (1972). *La psychanalyse révisée* [*Psychoanalysis Revisited*]. (J. Le Rider, Trans.). Paris: Éditions de l'Olivier, 2007.

Agamben, G. (1995). *Homo Sacer: Sovereign Power and Bare Life*. (D. Heller-Roazen, Trans.). Stanford, CA: Stanford University Press, 1998.

Agamben, G. (2002). *The Open: Man and Animal*. (K. Attell, Trans.). Stanford, CA: Stanford University Press, 2004.

Agamben, G. (2003). *State of Exception*. (K. Attell, Trans.). Chicago, IL: University of Chicago Press, 2005.

Alizadeh, A. (2017). Marx and art: Use, value, poetry. *Continental Thought & Theory*, *1*(4): 587–615.

Althusser, L. (1965). *For Marx*. (B. Brewster, Trans.). London: Verso, 1979.

Althusser, L. (1966). Three notes on the theory of discourses. In F. Matheron (Ed.), G. M. Goshgarian (Trans.), *The Humanist Controversy and Other Writings (1966–67)* (pp. 33–84). London: Verso, 2003.

Althusser, L. (1970). Ideology and ideological state apparatuses. In B. Brewster (Trans.), *On the Reproduction of Capitalism: Ideology and Ideological State Apparatuses* (pp. 232–272). London: Verso, 2014.

Althusser, L. (1973). Sur le transfert et le contre-transfert (petites incongruités portatives) [On transference and countertransference (little portable incongruities)]. In O. Corpet & F. Matheron (Eds.), *Écrits sur la psychanalyse: Freud et Lacan* (pp. 171–186). Paris: Stock/IMEC, 1993.

Althusser, L. (1976). *Positions (1964–1975)*. Paris: Éditions sociales.

Althusser, L. (1992). *The Future Lasts Forever: A Memoir*. (O. Corpet & Y. Moulier Boutang, Eds., R. Veasey, Trans.). New York: New Press, 1993.

Althusser, L. (1993). *Writings on Psychoanalysis: Freud and Lacan*. (O. Corpet & F. Matheron, Eds., J. Mehlman, Trans.). New York: Columbia University Press, 1996.

Anzieu, D. (1959). *Freud's Self-Analysis*. (P. Graham, Trans.). London: Hogarth and the Institute of Psycho-analysis, 1986.

Artaud, A. (1947a). From "Interjections." In C. Eshleman (Trans.), *Watchfiends & Rack Screams: Works From the Final Period* (pp. 243–274). Boston, MA: Exact Change, 1995.

Artaud, A. (1947b). To have done with the judgment of God: A radio play. In S. Sontag (Ed.), H. Weaver (Trans.), *Selected Writings* (pp. 555–574). New York: Farrar, Straus and Giroux, 1976.

Askofaré, S. (1989). *Les références de Jacques Lacan: Aristote, Descartes, Kant, Hegel, Marx [Jacques Lacan's References: Aristotle, Descartes, Kant, Hegel, Marx]*. Toulouse: Presses Universitaires du Mirail.

Augustine of Hippo. (400 CE). *The Trinity*. (J. E. Rotelle, Ed., E. Hill, Trans.). New York: New City Press, 1994.

Badiou, A. (1988). *Being and Event*. (O. Feltham, Trans.). London: Continuum, 2007.

Badiou, A. (1990). *Number and Numbers*. (R. Mackay, Trans.). Cambridge: Polity, 2008.

Bataille, G. (1933). The notion of expenditure. In A. Stoekl (Ed.), A. Stoekl, C. R. Lovitt, & D. M. Leslie Jr. (Trans.), *Visions of Excess: Selected Writings, 1927–1939* (pp. 116–129). Minneapolis, MN: University of Minnesota Press, 1985.

Bataille, G. (1961). *The Tears of Eros*. (P. Connor, Trans.). San Francisco, CA: City Lights, 1989.

Bataille, G. (1967). *The Accursed Share: An Essay on General Economy*. (R. Hurley, Trans.). New York: Zone Books, 1988.

Bataille, G. (1986). Georges Bataille: Writings on Laughter, Sacrifice, Nietzsche, Un-Knowing. (A. Michelson, Trans.). *October, 36*(Spring).

Baudelaire, C. (1857). The enemy. In R. Howard (Trans.), *Les Fleurs du Mal* (p. 20). Boston, MA: D.R. Godine, 1983.

Baudelaire, C. (1869). Dog and flask. In K. Waldrop (Trans.), *Paris Spleen: Little Poems in Prose* (p. 14). Middletown, CT: Wesleyan, 2009.

Baudelaire, C. (1897). *Intimate Journals*. (C. Isherwood, Trans.). Mineola, NY: Dover, 2006.

Baudry, J.-L. (1986). The apparatus. In P. Rosen (Ed.), *Narrative, Apparatus, Ideology: A Film Theory Reader* (pp. 299–318). New York: Columbia University Press.

Bausset, L.-F. de. (1817). *Histoire de Fénelon, archevêque de Cambrai [The History of Fénelon, Archbishop of Cambrai], Tome I*. Versailles: J. A. Lebel.

Beckett, S. (1954). *Waiting for Godot: A Tragicomedy in Two Acts*. New York: Grove, 2011.

Bénichou, P. (1948). *Morales du grand siècle [Morals of the Great Century]*. Paris: Gallimard.

Benjamin, W. (1950). Theses on the philosophy of history. In H. Arendt (Ed.), H. Zohn (Trans.), *Illuminations* (pp. 253–264). New York: Harcourt, Brace and World, 1968 [reprinted New York: Schocken, 2007].

Bentham, J. (1843). *The Panopticon Writings*. (M. Božovič, Ed.). London: Verso, 2011.

Binswanger, L. (1930). Dream and existence. (J. Needleman, Trans.). *Review of Existential Psychology and Psychiatry: Dream and Existence, XIX*(1, 1984–1985): 79–106.

Bion, W. R. (1965). *Transformations*. London: William Heinemann Medical [reprinted London: Karnac, 2002].

Boltanski, L., & Chiapello, È. (1999). *The New Spirit of Capitalism*. (G. Elliott, Trans.). London: Verso, 2007.

Borch-Jacobsen, M. (1990). *Lacan: The Absolute Master*. (D. Brick, Trans.). Stanford, CA: Stanford University Press, 1991.

Bousseyroux, M. (2001). Fondations du champ lacanien [Foundations of the Lacanian field]. *Héterité, 1*: 23–33.

Brecht, B. (1931). Saint Joan of the stockyards. In J. Willett (Ed.), R. Manheim (Trans.), *Collected Plays: 3* (pp. 201–311). London: Methuen Drama, 1980.

Brecht, B. (1932). The mother. In J. Willett (Ed. & Trans.), *Collected Plays: 3* (pp. 93–152). London: Methuen Drama, 1980.

Brecht, B. (1938). Life of Galileo. In R. Manheim & J. Willett (Eds.), J. Willett (Trans.), *Collected Plays: 5* (pp. 1–98). London: Methuen Drama, 1972.

Breuer, J., & Freud, S. (1895). Studies on hysteria. (J. Strachey, Trans.). *The Standard Edition of the Complete Psychological Works, 2*. London: Hogarth, 1957.

Briest, A., Le Fur, P., & Tajan, F. (Ed.). (2006). *Jacques Lacan, oeuvres graphiques et manuscrits [Catalogue for the Auction of Written Documents and Drawings by Jacques Lacan]: vente, 30 juin 2006 à 14h15, Hôtel Dassault, Paris.* Paris: Artcurial.

Bruno, P. (2000). *Papiers psychanalytiques: expérience et structure [Psychoanalytic Papers: Experience and Structure]*. Toulouse: Presses universitaires du Mirail.

Bruno, P. (2003a). *La passe: papiers psychanalytiques II [The Pass: Psychoanalytic Papers II]*. Toulouse: Presses universitaires du Mirail.

Bruno, P. (2003b). On the real father. (J. Holland, Trans.). *Journal for Lacanian Studies, 1*(2): 181–203.

Bruno, P., & Sauret, M.-J. (2006). *Problèmes de psychanalyse: symptôme et savoir [Psychoanalytic Issues: Symptom and Knowledge]*. Paris: Association de psychanalyse Jacques Lacan.

Camus, A. (1951). *The Rebel.* (A. Bower, Trans.). London: Penguin, 2000.

Canfora, L. (2004). *Democracy in Europe: A History of an Ideology.* (S. Jones, Trans.). Malden, MA: Blackwell, 2006.

Carmona, M. (1988). *Les diables de Loudun: sorcellerie et politique sous Richelieu [The Devils of Loudon: Witchcraft and Politics Under Richelieu]*. Paris: Fayard.

Cassou-Noguès, P. (2007). *Les démons de Gödel: logique et folie [Gödel's Demons: Logic and Madness]*. Paris: Seuil.

Chesnais, F. (Ed.). (2004). *La finance mondialisée: racines sociales et politiques, configuration, conséquences [Global Finance: Social and Political Origins, Configurations, Consequences]*. Paris: La Découverte.

Choderlos de Laclos, P.-A.-F. (1782). *Les liaisons dangereuses.* (D. Parmée, Ed. & Trans.). Oxford: Oxford University Press, 1995.

Clanchy, M. T. (1997). *Abelard: A Medieval Life.* Oxford: Blackwell.

Claudel, P. (1911). *The Hostage, a Drama.* (P. Chavannes, Trans.). New Haven, CT: Yale University Press, 1917.

Clément, C., & Kakar, S. (1993). *La folle et le saint [The Madwoman and the Saint]*. Paris: Seuil.

Daumal, R. (1938). *A Night of Serious Drinking.* (D. Coward & E. A. Lovatt, Trans.). Boston, MA: Shambhala, 1979.

Davis, B. W. (2010). Translator's foreword. In M. Heidegger & B. W. Davis (Trans.), *Country Path Conversations* (pp. vii–xxii). Bloomington, IN: Indiana University Press.

Debord, G. (1967). *The Society of the Spectacle.* (K. Knabb, Trans.). London: Rebel Press, 2005.

Deleuze, G., & Guattari, F. (1972). *Anti-Oedipus: Capitalism and Schizophrenia.* (R. Hurley, M. Seem, & H. R. Lane, Trans.). New York: Viking, 1977 [reprinted Minneapolis, MN: University of Minnesota Press, 1983].

Deleuze, G., & Guattari, F. (1980). *A Thousand Plateaus: Capitalism and Schizophrenia.* (B. Massumi, Trans.). Minneapolis, MN: University of Minnesota Press, 1987.

Delumeau, J. (1995). *Une histoire du paradis, vol 2: mille ans de bonheur [A History of Paradise, Volume 2: A Thousand Years of Happiness]*. Paris: Fayard.

Derrida, J. (1993). *Specters of Marx: The State of the Debt, the Work of Mourning and the New International.* (P. Kamuf, Trans.). New York: Routledge, 1994.

Derrida, J. (2000). Psychoanalysis searches the states of its soul: The impossible beyond of a sovereign cruelty. In P. Kamuf (Trans.), *Without Alibi* (pp. 238–280). Stanford, CA: Stanford University Press, 2002.

Derrida, J. (2002). *Marx & Sons.* Paris: Presses Universitaires de France.

Destutt de Tracy, A. L. C. (1817). *A Treatise on Political Economy: To Which Is Prefixed a Supplement to a Preceding Work on the Understanding, or, Elements of Ideology.* (T. Jefferson, Trans.). Washington, DC: Joseph Milligan.

Didier-Weill, A. (2003). *Lila et la lumière de Vermeer: la psychanalyse à l'école des artistes [Lila and Vermeer's Light: Psychoanalysis Goes to Art School]*. Paris: Denoël.

Dolar, M. (2013). Tyche, clinamen, den. *Continental Philosophy Review, 46*(2): 223–239.

Duras, M. (1964). *The Ravishing of Lol Stein*. (R. Seaver, Trans.). New York: Pantheon, 1986.

Dury, R. (2005). Introduction. In R. L. Stevenson (Ed.), *The Annotated Dr Jekyll and Mr Hyde* (pp. 1–78). Genoa: Edizioni Culturali Internazionali.

Engels, F. (1883). *Dialectics of Nature*. (C. P. Dutt, Trans.). New York: International Publishers, 1940.

Engels, F. (1886). Ludwig Feuerbach and the end of classical German philosophy. In K. Marx & F. Engels, *Collected Works, Volume 26: Engels 1882–89* (pp. 353–398). London: Lawrence & Wishart [Electric Book], 2010.

Fénelon, F. de S. de L. M. (1695). Articles arrêtés à Issy, sur les états d'oraison [Articles of Issy on the states of prayer]. In *Oeuvres complètes de Fénelon, Tome IV. Théologie et controverse. Quiétisme*. (pp. 11–19). Paris: Gauthier, 1830.

Fénelon, F. de S. de L. M. (1697a). Explication des maximes des saints sur la vie interieure [An explanation of the saints' maxims on the inner life]. In *Oeuvres de Fénelon . . . précédées d'études sur sa vie, par M. Aimé-Martin. Tome 2*. (pp. 1–40). Paris: Lefèvre, 1835.

Fénelon, F. de S. de L. M. (1697b). *Maxims of the Mystics*. (B. W. Randolph, Ed., W. W. Williams, Trans.). London: Mowbray, 1909.

Feynman, R. (1985). *QED: The Strange Theory of Light and Matter*. Princeton, NJ: Princeton University Press.

Fichtner, G. (Ed.). (2003). *The Sigmund Freud-Ludwig Binswanger Correspondence 1908–1938*. New York: Other Press.

Foucault, M. (1954). Dream, imagination, and existence. (F. Williams, Trans.). *Review of Existential Psychology and Psychiatry: Dream and Existence, XIX*(1, 1984–1985): 29–78.

Foucault, M. (1963). *Birth of the Clinic: An Archaeology of Medical Perception*. (A. M. Sheridan Smith, Trans.). New York: Pantheon, 1973.

Foucault, M. (1971). Appendix: The discourse on language. In R. Swyer (Trans.), *The Archaeology of Knowledge* (pp. 215–238). London: Tavistock, 1972.

Foucault, M. (1976). Le discours ne doit pas être pris comme. . . [Don't take discourse to be . . .]. In D. Defert & F. Ewald (Eds.), *Dits et ecrits 1954–1988: III, 1976–1979* (pp. 123–124). Paris: Gallimard, 1994.

Foucault, M. (1984). Le souci de la vérité (entretien avec F. Ewald) [Caring about truth (interview with F. Ewald)]. In D. Defert & F. Ewald (Eds.), *Dits et ecrits 1954–1988: IV, 1980–1988* (pp. 668–678). Paris: Gallimard, 1994.

Frege, G. (1892). On *Sinn* and *Bedeutung*. In M. Beaney (Ed. & Trans.), *The Frege Reader* (pp. 151–171). Oxford: Blackwell, 1997.

Freud, A. (1936). *The Ego and the Mechanisms of Defence*. (C. Baines, Trans.). London: Hogarth [reprinted London: Karnac, 1993].

Freud, E. L. (Ed.). (1975). *Letters of Sigmund Freud*. (T. Stern & J. Stern, Trans.). New York: Basic Books.

Freud, S. (1888). Hysteria. *The Standard Edition of the Complete Psychological Works, 1*: 39–62. London: Hogarth, 1966.

Freud, S. (1900). The interpretation of dreams (II). *The Standard Edition of the Complete Psychological Works, 5*: 339–722. London: Hogarth, 1953.

Freud, S. (1901). The psychopathology of everyday life. *The Standard Edition of the Complete Psychological Works, 6*: 1–289. London: Hogarth, 1960.

Freud, S. (1905a). Jokes and their relation to the unconscious. *The Standard Edition of the Complete Psychological Works, 8*: 3–238. London: Hogarth, 1960.

Freud, S. (1905b). Three essays on the theory of sexuality. *The Standard Edition of the Complete Psychological Works, 7*: 125–243. London: Hogarth, 1953.

Freud, S. (1909). Notes upon a case of obsessional neurosis. *The Standard Edition of the Complete Psychological Works, 10*: 153–318. London: Hogarth, 1955.

Freud, S. (1912–13). Totem and taboo. *The Standard Edition of the Complete Psychological Works, 23*: 1–163. London: Hogarth, 1964.
Freud, S. (1914). Remembering, repeating and working-through (further recommendations on the technique of psycho-analysis II). *The Standard Edition of the Complete Psychological Works, 12*: 145–156. London: Hogarth, 1958.
Freud, S. (1915a). Instincts and their vicissitudes. *The Standard Edition of the Complete Psychological Works, 14*: 109–140. London: Hogarth, 1957.
Freud, S. (1915b). Observations on transference-love (further recommendations on the technique of psycho-analysis III). *The Standard Edition of the Complete Psychological Works, 12*: 157–171. London: Hogarth, 1958.
Freud, S. (1916–1917). Introductory lectures on psycho-analysis. *The Standard Edition of the Complete Psychological Works, 16*: 3–463. London: Hogarth, 1961.
Freud, S. (1917). Mourning and melancholia. *The Standard Edition of the Complete Psychological Works, 14*: 237–259. London: Hogarth, 1957.
Freud, S. (1918). From the history of an infantile neurosis. *The Standard Edition of the Complete Psychological Works, 17*: 3–122. London: Hogarth, 1955.
Freud, S. (1919). A child is being beaten. *The Standard Edition of the Complete Psychological Works, 17*: 179–204. London: Hogarth, 1955.
Freud, S. (1920). Beyond the pleasure principle. *The Standard Edition of the Complete Psychological Works, 18*: 3–66. London: Hogarth, 1955.
Freud, S. (1921). Group psychology and the analysis of the ego. *The Standard Edition of the Complete Psychological Works, 18*: 67–143. London: Hogarth, 1955.
Freud, S. (1923). A seventeenth-century demonological neurosis. *The Standard Edition of the Complete Psychological Works, 19*: 67–105. London: Hogarth, 1961.
Freud, S. (1924). The economic problem of masochism. *The Standard Edition of the Complete Psychological Works, 19*: 155–170. London: Hogarth, 1961.
Freud, S. (1925). Negation. *The Standard Edition of the Complete Psychological Works, 19*: 235–242. London: Hogarth, 1961.
Freud, S. (1926a). Inhibitions, symptoms and anxiety. *The Standard Edition of the Complete Psychological Works, 20*: 77–178. London: Hogarth, 1959.
Freud, S. (1926b). The question of lay analysis. *The Standard Edition of the Complete Psychological Works, 20*: 179–258. London: Hogarth, 1959.
Freud, S. (1928). Dostoevsky and parricide. *The Standard Edition of the Complete Psychological Works, 21*: 175–198. London: Hogarth, 1961.
Freud, S. (1930). Civilization and its discontents. *The Standard Edition of the Complete Psychological Works, 21*: 57–146. London: Hogarth, 1961.
Freud, S. (1931). Female sexuality. *The Standard Edition of the Complete Psychological Works, 21*: 223–246. London: Hogarth, 1961.
Freud, S. (1933). New introductory lectures on psycho-analysis. *The Standard Edition of the Complete Psychological Works, 22*: 3–184. London: Hogarth, 1964.
Freud, S. (1936). A disturbance of memory on the Acropolis. *The Standard Edition of the Complete Psychological Works, 22*: 239–248. London: Hogarth, 1964.
Freud, S. (1937). Analysis terminable and interminable. *The Standard Edition of the Complete Psychological Works, 23*: 209–254. London: Hogarth, 1964.
Freud, S. (1940a). Medusa's head. *The Standard Edition of the Complete Psychological Works, 18*: 273–274. London: Hogarth, 1955.
Freud, S. (1940b). Splitting of the ego in the process of defence. *The Standard Edition of the Complete Psychological Works, 23*: 275–278. London: Hogarth, 1964.
Freud, S. (1950). A project for a scientific psychology. *The Standard Edition of the Complete Psychological Works, 1*: 283–398. London: Hogarth, 1966.

Freud, S., & Bullitt, W. C. (1966). *Thomas Woodrow Wilson – Twenty-Eighth President of the United States – A Psychological Study*. Boston, MA: Houghton Mifflin.

Goethe, J. W. von. (1808). *Faust: A Tragedy*. (C. Hamlin, Ed., W. W. Arndt, Trans.). London: Norton, 1976.

Gorday, P. (2012). *François Fénelon: A Biography – The Apostle of Pure Love*. Brewster, MA: Paraclete.

Goux, J.-J. (1973). *Symbolic Economies: After Marx and Freud*. (J. C. Gage, Trans.). Ithaca, NY: Cornell University Press, 1990.

Goux, J.-J. (2000). *Frivolité de la valeur: Essai sur l'imaginaire du capitalisme* [*The Frivolity of Value: An Essay on the Imaginary Dimension of Capitalism*]. Paris: Blusson.

Guillen, F. (2007). La querelle du phallus [The quarrel about the phallus]. *Psychanalyse*, *8*(1): 73–79.

Hegel, G. W. F. (1807). *Phenomenology of Spirit*. (A.V. Miller, Trans.). Oxford: Clarendon, 1977.

Hegel, G. W. F. (1832). *Science of Logic*. (A. V. Miller, Trans.). London: Routledge, 1969 [reprinted 2002].

Henley, W. E., & Stevenson, R. L. (1892). Deacon Brodie, or the double life. In *Three Plays* (pp. 1–110). New York: C. Scribner's Sons.

Hibbard, A. (Ed.). (1961). Interview with William Burroughs, Gregory Corso and Allen Ginsberg. In *Conversations With William S. Burroughs* (pp. 1–5). Jackson, MS: University Press of Mississippi, 1999.

Hölderlin, F. (1801). *Dichterberuf*/The poet's vocation. In E. L. Santner (Ed.), C. Middleton (Trans.), *Hyperion and Selected Poems* (pp. 153–157). New York: Continuum, 1990.

Janet, P. (1928). *De l'angoisse à l'extase* [*From Anxiety to Ectasy*]. Paris: F. Alcan.

Jones, E. (1957). *The Life and Work of Sigmund Freud, Volume 3: The Last Phase 1919–1939*. London: Hogarth.

Joyce, J. (1957). *Finnegans Wake*. New York: Viking.

Kakar, S. (1982). *Shamans, Mystics, and Doctors: A Psychological Inquiry into India and Its Healing Traditions*. New York: Knopf Doubleday.

Kakar, S. (1991). *The Analyst and the Mystic: Psychoanalytic Reflections on Religion and Mysticism*. Chicago, IL: University of Chicago Press.

Kant, I. (1781). *Critique of Pure Reason*. (P. Guyer & A. W. Wood, Trans.). Cambridge: Cambridge University Press, 1998.

Kierkegaard, S. (1843). *Either/Or: A Fragment of Life*. (V. Eremita, Ed., A. Hannay, Trans.). London: Penguin, 1992.

Klein, É. (2004). *Petit voyage dans le monde des quanta* [*A Visit to the Realm of the Quants*]. Paris: Flammarion.

Klein, M. (1957). Envy and gratitude. In M. R. Khan (Ed.), *Envy and Gratitude, and Other Works, 1946–1963* (pp. 176–235). New York: Free Press, 1984.

Klein, N. (2000). *No Logo: Taking Aim at the Brand Bullies*. New York: Picador.

Kleist, H. von. (1808). *Penthesilea: A Tragic Drama*. (J. Agee, Trans.). New York: Harper Perennial, 2000.

Kripke, S. A. (1980). *Naming and Necessity*. Cambridge, MA: Harvard University Press.

Krutzen, H. (2003). *Jacques Lacan, le séminaire 1952–1980: index référentiel* [*A Concordance to the Seminar of Jacques Lacan, 1953–1980*]. Paris: Anthropos.

Lacan, J. (1937). Intervention sur l'exposé de J. Picard, "Mécanismes névrotiques dans les psychoses: Œdipe, homosexualité, théâtralisme hystérique et perversité" [Response to J. Picard's presentation on "Neurotic mechanisms in psychosis: Oedipus, homosexuality, hysterical theatricality and perverseness"]. *Évolution Psychiatrique*, (Fasicule IV): 87–89.

Lacan, J. (1945). Logical time and the assertion of anticipated certainty. In B. Fink (Trans.), *Écrits: The First Complete Edition in English* (pp. 161–175). New York: Norton, 2006.

Lacan, J. (1947a). La psychiatrie anglaise et la guerre [English psychiatry and the war]. In *Autres écrits* (pp. 101–120). Paris: Seuil, 2001.

Lacan, J. (1947b). Presentation on psychical causality. In B. Fink (Trans.), *Écrits: The First Complete Edition in English* (pp. 123–158). New York: Norton, 2006.

Lacan, J. (1949). The mirror stage as formative of the *I* function as revealed in psychoanalytic experience. In B. Fink (Trans.), *Écrits: The First Complete Edition in English* (pp. 75–89). New York: Norton, 2006.

Lacan, J. (1956a). Response to Jean Hyppolite's commentary on Freud's "Verneinung." In B. Fink (Trans.), *Écrits: The First Complete Edition in English* (pp. 318–333). New York: Norton, 2006.

Lacan, J. (1956b). The function and field of speech and language in psychoanalysis. In B. Fink (Trans.), *Écrits: The First Complete Edition in English* (pp. 197–268). New York: Norton, 2006.

Lacan, J. (1957a). La psychanalyse et son enseignement [Psychoanalysis and its teaching]. *Bulletin de la Société française de philosophie, 49*(2): 65–101.

Lacan, J. (1957b). The Freudian thing, or the meaning of the return to Freud in psychoanalysis. In B. Fink (Trans.), *Écrits: The First Complete Edition in English* (pp. 334–363). New York: Norton, 2006.

Lacan, J. (1957c). The instance of the letter in the unconscious, or reason since Freud. In B. Fink (Trans.), *Écrits: The First Complete Edition in English* (pp. 412–441). New York: Norton, 2006.

Lacan, J. (1958). The signification of the phallus. In B. Fink (Trans.), *Écrits: The First Complete Edition in English*. New York: Norton, 2006.

Lacan, J. (1959). On a question prior to any possible treatment of psychosis. In B. Fink (Trans.), *Écrits: The First Complete Edition in English* (pp. 445–488). New York: Norton, 2006.

Lacan, J. (1960). The subversion of the subject and the dialectic of desire in the Freudian unconscious. In B. Fink (Trans.), *Écrits: The First Complete Translation in English* (pp. 671–702). New York: Norton, 2006.

Lacan, J. (1961). Remarks on Daniel Lagache's presentation: "Psychoanalysis and personality structure." In B. Fink (Trans.), *Écrits: The First Complete Edition in English* (pp. 543–574). New York: Norton, 2006.

Lacan, J. (1962). Guiding remarks for a convention on female sexuality. In B. Fink (Trans.), *Écrits: The First Complete Translation in English* (pp. 610–620). New York: Norton, 2006.

Lacan, J. (1963). Kant with Sade. In B. Fink (Trans.), *Écrits: The First Complete Edition in English* (pp. 645–668). New York: Norton, 2006.

Lacan, J. (1964). On Freud's "Trieb" and the psychoanalyst's desire. In B. Fink (Trans.), *Écrits: The First Complete Edition in English* (pp. 722–725). New York: Norton, 2006.

Lacan, J. (1965). Homage to Marguerite Duras, on *Le ravissement de Lol V. Stein*. In P. Connor (Trans.), *Marguerite Duras* (pp. 122–129). San Francisco, CA: City Lights, 1987.

Lacan, J. (1965–1966). *Le séminaire XIII: L'objet de la psychanalyse* [*The Object of Psychoanalysis*], *1965–1966*. Retrieved from http://staferla.free.fr/S13/S13%20L'OBJET.pdf

Lacan, J. (1966–1967). *Le séminaire XIV: Logique du fantasme* [*The Logic of Fantasy*], *1966–1967*. Paris. Retrieved from http://staferla.free.fr/S14/S14%20LOGIQUE.pdf

Lacan, J. (1966a). Bibliographical references in chronological order. In B. Fink (Trans.), *Écrits: The First Complete Edition in English* (pp. 864–868). New York: Norton, 2006.

Lacan, J. (1966b). Index of proper names. In B. Fink (Trans.), *Écrits: The First Complete Edition in English* (pp. 871–878). New York: Norton, 2006.

Lacan, J. (1966c). On my antecedents. In B. Fink (Trans.), *Écrits: The First Complete Edition in English* (pp. 51–57). New York: Norton, 2006.

Lacan, J. (1966d). On the subject who is finally in question. In B. Fink (Trans.), *Écrits: The First Complete Edition in English* (pp. 189–196). New York: Norton, 2006.

Lacan, J. (1966e). Position of the unconscious. In B. Fink (Trans.), *Écrits: The First Complete Edition in English* (pp. 703–721). New York: Norton, 2006.

Lacan, J. (1966f). Responses to students of philosophy concerning the object of psychoanalysis. In J. Copjec (Ed.), D. Hollier, R. Krauss, A. Michelson, & J. Mehlman (Trans.), *Television: A Challenge to the Psychoanalytic Establishment* (pp. 107–114). New York: Norton, 1990.

Lacan, J. (1966g). Science and truth. In B. Fink (Trans.), *Écrits: The First Complete Edition in English* (pp. 726–745). New York: Norton, 2006.

Lacan, J. (1967–1968). *Le séminaire XV: L'acte psychanalytique* [*The Psychoanalytic Act*], *1967–1968*. Retrieved from http://staferla.free.fr/S15/S15%20L%27ACTE.pdf

Lacan, J. (1968a). La psychanalyse, raison d'un échec [Psychoanalysis, the reason for a failure]. In *Autres écrits* (pp. 361–371). Paris: Seuil, 2001.

Lacan, J. (1968b). Proposition of 9 October 1967 on the psychoanalyst of the school. (R. Grigg, Trans.). *Analysis*, *6*: 1–13, 1995.

Lacan, J. (1969). On a reform in its hole (J. Holland, Trans.). *S: Journal of the Circle for Lacanian Ideology Critique*, *8*: 14–21, 2015.

Lacan, J. (1970). Radiophonie [Radiophony]. In *Autres écrits* (pp. 403–447). Paris: Seuil, 2001.

Lacan, J. (1971). Lituraterre. (D. Nobus, Trans.). *Continental Philosophy Review*, *46*(2): 327–334, 2013.

Lacan, J. (1973a). L'acte psychanalytique: compte rendu du séminaire 1967–1968 [The psychoanalytic act: Summary of the 1967–1968 seminar]. In *Autres écrits* (pp. 375–386). Paris: Seuil, 2001.

Lacan, J. (1973b). L'étourdit [Blunderings]. In *Autres écrits* (pp. 449–495). Paris: Seuil, 2001.

Lacan, J. (1973c). Postface au *séminaire XI* [Postface to seminar XI]. In *Autres écrits* (pp. 503–508). Paris: Seuil, 2001.

Lacan, J. (1973d). *The Four Fundamental Concepts of Psycho-Analysis* [*Seminar XI*]. (J.-A. Miller, Ed., A. Sheridan, Trans.). New York: Norton, 1977.

Lacan, J. (1974–1975). *Le séminaire XXII: R.S.I., 1974–1975*. Retrieved from http://staferla.free.fr/S22/S22%20R.S.I.pdf

Lacan, J. (1974a). Spring awakening. (S. Rodríguez, Trans.). *Analysis*, *6*: 32–34, 1995.

Lacan, J. (1974b). Television. In J. Copjec (Ed.), D. Hollier, R. Krauss, A. Michelson, & J. Mehlman (Trans.), *Television: A Challenge to the Psychoanalytic Establishment* (pp. 1–48). New York: Norton, 1990.

Lacan, J. (1975a). Conférences dans les universités nord-américaines: le 2 décembre 1975 au [Lectures Given at North American Universities: 2 December 1975] Boston, MA: Massachusetts Institute of Technology. *Scilicet*, (6–7): 53–63.

Lacan, J. (1975b). La troisième [The third]. *Lettres de l'Ecole freudienne*, *16*: 177–203.

Lacan, J. (1975c). *On Feminine Sexuality, the Limits of Love and Knowledge: The Seminar of Jacques Lacan, Book XX Encore, 1972–1973*. (J.-A. Miller, Ed., B. Fink, Trans.). New York: Norton, 1998.

Lacan, J. (1976–1977). *Le séminaire XXIV: L'insu que sait de l'une-bévue s'aile à mourre* [*The Unawareness Known by the One-Blunder: That's Love/Death/Chance!*], *1976–1977*. Retrieved from http://staferla.free.fr/S24/S24%20L'INSU. . . . pdf

Lacan, J. (1977–1978). Le séminaire XXV: Le moment de conclure [The moment of concluding], 1977–1978. Retrieved from http://staferla.free.fr/S25/S25.pdf

Lacan, J. (1978a). Annex: premiere version de la "Proposition du 9 octobre 1967 sur le psychanalyste de l'école" [Appendix: First version of the "Proposition of 9 October 1967 on the psychoanalyst of the school"]. In *Autres écrits* (pp. 575–591). Paris: Seuil, 2001.

Lacan, J. (1978b). Du discours psychanalytique [On psychoanalytic discourse]. In G. Contri (Ed.), *Lacan in Italia/Lacan en Italie (1953–1978)* (pp. 32–55). Milan: La Salamandra.

Lacan, J. (1979). Joyce le Symptôme (II). In *Autres écrits* (pp. 565–570). Paris: Seuil, 2001.

Lacan, J. (1980a). Letter of dissolution. In J. Copjec (Ed.), D. Hollier, R. Krauss, & A. Michelson (Trans.), *Television/A Challenge to the Psychoanalytic Establishment* (pp. 129–132). New York: Norton, 1990.

Lacan, J. (1980b). Monsieur A., 18 mars 1980. *Ornicar?* (20–21): 18–19.

Lacan, J. (1980c). The other is missing. In J. Copjec (Ed.), D. Hollier, R. Krauss, & A. Michelson (Trans.), *Television/A Challenge to the Psychoanalytic Establishment* (pp. 133–135). New York: Norton, 1990.

Lacan, J. (1981a). Jacques Lacan: conférence de Louvain (13 octobre 1972) [Louvain Lecture (13 October 1972)]. *Quarto, 3*: 5–20.

Lacan, J. (1981b). Overture to the first international encounter of the Freudian field, Caracas, 12 July 1980. (A. R. Price, Trans.). *Hurly-Burly, 6*(September): 17–20, 2011.

Lacan, J. (1982a). Joyce the symptom (I). In A. R. Price (Trans.), *The Sinthome: The Seminar of Jacques Lacan, Book XXIII* (pp. 141–148). Cambridge: Polity, 2016.

Lacan, J. (1982b). Note italienne [Letter to the Italians]. In *Autres écrits* (pp. 307–311). Paris: Seuil, 2001.

Lacan, J. (1986). *The Ethics of Psychoanalysis, 1959–1960* [*Seminar VII*]. (J.-A. Miller, Ed., D. Porter, Trans.). New York: Norton, 1992.

Lacan, J. (1991). *The Other Side of Psychoanalysis* [*Seminar XVII*]. (J.-A. Miller, Ed., R. Grigg, Trans.). New York: Norton, 2007.

Lacan, J. (1994). *Le séminaire de Jacques Lacan, livre IV: La relation d'objet* [*Object Relations*], *1956–1957*. (J.-A. Miller, Ed.). Paris: Éditions du Seuil.

Lacan, J. (2001a). Index des noms cités [Index of cited names]. In *Autres écrits* (pp. 597–601). París: Éditions du Seuil.

Lacan, J. (2001b). *Transference: The Seminar of Jacques Lacan, Book VIII*. (J.-A. Miller, Ed., B. Fink, Trans.). Cambridge: Polity, 2015.

Lacan, J. (2004). *Anxiety: The Seminar of Jacques Lacan, Book X*. (J.-A. Miller, Ed., A. R. Price, Trans.). Cambridge: Polity, 2014.

Lacan, J. (2005a). *On the Names-of-the-Father*. (B. Fink, Trans.). Cambridge: Polity, 2013.

Lacan, J. (2005b). *The Sinthome: The Seminar of Jacques Lacan, Book XXIII*. (A. R. Price, Trans.). Cambridge: Polity, 2016.

Lacan, J. (2006a). *Le séminaire de Jacques Lacan. livre XVI: D'un Autre à l'autre* [*From an Other to the Other*], *1968–1969*. (J.-A. Miller, Ed.). Paris: Seuil.

Lacan, J. (2006b). *Le séminaire de Jacques Lacan. Livre XVIII, D'un discours qui ne serait pas du semblant* [*On a Discourse That Would Not Be of a Semblance*]*: 1971*. (J.-A. Miller, Ed.). Paris: Seuil.

Lacan, J. (2011a). *Le séminaire de Jacques Lacan. Livre XIX, . . .ou pire . . .or Worse*]*: 1971–1972*. (J.-A. Miller, Ed.). Paris: Seuil.

Lacan, J. (2011b). *Talking to Brick Walls: A Series of Presentations in the Chapel at Sainte-Anne Hospital*. (A. R. Price, Trans.). Cambridge: Polity, 2017.

Lacan, J. (2013). *Le séminaire de Jacques Lacan. Livre VI, Le désir et son interprétation* [*Desire and its Interpretation*]*: 1958–1959*. Paris: Éditions de la Martinière.

Lamartine, A. de. (1820). *Solitude, and Other Poems, With Translations From the "Méditations Poétiques" of Lamartine, and From Metastasio*. (J. Churchill, Trans.). London: Hookham, 1830.

Laplanche, J. (1970). *Life and Death in Psychoanalysis*. (J. Mehlman, Trans.). Baltimore, MD: Johns Hopkins University Press, 1976.

Laplanche, J., & Pontalis, J. B. (1974). *The Language of Psycho-analysis*. (D. Nicholson-Smith, Trans.). New York: Norton.

Laval, C. (2007). *L'homme économique: essai sur les racines du néolibéralisme* [*Homo Oeconomicus: An Essay on the Roots of Neoliberalism*]. Paris: Gallimard.

Leach, E. R. (1961). *Rethinking Anthropology*. London: Athlone.

Le Brun, J. (2002). *Le pur amour de Platon à Lacan* [*Pure Love: From Plato to Lacan*]. Paris: Seuil.

Lebrun, J.-P. (Ed.). (2001). *Les désarrois nouveaux du sujet: prolongements théorico-cliniques au "Monde sans limite" [The New Sorrows of the Subject: Theoretical and Clinical Additions to "A World Without Limits"]*. Ramonville Saint-Agne: Erès.

Legendre, P. (1989). *Le crime du caporal Lortie: traité sur le père [The Crime of Corporal Lortie: A Treatise on the Father.]*. Paris: Fayard.

León-Lopez, P. (1999). *Le réel n'est pas le monde: études psychanalytiques sur le théâtre [The Real is not the World: Psychoanalytic Explorations of the Theatre]* (Thèse de doctorat en Psychanalyse). Paris: University of Paris VIII.

Lesourd, S. (2006). *Comment taire le sujet?: des discours aux parlottes libérales [How Can the Subject be Silenced? From Discourses to Liberal Chitchat]*. Ramonville Saint-Agne, France: Érès.

Levinas, E. (1961). *Totality and Infinity: An Essay on Exteriority*. (A. Lingis, Trans.). Pittsburgh, PA: Duquesne University Press, 1969.

Lévi-Strauss, C. (1969). *The Elementary Structures of Kinship*. (R. Needham, Ed., J. H. Bell & J. R. von Sturmer, Trans.). Boston, MA: Beacon Press.

Lewis, C. S. (1966). *Surprised by Joy: The Shape of My Early Life*. New York: Harcourt, Brace, Jovanovich.

Maleval, J.-C. (2003). Elements pour une apprehension clinique de la psychose ordinaire [Towards a clinical understanding of ordinary psychosis]. Presented at the Séminaire de la découverte freudienne, Toulouse. Retrieved from www.psychaanalyse.com/pdf/psychose_ordinaire_apprehension_clinique.pdf

Mandrou, R. (Ed.). (1979). *Possession et sorcellerie au XVIIe siècle [Possession and Witchcraft in the Seventeenth Century]*. Paris: Fayard.

Mao, Z. (2007). *On Practice and Contradiction*. (S. Žižek, Ed.). London: Verso.

Marx, K. (1843). A contribution to the critique of Hegel's philosophy of right. In R. Livingstone & G. Benton (Trans.), *Early Writings* (pp. 243–250). London: Penguin, 2005.

Marx, K. (1852). The eighteenth Brumaire of Louis Bonaparte. In K. Marx & F. Engels, *Collected Works, Volume 11: Marx and Engels 1851–53* (pp. 99–197). London: Lawrence & Wishart [Electric Book], 2010.

Marx, K. (1856). Speech at the anniversary of the *People's Paper*. In D. Fernbach (Ed.), *Surveys from Exile: Political Writings, Volume 2* (pp. 299–300). London: Verso, 2010.

Marx, K. (1865). Value, price and profit. In K. Marx & F. Engels, *Collected Works, Volume 20: Marx and Engels 1864–68*. London: Lawrence & Wishart [Electric Book], 2010.

Marx, K. (1867). *Capital: A Critique of Political Economy*. (B. Fowkes, Trans.). London: Penguin, 1976.

Marx, K. (1875). Critique of the Gotha Programme. In D. Fernbach (Ed.), J. de Bres (Trans.), *The First International and After: Political Writings, Volume 3* (pp. 339–359). London: Verso, 2010.

Marx, K. (1877). Letter to *Otechestvenniye Zapiski*. In K. Marx & F. Engels, *Collected Works, Volume 24: Marx and Engels 1874–83* (pp. 196–201). London: Lawrence & Wishart [Electric Book], 2010.

Marx, K. (1894). *Capital: Critique of Political Economy, Volume III*. (E. Mandel, Ed., D. Fernbach, Trans.). New York: Pelican, 1981 [reprinted London: Penguin, 1991].

Marx, K. (1924). *Oeuvres complètes [Complete Works]*. (J. Molitor, Trans.). Paris: Costes.

Marx, K. (1939). *Grundrisse: Foundations of the Critique of Political Economy (Rough Draft)*. (M. Nicolaus, Trans.). London: Penguin, 1973.

Marx, K. (1994). *Œuvres. IV, Politique. I [Political Works]*. (M. Rubel, Ed.). Paris: Gallimard.

Marx, K., & Engels, F. (1932). The German ideology. In C. Dutt (Trans.), *Marx and Engels Collected Works, Volume 5: Marx and Engels 1845–47* (pp. 19–540). London: Lawrence & Wishart [Electric Book], 2010.

Melman, C. (2002). *L'homme sans gravité: jouir à tout prix [Lightweight Man: Jouissance at Any Price]*. Paris: Gallimard.

Meng, H., & Freud, E. L. (Eds.). (1963). *Psycho-Analysis and Faith: The Letters of Sigmund Freud and Oskar Pfister*. (E. Mosbacher, Trans.). London: Hogarth.

Meyer, C. (Ed.). (2005). *Le livre noir de la psychanalyse: vivre, penser et aller mieux sans Freud* [*The Black Book of Psychoanalysis: Live, Think and Feel Better Without Freud*]. Paris: Éditions des Arènes.

Michaux, H. (1997). *Darkness Moves: An Henri Michaux Anthology, 1927–1984*. (D. Ball, Trans.). Berkeley, CA: University of California Press.

Michelet, J. (1862). *Satanism and Witchcraft: A Study in Medieval Superstition*. (A. R. Allinson, Trans.). New York: Citadel, 1965.

Mill, J. S. (1863). *Utilitarianism*. London: Parker, Son, & Bourn, West Strand.

Miller, J.-A. (1990). L'école et son psychanalyste (Conférence donnée à Grenade le 27 octobre 1990) [The school and its psychoanalyst (Lecture delivered in Grenada on 27 October 1990)]. (A. Bukschtein. Trans.). Retrieved from www.causefreudienne.net/lecole-et-son-psychanalyste-2/

Miller, J.-A. (2005). Foreward. In J. Lacan & B. Fink (Trans.), *On the Names-of-the-Father* (pp. vi–viii). Cambridge: Polity, 2013.

Millot, C. (2001). *Abîmes ordinaires* [*Ordinary Abysses*]. Paris: Gallimard.

Millot, C. (2012). La belle indifférence de [The beautiful indifference of] Madame Guyon. *Insistance, 1*(7): 89–97.

Morin, F. (2006). *Le nouveau mur de l'argent: essai sur la finance globalisée* [*The New Money Wall: An Essay on Global Finance*]. Paris: Seuil.

Morin, I. (2009). *La phobie, le vivant, le féminin* [*Phobia, the Living Being, and the Feminine*]. Toulouse: Presses universitaires du Mirail.

Müller, H. (1980). Quartet. In C. Weber (Trans.), *Hamlet-Machine and Other Texts for the Stage* (pp. 103–122). New York: Performing Arts Journal, 2001.

Müller, H. (1982). I am interested in the Althusser case. In S. Lotringer (Ed.), B. Schütze & C. Schütze (Trans.), *Germania* (pp. 184–189). New York: Semiotext[e], 1990.

Musil, R. (1930). *The Man Without Qualities*. (S. Wilkins & B. Pike, Trans.). New York: Vintage International, 1996.

Nagel, E., & Newman, J. R. (1986). *Gödel's Proof*. New York: New York University Press.

Nancy, J.-L. (2005). *Dis-Enclosure: The Deconstruction of Christianity*. (B. Bergo, G. Malenfant, & M. B. Smith, Trans.). New York: Fordham University Press, 2008.

Naugrette, J.-P. (1994). Présentation [Preface]. In R. L. Stevenson & T. Varlet (Trans.), *Le cas étrange du Dr Jekyll et de M. Hyde* (pp. 6–39). Paris: Flammarion.

Nerval, G. de. (1851). *Journey to the Orient*. (C. Elphinstone, Trans.). Plimmerton: Antipodes, 2013.

Nerval, G. de. (1855). Aurélia. In R. Sieburth (Trans.), *Selected Writings* (pp. 265–316). London: Penguin, 1999.

Nicole, P. (1671). De la charité et de l'amour-propre [On Charity and Self-Worth]. In L. Thirouin (Ed.), *Essais de Morale* (pp. 381–416). Paris: Les Belles Lettres, 2016.

Noth, I. (2014). *Sigmund Freud – Oskar Pfister: Briefwechsel 1909–1939*. Zürich: Theologischer Verlag.

Onfray, M. (1993). *La sculpture de soi: la morale esthétique* [*Sculpting the Self: Aesthetic Ethics*]. Paris: B. Grasset.

Orwell, G. (1949). *Nineteen Eighty-Four*. London: Penguin, 2004.

Politzer, G. (1939). La fin de la psychanalyse [The End of Psychoanalysis]. *La Pensée, 3*(octobre-novembre-décembre): 13–23 [Published under the pseudonym Th. W. Morris].

Popper, K. (1974). The problem of demarcation. In N. Warburton (Ed.), *Philosophy: The Basic Readings* (pp. 247–257). London: Routledge, 1999.

Praz, M. (1933). *The Romantic Agony*. (A. Davidson, Trans.). Oxford: Oxford University Press, 1978.

Rancière, J. (2005). *Hatred of Democracy*. (S. Corcoran, Trans.). London: Verso, 2006.

Reich, W. (1933). *The Mass Psychology of Fascism*. (V. R. Carfagno, Trans.). New York: Farrar, Straus and Giroux, 1980.

Rimbaud, A. (1871). Letter: Rimbaud to Paul Demeny. In P. Schmidt (Trans.), *Complete Works* (pp. 114–119). New York: Harper Perennial, 2008.

Roazen, P. (2001). The exclusion of Erich Fromm from the IPA. *Contemporary Psychoanalysis*, *37*: 5–42.

Robinson, D., & Groves, J. (2002). *Introducing Bertrand Russell: A Graphic Guide*. Cambridge: Icon Books.

Russell, B. (1902). Letter to Frege. In J. van Heijenoort (Ed.), *From Frege to Gödel: A Source Book in Mathematical Logic, 1879–1931* (pp. 124–125). Cambridge, MA: Harvard University Press, 1967.

Russell, B. (1905). On denoting. *Mind*, *14*(56): 479–493.

Sartre, J.-P. (1947). *No Exit*. (P. Bowles, Trans.). New York: Samuel French, 1972.

Sauret, M.-J. (2009). Figure des *états limites* – les *hommes aux loupes* [*Borderline* figure: The *wolf men*]. In *Malaise dans le capitalisme* [*Capitalism and Its Discontents*] (pp. 171–213). Toulouse: Presses Universitaires du Mirail.

Saussure, F. de. (1911). *Course in General Linguistics*. (C. Bally, A. Sechehaye, & A. Riedlinger, Eds., R. Harris, Trans.). LaSalle, IL: Open Court, 1986.

Schiller, F. (1781). The robbers. In F. J. Lamport (Trans.), *The Robbers and Wallenstein* (pp. 21–160). Harmondsworth: Penguin, 1979.

Schiller, F. (1801). *The Maid of Orleans*. (A. Swanwick, Trans.). Philadelphia, PA: D. McKay, 1899.

Schiller, F. von. (1797). The diver. (Lord E. Bulwer-Lytton, Trans.). In Bliss Carman et al. (ed.), *The World's Best Poetry*, Volume IX (pp. 44–52). Philadelphia, PA: John D. Morris & Co., 1904.

Schmitt, C. (1950). *The* Nomos *of the Earth in the International Law of the* Jus Publicum Europaeum. (G. L. Ulmen, Trans.). New York: Telos, 2006.

Schmitt, C. (1955). The planetary tension between orient and occident and the opposition between land and sea. (J. D. Blanco, Trans.). *Política Común*, *5*, 2014 [Originally published in *Revista de Estudios Políticos*, *81*: 3–28].

Schnurmann, A. (1947). Observation of a phobia. *The Psychoanalytic Study of the Child*, *3*(1): 253–270.

Seife, C. (2000). *Zero: The Biography of a Dangerous Idea*. London: Penguin.

Sloterdijk, P. (2007). *The Aesthetic Imperative: Writings on Art*. (K. Margolis, Trans.). Cambridge: Polity, 2017.

Soler, C. (2002). Le savoir, sans la fatalité [Knowledge, Without the Inevitability]. *Link*, *14–15*: 168–175.

Stendhal. (1822). *On Love*. (S. Lewis, Trans.). London: Hesperus, 2009.

Stevenson, R. L. (1886). *Strange Case of Dr. Jekyll and Mr. Hyde*. London: Longmans, Green.

Stevenson, R. L. (1887). Markheim. In *The Merry Men and Other Tales and Fables* (pp. 117–143). New York: Charles Scribner's Sons.

Stevenson, R. L. (1892). A chapter on dreams. In *Across the Plains* (pp. 229–252). London: Chatto and Windus.

Strachey, J. (1962). Appendix: The emergence of Freud's fundamental hypotheses. *The Standard Edition of the Complete Psychological Works*, *3*: 62–69. London: Hogarth.

Surya, M. (2002). *Georges Bataille: An Intellectual Biography*. (K. Fijałkowski & M. Richardson, Trans.). London: Verso.

Tort, M. (2005). *Fin du dogme paternel* [*The End of Paternal Dogma*]. (J.-F. de Sauverzac, Ed.). Paris: Aubier.

Turnheim, M. (2001). *L'autre dans le même: réflexions psychanalytiques sur le deuil, le mot d'esprit et la politique* [*The Other in the Same: Psychoanalytic Reflections on Mourning, Jokes, and Politics*]. Paris: Éditions du Champ lacanien.

Vasse, D. (1978). *Un parmi d'autres* [*One Among Others*]. Paris: Seuil.

Weber, M. (1905). *The Protestant Ethic and the Spirit of Capitalism: With Other Writings on the Rise of the West*. (S. Kalberg, Trans.). Oxford: Blackwell, 2002.

Wilde, L.W. (2000). *On the Trail of the Women Warriors: The Amazons in Myth and History*. New York: Thomas Dunne.

Wittgenstein, L. (1921). *Tractatus Logico-Philosophicus*. (D. F. Pears & B. F. McGuinness, Trans.). London: Routledge, 1974.

Wittgenstein, L. (1953). *Philosophical Investigations*. (G. E. M. Anscombe, P. M. S. Hacker, & J. Schulte, Trans.). Chichester: Wiley-Blackwell, 2009.

Žižek, S. (1993a). *Subversions du sujet: psychanalyse, philosophie, politique* [*Subversions of the Subject: Psychoanalysis, Philosophy, Politics*]. (É. Doisneau-Guéguen & A. Abelhauser, Trans.). Rennes: Presses Universitaires de Rennes, 1999.

Žižek, S. (1993b). *Tarrying With the Negative: Kant, Hegel, and the Critique of Ideology*. Durham, NC: Duke University Press.

Žižek, S. (1995). Hegel avec Lacan [Hegel with Lacan]. In P. Verstraeten (Ed.), *Hegel aujourd'hui* (pp. 107–118). Paris: J. Vrin.

Žižek, S. (2003). *The Puppet and the Dwarf: The Perverse Core of Christianity*. Cambridge, MA: MIT Press.

INDEX

For Product Safety Concerns and Information please contact our EU representative GPSR@taylorandfrancis.com
Taylor & Francis Verlag GmbH, Kaufingerstraße 24, 80331 München, Germany

www.ingramcontent.com/pod-product-compliance
Lightning Source LLC
LaVergne TN
LVHW021123300926
849160LV00010B/843
9780367334017